# OSTOMIES AND
# CONTINENT DIVERSIONS

## NURSING MANAGEMENT

# OSTOMIES AND CONTINENT DIVERSIONS

## NURSING MANAGEMENT

*Edited by*

### BEVERLY G. HAMPTON, MSN, RN, CETN, OCN

Director,
ET Nursing Education Program
M.D. Anderson Cancer Center
Houston, Texas

### RUTH A. BRYANT, MS, RN, CETN

Former Director,
ET Nursing Education Program
Abbott Northwestern Hospital
Minneapolis, Minnesota

Private Practice,
Oklahoma City, Oklahoma

With *115* illustrations
including *24* color plates

Coordinated with assistance from the
International Association for Enterostomal Therapy

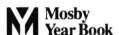
Mosby
Year Book

St. Louis  Baltimore  Boston  Chicago  London  Philadelphia  Sydney  Toronto

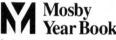

**Mosby
Year Book**

Dedicated to Publishing Excellence

Publisher: Alison Miller
Editor: Terry Van Schaik
Developmental Editor: Jeanne Rowland
Project Manager: Patricia Tannian
Production Editor: Mary McAuley
Book and Cover Design: Gail Morey Hudson

Printed in the United States of America

Mosby–Year Book, Inc.
11830 Westline Industrial Drive, St. Louis, Missouri 63146

**Library of Congress Cataloging in Publication Data**

Ostomies and continent diversions: nursing management/edited by
   Beverly G. Hampton, Ruth A. Bryant.
        p.      cm.
      "Coordinated with assistance from the International Association
for Enterostomal Therapy."
      Includes bibliographical references and index.
      ISBN 0-8016-2041-4
      1. Enterostomy—Nursing.      2.Urinary diversion—Nursing.
   3. Ostomates—Rehabilitation.      4. Gastrointestinal system—Diseases—
   Treatment.      5. Genitourinary organs—Diseases—Treatment.
   I. Hampton, Beverly G.      II. Bryant, Ruth A.      III. International
   Association for Enterostomal Therapy.
      [DNLM:      1. Ostomy—nursing.      2. Urinary Diversion—nursing.      WY
   156.5 085]
   RD540.086   1992
   617.5'54—dc20
   DNLM/DLC
   for Library of Congress                                          92-8482
                                                                        CIP

92  93  94  95  96  CL/UN/MY  9  8  7  6  5  4  3  2  1

# Editorial Board

# Contributors

**RUTH A. BRYANT, MS, RN, CETN**

Private Practice
Oklahoma City, Oklahoma

**JOHN G. BULS, MD, BS, FRACS**

Clinical Associate Professor, Department of Surgery
Division of Colon and Rectal Surgery
University of Minnesota
Minneapolis, Minnesota

**DOROTHY B. DOUGHTY, MN, RN, CETN**

Director, ET Nursing Education Program
Emory University
Atlanta, Georgia

**PAULA ERWIN-TOTH, MSN, RN, CETN**

Manager, ET Nursing
Director, ET Nursing Education Program
Cleveland Clinic Foundation
Cleveland, Ohio

**KATHLEEN A. FITZGERALD, MS, RN, CETN**

Clinical Nurse Specialist
Northwestern Memorial Hospital
Chicago, Illinois

**BEVERLY G. HAMPTON, MSN, RN, CETN, OCN**

Director, ET Nursing Education Program
M. D. Anderson Cancer Center
The University of Texas
Houston, Texas

**KATHRYN HOYMAN, MSN, RN, CETN**

Clinical Nurse Specialist
University of Minnesota Hospitals and Clinics
Minneapolis, Minnesota

**SALLY J. IRRGANG, MA, RN, CETN**

Quality Assessment Manager
MedCenters Health Plan
Minneapolis, Minnesota

**DEBORAH J. LIGHTNER, MD**

Staff Urologist, Twin Cities Urology, PA
Minneapolis, Minnesota

**KEN McCALLA, MD**

Staff Urologist, Group Health, Inc.
Minneapolis, Minnesota

**WILLIAM C. McGARITY, MD**

Chief of Surgery, Emory University Hospital
Professor of Surgery, School of Medicine
Medical Director, ET Nursing Education Program
Emory University
Atlanta, Georgia

**CATHERINE R. RATLIFF, MS, RNCS, CETN**

Clinical Nurse Specialist
University of Virginia Hospitals
Charlottesville, Virginia

**BONNIE SUE ROLSTAD, BA, RN, CETN**

Director and Clinical Consultant
ET Nurse Consultants, PA
St. Paul, Minnesota

**DOROTHY B. SMITH MS, RN, ET, OCN**

Director of Nursing Staff Development
M.D. Anderson Cancer Center
The University of Texas

# Preface

Ostomy and continent diversion surgical procedures are integral to the management of many gastrointestinal (GI) and genitourinary (GU) tract diseases (malignant and benign) and may be required at any age from neonate to adult. Although the precise number of individuals who require such surgery is not known, the impact on an individual and a family is well known. Because ostomy surgery alters external appearance and renders an individual incontinent, it can have a negative impact on life-style, interpersonal relationships, marriage, self-esteem, and sexuality. Therefore an individualized and comprehensive care plan with the objective of restoring not only the patient's physical health but also the patient's quality of life must be a mutual goal of the health care team.

Ostomy surgery will always pose many psychosocial and physical challenges; however, new advances in care better enable the patient to meet these challenges. These advances include enhanced patient and family education, expanded outpatient follow-up, and improved ostomy products, surgical techniques, perioperative management, and pharmacotherapy. This book will equip nurses to collaborate in the comprehensive, long-term effort required from the health care team to effectively address the constellation of concerns the patient with an ostomy or continent diversion may have.

Care of the patient with an ostomy or a continent diversion is complicated and challenging. Complete physical recuperation with psychosocial adaptation is a lengthy process. Nurses have long recognized that although the patient may recover physically, the psychosocial hurdles posed by ostomy surgery may be even more significant to the patient and family. Chapter 1 prepares the nurse to assess the patient's psychologic status, to counsel the patient regarding sexual implications, and to educate the patient and family about ongoing care through home health services and other outpatient resources. Recognition of the importance of patient education underscores the need for teaching programs that provide information before surgery, during the hospital stay, and after discharge. A visit with another person who has had similar surgery is often beneficial. Chapter 1 discusses the many types of support that various sources can provide to facilitate the patient's adaptation.

A technologic explosion has resulted in a new generation of superior, more effective ostomy care products. Chapter 2 discusses procedures for ostomy management and explains how to use all the available products so that a pouching system can be tailored to the needs of the individual. Management-related issues such as diet, colostomy irrigations, specific considerations for the infant, and urostomy night drainage are discussed. Follow-up care is emphasized as a means of providing continued instructions, monitoring complications, and evaluating adaptation. Because long after the original surgical procedure patients experience many changes such as weight gain or loss, pregnancy, trauma, or illness, continued outpatient follow-up is essential.

Chapter 3 explains the assessment and management of peristomal and stomal complications. Color illustrations of many complications are included.

Improvements in the construction of continent diversions and intriguing advances in surgical techniques that preserve sphincter function, as well as specific management issues, are explored in Chapter 4. The added challenge of managing the care of the patient who has an ostomy or a continent reservoir and is receiving cancer therapy is addressed in Chapter 5. Chapters 6 through 11 provide a foundation of information that is essential to competent nursing care of the patient with an ostomy or a continent diversion: GI and GU physiology, disorders, and surgical techniques.

In addition to knowledge, the nurse must possess specific clinical skills to manage the care of the patient with an ostomy or a continent reservoir. This book teaches these techniques, when to use them, and how to interpret the results.

With all these thoughts in mind we have developed *Ostomies and Continent Diversions: Nursing Management.* Initially conceptualized as a resource for nurses preparing for board certification or attending ET nursing education programs, the book will be valuable and relevant to any health care provider responsible for the complex care of patients who have ostomies or continent diversions.

Beverly G. Hampton
Ruth A. Bryant

# Acknowledgments

A book is developed and created as a result of the help, support, reviewing, and guidance of many people.

We extend sincere appreciation to the editorial board, Donna Brewer, Paula Erwin-Toth, Michiko Ooka, Joan Van Niel, and particularly Dorothy Doughty, who provided editorial assistance and rewriting; Jeanne Rowland, nursing developmental editor, who was ever available for direction and suggestions; our husbands, Herman Hampton and Dennis Confer, who tolerated neglect and being placed in secondary roles over many months; the M. D. Anderson Cancer Center, Houston, Texas, and Abbott Northwestern Hospital, Minneapolis, Minnesota, for providing favorable environments for our professional development; and ConvaTec, for generous financial support of the project.

Beverly G. Hampton
Ruth A. Bryant

# Contents

# OSTOMIES AND CONTINENT DIVERSIONS

## NURSING MANAGEMENT

# 1

# Psychosocial Adaptation

DOROTHY B. SMITH

## OBJECTIVES

1. Identify factors that affect the patient during the preoperative assessment process.
2. Discuss physical conditions of the patient that influence the learning of self-care.
3. Discuss the influence of culture and educational level on learning self-care.
4. Review the reasons for stoma site selection.
5. Identify physical conditions that affect the stoma site placement.
6. Discuss the principles of adult learning.
7. Present guidelines for teaching children ostomy self-care.
8. Address theories useful in patient counseling.
9. Identify components of normal sexual functioning.
10. Describe changes in sexual functioning related to the disease.
11. Describe the use of the PLISSIT model in the teaching of ostomy patients.
12. Review the discharge teaching and planning appropriate for the patient.

The patient who has an ostomy presents the health care team with a full cycle of physiologic and psychosocial needs. The physical alterations in the patient's elimination pattern caused by the stoma not only demand immediate and long-term attention but also affect the patient's psychologic nature and social relationships for the duration of the stoma. It is just this challenging cycle of needs that makes nursing care of patients with an ostomy so rewarding. All aspects of acute nursing care plus long-term rehabilitation planning are required, and none of them is successful by chance. Goals and objectives must be identified, and care plans established.

Nursing care of the patient who has an ostomy is part of a structured process, whether or not it is consciously recognized as such. Specific structural components are called into play regardless of when the nurse first meets the patient and family—whether before or after surgery. The components include assessment, relationship building, education, developing and implementing a care plan, counseling, and follow-up evaluation and care. These components are not independent of each other but, rather, overlap in an interactive manner as patient and family care evolves from acute nursing care. This chapter deals with each of these components, theoretically and practically, as they relate to the patient with an ostomy.

## PREOPERATIVE MANAGEMENT

Both patient and family are most vulnerable, as well as most receptive, to preparatory information during the interval after the patient learns of the need for an ostomy and before the actual surgery. This is a time when the patient and family are seeking information, dealing with the fear and anxiety of the unknown, and activating coping strategies. It is an excellent time for nursing intervention, beginning with assessment and including education, counseling, stoma site selection, and team building.[30]

### Assessment

Before needs can be determined and care planned, the patient's status and resources must be carefully assessed. Although this assessment requires some deliberate questioning and investigation that may upset the patient, these initial questions will, in the long run, save both patient and nurses time and frustration. The primary goal is to determine the patient's ability to perform ostomy self-care and resume normal life habits; a secondary goal is to identify any adverse factors that could be modified to facilitate learning during rehabilitation. The assessment must be comprehensive and must include physical, psychologic, social, cultural, and educational components. This multifocal approach requires the nurse to have a broad knowledge base in these disciplines. Assessment as a process is ongoing, involves the patient and family, and occurs throughout the nurse's every interaction with them. The nurse can collect data for assessment by interview, observation, physical examination, review of medical records, and collaboration with other health care team members.[8] The nurse should be aware that numerous factors affecting both the patient and the nurse may influence the assessment process and the interpretation of data. Christensen[9] has identified some of these specific factors as the following:
1. Physical, psychologic mental, and emotional status
2. Cultural, social, and philosophic backgrounds
3. Sensory capabilities
4. Past experiences relevant to the present situation
5. Actual meaning of the event
6. Interests, preoccupations, preconceptions, and motivational levels
7. Knowledge of the situation
8. Environmental conditions and distractions
9. Presence, attitudes, and reactions of others

**Physical Status.** The patient's overall physical condition is a factor in determining the risk of the surgical procedure and the individual's ability to accept it. The physical assessment components that affect the nursing plan of ostomy care are highly specific.

*Vision.* The visual capability of the patient affects the goals of ostomy care, the type of equipment selected, and the teaching plan. Patients with visual limitations may have adopted satisfactory compensatory methods. By interviewing the patient and family, the nurse can determine the type of activities suitable for patient participation and can ascertain the visual aids already in use. Does the patient wear trifocal glasses? Contact lenses? Can the patient read a newspaper? Where is the visual point of clarity obtained through glasses? Sometimes looking down on the abdomen at a specific site (stoma) is difficult through bifocal or trifocal lenses. The patient may have better visual acuity looking into a mirror. A lighted makeup mirror may offer sufficient magnification and an angle appropriate for satisfactory viewing. Collecting data by observation, the nurse can mark a circle on the patient's abdomen and have the person practice placing a pouch, using various positions or placement of mirrors. This method can give the nurse actual assessment data concerning the patient's visual capability without relying solely on the individual's self-perception of vision. Frequently patients overestimate their actual auditory and visual capabilities and are sensitive to any discovery of their limitation. If vision is markedly impaired, the patient may be taught to apply the ostomy equipment by touch, using the stoma as a landmark for positioning. Selection of a nonadhesive model or a pouching system with an oversized stoma opening can help reduce leakage relative to positioning. This approach may not provide complete skin protection but may be preferable when pouch application is too difficult for the patient to manage independently.

*Dexterity.* Has the patient had a stroke, with residual immobility? Does the patient have a tremor that increases with intentional effort, painful or limiting arthritis in the joints, missing fingers, or a missing arm? Through interview the nurse determines which activities the patient is capable of performing at home. Does the patient sew, knit, quilt, or do carpentry work requiring coordination? By observation the nurse determines whether the patient can open a clamp closure or drain valve, remove adhesive backing from a pouch, or apply a pouch to a faceplate. The patient's capability influences the goals of care and selection of equipment. A one-piece, precut pouch is much less complicated than a two-piece sizable pouch. Applying surgical adhesive to a reusable faceplate may be less challenging than positioning a disposable adhesive disk. A nonadhesive pouching system that requires only connecting the preset belt to the pouch may be the choice for the patient with minimal fine-motor capabilities. Numerous available alternatives can be matched to the patient's dexterity. Assessment and practice before surgery can help narrow the choices and minimize the frustration of leakage during the postsurgery learning phase.

*Hearing.* Although hearing loss is not usually considered an impediment to ostomy care, it can cause a frustrating breach of communication during patient teaching. It is important for the nurse to confirm that the patient actually is hearing what is being said, not just agreeing with it. Elderly patients whose hearing loss has occurred gradually frequently can conceal their actual loss through their socializing skills. A good check of the effectiveness of verbal communication is to have the patient repeat what he or she has understood or perform a task after receiving verbal instructions. If hearing is a problem, ostomy care can be taught through written and visual instruction. A slide-tape or video presentation showing the steps of ostomy care can, in effect, be "worth a thousand words." The video does not have to be professionally made; it can be a candid demonstration using the familiar nursing staff.

*Skin condition.* Because skin adhesives are used frequently with ostomy pouching systems, a careful assessment of the patient's skin condition and history of allergies or skin disorders is important. By physical examination the nurse checks the skin area where the stoma will be located. Is the skin dry, oily, slick, scaly, irritated? Does the patient have a history of any localized or systemic skin disorders such as psoriasis, atopic dermatitis, pemphigus, pyoderma gangrenosum, or mycosis fungoides? Has the patient had any skin reactions to adhesive bandages? If any clues suggest adhesive intolerance, preoperative patch tests with various adhesives should be considered. If systemic skin disorders are present, preoperative consultation with a dermatologist is necessary to provide comprehensive planning before the ostomy pouch is required. The advances made in the quality of hypoallergenic pouches and adhesives have reduced the number of problems with skin care over the years, but prevention, involving proper assessment and identification of potential problems, is more effective than treatment.

**Psychologic, Mental, and Emotional Status.** Assessment of the patient's psychologic and mental status is important because it determines the patient's ability to learn and to adapt to stress and changes in body image and life habits. Is the patient having problems with memory, with comprehension, with retention? Does the patient have a known learning disability or emotional disorder? If these are identified preoperatively, additional instructional time can be provided before surgery and before the patient's mental status is clouded with medications and pain.

The preoperative period also is a time when the patient demonstrates coping behaviors. Illness, which is a stressor that threatens a person's sense of wholeness, inevitably creates anxiety. The threat of helplessness, the loss of control, a sense of lost function and self-esteem, the failure of former defenses, a sense of isolation, and a fear of dying[6] are all components of an illness that can contribute to this anxiety. Cognitive behavior in response to threatened body image may include but may not be limited to anger, denial, hostility, sarcasm, withdrawal, humor, depression, apathy, hopelessness, and restlessness.[21] The nurse, who probably cannot remove the source of the anxiety, can identify coping behaviors and support them. For example, a patient's sense of control can be increased by the nurse who provides predictability, allows choices whenever possible, and includes the patient in decisions. Simple things such as the nurse explaining the schedule for the afternoon—for example, "You will see the doctor in the urology clinic, then go from there to radiology"—contribute to the patient's feeling of confidence. Expecting something to happen and having it happen provide order and predictability and increase confidence in the person who made the "prediction," even though the nurse's contribution is as simple as explaining an afternoon schedule.

Providing information and guidance are other forms of intervention that can enhance the patient's coping capacity. Sometimes patients feel apologetic about asking questions and taking the nurse's time. A planned session during which the nurse provides information, answers questions, and leaves educational material if appropriate can give the patient needed information, correct many misconceptions, and relieve unfounded fears.

Sharing concerns is another way the nurse can help the patient cope. The nurse can accomplish this by acknowledging the seriousness of the ostomy surgery and letting the patient know that fears relating to it are normal. Introducing a visitor with an ostomy also can provide encouragement. Such a person shows the patient that he or she is not alone and that someone else has had the same surgery and possibly the same feelings. The visitor provides the patient an ally who is nonprofessional yet "experienced" in the event that is producing the anxiety.

**Cultural Background.** A frequently overlooked component of nursing assessment is cultural history. Cultural differences between the nurse and the patient may not be a factor when their cultures are similar but can be significant when cultures differ. If the nurse does not understand the reason behind a patient's or family's behavior, the nurse finds it difficult to determine the real problem, plan to meet the patient's needs, or resolve any conflicts. For example, a problem with noncompliance or lack of cooperation from a patient who is a Gypsy might be better understood if the nurse were aware that Gypsy families tend not to trust medical personnel and believe that hospital and medical personnel carry germs.[29] Similarly the Islamic religion greatly influences most Arabs during illness.[18] They refrain from touching anything they consider contaminated, which could create a cultural conflict for the nurse trying to teach colostomy self-care to an Arabian patient. Patients from Asian cultures may employ self-control and self-reliance as coping strategies and may be reluctant to express their emotions or to request assistance.[25] Relationships, communication, beliefs, values, practices, hygiene, food habits, and health care are all affected by one's culture. To plan effective nursing care based on the patient's needs, the nurse should consider data from a cultural assessment of the patient and family.

**Educational Status.** An assessment of the patient's educational background should include the amount of formal schooling. Determining the literacy skills of the patient is important if written instructions are to be considered a part of teaching.[31] The patient may be able to speak two or more languages but read only one. Literacy level should be determined before plans are made. The patient who is illiterate may in fact be an exceptional learner of ostomy care. Some persons who have faced a lifetime of compensation for not being able to read are adept at working with their hands or with equipment. At the other extreme a patient whose profession has focused on mental processes may fear trying to work with pouching systems and gadgets. Past experiences and accomplishments are important to consider in assessing the patient's capabilities to learn self-care.

Assessment may appear to be a formidable, time-consuming task. It is, however, an ongoing activity that occurs throughout every encounter with the patient and family. A formal assessment interview may be appropriate initially,[24] and documentation is essential if the information is intended to shape the total plan of care for the patient.

## Stoma Site Selection

The preoperative visit with the patient receiving ostomy surgery is a critical interaction that serves several purposes: identification of the role of the ET (enterostomal therapy) nurse, assessment of physical and psychosocial factors, initiation of patient teaching, and selection and marking of a stoma site or sites.[5a] Stoma site selection must be a priority for the health care team. An improperly placed stoma complicates the patient's self-care (by adding time and expense to the pouch change routine) and may have a negative effect on adaptation. Six factors must be assessed when selecting a stoma site (see the box on p. 6).

The *type of ostomy surgery* must be known; this information reveals the portion of the bowel or urinary tract to be fashioned into a stoma. Understanding the patient's disease, talking with the surgeon, or reading the chart provides this information. The abdominal quadrant that correlates with the appropriate underlying organ(s) is then identified.

---

## FACTORS TO BE ASSESSED IN STOMA SITE SELECTION

1. Type of ostomy surgery
2. Location of rectus muscle
3. Adequate adhesive surface on abdomen
4. Avoidance of skin folds, scars, umbilicus, belt line, and any bony prominence

5. Visibility to patient
6. Presence of supportive devices

---

The *location of the rectus muscle* must be assessed. The rectus abdominus is a striated muscle that runs vertically from the xyphoid process to the pubic symphysis (Fig. 1-1). This muscle can be identified by inspection and palpation. Lifting the head while the patient is in a reclining position makes the rectus abdominus more prominent. To determine the width of the muscle, the nurse should begin palpation at the midline below the umbilicus and "walk" the fingers toward the side of the abdomen. When the stoma is within the rectus muscle, the potential for prolapse is reduced.

*Adequate adhesive surface area* must be determined. Ideally, adequate adherence of an adhesive pouching system on an adult requires approximately 2 to 2½ inches of smooth abdominal surface. In the child the pouching system may require only 1½ inches of smooth surface.

The stoma site should *avoid* skin folds, scars, the umbilicus, the belt line, and any bony prominence (such as the anterior iliac crest or ribs). With the patient in the supine position a possible stoma site is marked with an ink pen. This site is then assessed while the patient is sitting, standing, and bending. Suddenly, previously unnoticed abdominal wrinkles may appear or flat scars retract. Reduced subcutaneous tissue support becomes more apparent when the patient is standing and can alter abdominal contours dramatically. Ideally the stoma should be located below the beltline; since this location seldom interferes with clothing styles, the need to alter the wardrobe is minimized.

The stoma site must also be *visible to the patient.* When the patient cannot see a stoma, it is quite difficult for the patient to become independent in self-care. Most often the infraumbilical bulge is the location visible to the patient. The nurse can assess the patient's ability to see the stoma site (while the patient is in a relaxed, sitting position) by placing the fifth finger on the stoma site and asking the patient whether he or she can see the nurse's fingernail.

Finally the nurse must assess the patient for the *presence of supportive devices* such as an abdominal back support. Consultation with a prosthetic technician may be warranted to determine whether equipment modifications are feasible.

Many situations provide extenuating circumstances to these assessment factors.[35] For example, patients who are in wheelchairs need to be assessed only while sitting in the wheelchair to ensure that the stoma site is visible and avoids a lap tray or lap belt. Abdominal contours distorted by abdominal distention complicate site selection. Irradiated abdominal fields (or potential fields) must be avoided. When two stomas are required, they should be located far enough apart to allow for two separate pouching systems, generally on opposite sides of the abdomen.

After considering these factors, the nurse marks the selected stoma site, using one of the techniques described in the box on p. 7. The technique used should be indelible, safe to the

## STOMA SITE MARKING TECHNIQUE

**OPTION 1**

Cleanse abdominal site with alcohol swab. Administer intradermal injection of sterile methylene blue using a tuberculin syringe. This technique creates a permanent mark (tattoo), so it should not be used when there is a possibility that the site may not be used or when the patient objects to the permanent mark.

**OPTION 2**

Using an indelible pen or marker, draw a circle or an X at the preferred stoma site. This site may be protected by covering the indelible ink mark with a skin sealant spray.

**OPTION 3**

Cleanse abdominal site with alcohol swab. Using a sterile 25-gauge needle, scratch the epidermis in a cruciate fashion. This technique does create a break in the skin, introducing the *potential* for an infection at the site.

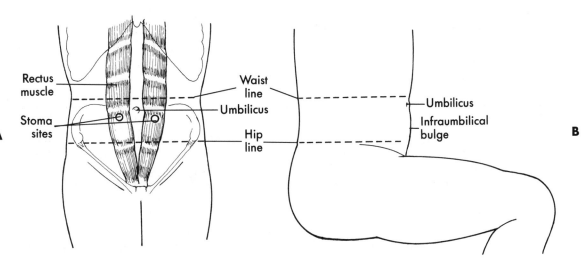

**A**

Rectus muscle
Stoma sites
Waist line
Umbilicus
Hip line
Umbilicus
Infraumbilical bulge

**B**

**Fig. 1-1    A,** Preferred location of stoma is identified in right and left lower quadrants with patient in supine or standing position. Landmarks such as beltline, umbilicus, and iliac crest are evident. **B,** Preferred location for stoma site with patient in sitting position. (Modified from Schrock TR: Ileostomy and colostomy. In Fromm D, editor: *Gastrointestinal surgery,* vol 2, New York, 1985, Churchill Livingstone.)

patient and nurse, and recognizable by the surgeon and should cause minimal discomfort. When the topographically correct site for a particular ostomy surgery (for example, the right lower quadrant for an ileostomy) is not the preferred stoma site, it is wise for the nurse to inform the surgeon of the situation before surgery. The surgeon may be aware of other factors that will impede the ability to use such a site, in which case the nurse and surgeon must identify other site options.

**Table 1-1**   Stoma site selection in the infant

| Principle | Rationale |
| --- | --- |
| Select a site away from umbilical cord | Adhesives interfere with cord care required during first 10 to 14 days after birth; once cord falls off, resulting irregular surface area interferes with effective pouching |
| Avoid low abdominal site | Baby's kicking dislodges pouch |
| Separate two limbs if double barrel stoma is needed (if possible) | Facilitates pouching functional stoma with a small pediatric pouch |
| Select a site away from incision | Reduces potential of contaminating incision with stool and creating dehiscence; as incision heals, scar retracts with baby's movements and creates irregular pouching surface |

Modified from Boarini JH: Principles of stoma care for infants, *J Enterostom Ther* 16(1):21, 1989.

Ostomy surgery in infants is typically required in emergency situations within the first few days of life. For this reason and because it is difficult to predict physical growth in the baby, stoma site marking in the infant or neonate is uncommon. However, the criteria listed in Table 1-1 should guide the placement of the stoma.

## EDUCATION

Patient and family teaching plans can begin before surgery and continue throughout acute recovery and rehabilitation. The assessment data are used to determine the patient's and the family's present level of knowledge about the surgical procedure, ostomy care and pouching equipment, sexual consequences, and hospital experience; to identify what the patient and family feel is important to learn; and to specify any particular concerns related to culture, finances, or other areas.

Patient teaching is a major part of the nurse's role. It is the single most important action toward independence, confidence, and rehabilitation for the patient. Some basic principles of education should be applied in the teaching-learning process. Because adult learners differ from child learners, the two groups are discussed separately.

### Adult Learning

**Characteristics.** *Andragogy* is the theory of education that deals with adult education.[4] Knowles,[15] an early proponent of adult education theories, identified four areas in which adults differ from children in their learning.

*Self-direction.* Adults are capable of self-direction. Their self-concepts have changed from dependence to independence, and they have defined roles in their careers and families. The presence of an ostomy may threaten the patient's self-concept as a producer, whether it be as breadwinner or homemaker of the family.

*Resources.* Because of their life experiences, adults have a large base of resources for learning. These experiences may enhance the learning process or may be detrimental to it. The nurse must be aware of how these experiences are influencing the patient. For example, a male patient who is a urologist and has been performing ileal conduit surgery and serving as head of the surgical health care team may have difficulty moving into the role of patient and "learner" when he himself needs a cystectomy and urinary diversion.

*Motivation.* Many adults have passed the stage of learning for the sake of learning and require specific motivation; however, they frequently respond to problems or identified needs. The teacher can encourage an adult to view learning ostomy care as a specific response to the need to know something to remain independent in personal hygiene. Not to learn self-care would result in losing independence and self-control.

*Application.* Adults expect to be able to apply what they have learned immediately. They participate more responsively if they have a "need" to learn. This is particularly applicable for ostomy patients. For example, before surgery the patient may be too preoccupied with other concerns to concentrate on disconnecting a urinary drainage adapter on a pouching system he or she does not yet have to wear. Four days after surgery, however, when the patient is interested in getting out of bed and moving about the room, attention can be more focused on learning how to disconnect the drainage adapter.

**Principles.** One of the most important considerations in teaching a patient to care for an ostomy is the awareness that teaching cannot be left to chance. A teaching plan must be based on assessment data, patient needs, and nursing diagnoses. Several members of the health care team and the family may share in the teaching, but it is vital that one person assume responsibility for the outcomes and for evaluation. This role usually is assumed by the nurse. For example, a patient with multiple sclerosis and motor disabilities requires a urinary diversion. Because the patient has impaired dexterity, the nurse improvises a pouch to attach the adapter of the drainage bag to the leg bag. The nurse secures and applies the equipment, evaluates its potential, sets up a teaching plan, and demonstrates the technique to the patient, the family, and the unit staff. The family and the unit staff can then assist the patient with practice sessions throughout the day, whereas the nurse provides follow-up lessons and reinforcement and makes adjustments if necessary. The nurse assumes the responsibility for the overall effectiveness of the teaching plan.

A second important principle in teaching is that learning requires some activity (mental or physical, or both) on the part of the learner. The learner must be active rather than passive in the process. Practice sessions make use of this theoretic principle.

**Learning Domains.** Three domains or types of learning are important to considerations in patient education. They are cognitive, which includes fact, concept, and problem solving; psychomotor; and affective, or attitude.[5,7,16,33] Different learning activities are appropriate for different types of learning.

*Cognitive.* For cognitive learning the patient must be motivated to learn and must believe that the new information is meaningful. The nurse can explain why the information should be learned and can use examples that are meaningful to the patient. For example, in explaining the potential for a cutaneous yeast infection around a urinary stoma and the need for an antifungal medication, the nurse might ask a woman whether she has ever had a vaginal yeast infection that required treatment; if so, she can correlate the two similar conditions. The nurse should give verbal instruction and follow it with written instruction to reinforce cognitive learning. Providing realistic situations that may occur at home helps challenge the patient to think through the steps of problem solving. The situations should move from the simple to the complex and incorporate positive feedback throughout the process. Written instructions should be simple yet include all necessary information.

*Psychomotor.* Psychomotor learning is a large part of the process for the ostomy patient. This is motor-skill learning and requires some coordinated muscular activity and practice. A highly effective method of teaching psychomotor skills is to break the procedure to be taught into small steps and use the demonstration and return-demonstration technique. In the first demonstration the nurse should review the steps of the procedure with the patient and then select one task for the patient to focus on. Depending on the patient's level of emotional adjustment to the ostomy, it may help if the task is one of low emotional charge. For example, some patients may be able to focus on cutting out a pattern of a skin barrier but not yet be ready to clean bloody mucus from fresh stomas on their own abdomens. Other patients, depending on their readiness, are quickly ready to remove an old pouch and cleanse their skin. The nurse should continually be assessing readiness, both emotional and mental. The nurse should stay with the patient while he or she initially performs the steps. Verbal guidance and support are necessary throughout practice. The nurse should be patient, taking time to let the patient actually practice, even though the patient's best efforts do not match the nurse's efficiency. Practice is necessary for the development of skill and confidence. If the patient makes mistakes, the nurse should provide gentle, positive correction. Negative correction such as, "Don't do it that way; it won't work," can be discouraging. A positive correction might be, "I think it will work better if you do it this way. Let me show you again, and then you try it." Feedback and encouragement are essential at every step and help patients develop confidence in their capability.

*Affective.* The third domain or type of learning is affective, or attitude learning. This also is very much a part of learning ostomy care. Attitude can be a powerful asset or a major deterrent to learning. The nurse may spend half of the visits helping to mold the patient's and family's attitudes and preparing them to accept what they need to learn. "Attitude therapy" is contagious. A patient responds to attitudes from the nurse, the physician, the unit staff, the family, and other patients. This is evident in a patient's response to visits by someone who has recovered from ostomy surgery; patients respond favorably to positive attitudes and confidence.

A word of caution: the nurse should make sure the attitudes presented are sincere, not false. The patient can detect a faked expression and turn it into a doubt. If the situation is complicated, for example, if a stoma is recessed, it should be acknowledged: "It may take several applications to find the pouching system that suits you the best, so I don't want you to feel discouraged during this period. We want to make sure the pouch fits accurately." It is not helpful to say, "Umm! This looks bad. I don't know if we will have anything to fit this stoma." The patient needs confident reassurance that the problem will be addressed, although several efforts may be required.

**Techniques.** In using various teaching principles and techniques with a patient, the nurse must remember to factor in the variable of illness. Consider whether the teaching is taking place on the day before surgery, when the patient's attention is elsewhere; whether the patient is being given postoperative narcotics or antiemetics, which affect memory and ability to retain knowledge; whether the patient's focus is on the nasogastric tube, the infiltrated intravenous catheter, pain, or fears. The presentation of four lessons does not necessarily mean that four lessons were received. Many home-care nurses can attest that, although the patient received good ostomy care and lessons in the hospital, home-care practices do not always reflect that care. Watson[33] states that little learning can take place in the first phase of illness, during the diagnosis and initial treatment phase. She says that patients see themselves as sick during that phase, and their energies are focused on dealing with the disease, the hospitalization, and the treatment. Teaching in this phase should focus on the patient's understanding of the disease and on alleviating anxiety. Unfortunately, much of the teaching a nurse does must occur in this stage of illness, either before surgery or in the immediate postoperative period. As patients move into recovery or even into subsequent therapy, they begin to see themselves as becoming well; they resume self-care activities and are better able to focus on learning activities. This phase usually occurs after discharge from the hospital.

A variety of other factors are involved in an adult's ability to learn, including environment, personality, cultural orientation, and family and community resources. All these factors must be acknowledged. To prevent becoming overwhelmed by influencing factors, however, the nurse should focus on what the patient needs to learn and which types of learning activities can accomplish the goals of the teaching-learning process.

## Child Learning

Very young children need to be taught in terms with which they can identify, using things they have experienced in their young lives, such as cartoon characters or coloring books. It is important to keep tasks simple so that the child does not become overwhelmed or frustrated with failure. The nurse should be aware of psychosocial and cognitive developmental factors that influence the child's capacity to learn. As children enter the toddler stage, they can begin to participate in parts of their care, such as washing the stoma while being supervised during bath time, holding the tape or other components of the pouching system, or working the drainage closure device. The child should be taught to say, like other toddlers, "I'm going to the potty" rather than "I'm going to empty my bags."

As motor skills develop during the preschool years, children can undertake more tasks. At this stage children are curious; therefore this is a natural time to involve them in learning independence in their personal hygiene. As children begin using scissors and crayons with some success, they are able to cut out adhesives, peel off adhesive backings, and assemble some of the equipment. Because dolls or stuffed animals are helpful teaching aids, infant-sized ostomy pouching systems can be given to children to apply to the dolls. This provides an aspect of "play" to the lesson and helps keep enthusiasm for learning. The steps of care are more easily learned if they are introduced during children's natural developmental phases. If children move through these growth and development processes without learning the steps in their care, dependency patterns begin developing that are hard to erase. For example, at the age for potty training, children can be taught to empty their pouches; when they are learning to bathe themselves, they can be taught basic stoma and skin cleanliness.

It is important first to assign simple tasks so that the child can begin with some measure of success and develop confidence. A sense of pride and accomplishment that results from succeeding in a task develops and increases the child's desire for more exploration and growth.[12] If at all possible, it is helpful for the child to be independent in ostomy care before beginning school. If the pouch leaks and the child has to leave school for a change, the disruption increases the embarrassment and calls attention to the stoma as a "handicap." The child who is confident in his or her ability to change the pouch can take an extra set of supplies to school and correct a pouch leak in a matter of minutes. If necessary, the school nurse can be taught to provide assistance and support.

The nurse who is teaching a child also must direct attention to the parents and their attitudes. Parental attitudes influence the child, and some parents tend to promote dependency because they fear the child cannot manage alone and must be protected. The nurse should encourage parents to support the child's efforts to learn and become independent. A parent is not normally needed to assist a 6-year-old with elimination functions; therefore the goal should be that the child with an ostomy handle ostomy care with the same minimal amount of parental assistance. The child who views ostomy care as a normal part of the daily toilet is more adept at integrating the ostomy into his or her self-image.

Documentation of the teaching plan and the patient's progress should be a part of the patient's record and discharge plan. Medical, nursing, and teaching plans must be coordinated to avoid last-minute and ineffective lessons that promote frustration, anxiety, and pouch leakage. The teaching plan for learning self-care is every bit as important in the patient's estimation as the surgery. No matter how skillfully the surgery was performed, if the patient cannot care for the ostomy, the operation was not a success.

## COUNSELING

The patient receiving ostomy surgery has myriad concerns to address emotionally: the cause of the surgery, that is, illness or trauma; the surgery itself; an altered body image resulting from a stoma; a change in lifelong elimination patterns; potential sexual dysfunction; threat of loss of life; and demands of the recovery process (including financial, personal, and work-related issues). Any one of these concerns could be viewed as a situational (or unexpected) crisis.

### Search for Balance

Aguilera and Messich have described three balancing factors that, if present in a threatening situation, can avert a crisis.[14] These are realistic perception of the event, adequate situational support or resources, and effective coping mechanisms. The nurse attempts to provide balance to the patient with an ostomy by helping the patient acquire accurate knowledge, soliciting available support resources, and identifying coping mechanisms that effectively serve the patient. Roy[22] suggests an adaptation model that interrelates a physiologic mode with three psychosocial adaptive modes: self-concept, role function, and interdependence. According to Roy, the nurse can help the patient's adaptive process by responding to the physiologic needs of ostomy care and to the psychosocial needs of self-esteem, role security, and individual worth. Theoretically, this concept of holistic assessment and response to the patient's needs is consistent with most models of adaptation.

### Reactive Phases

The presence of an ostomy presents special problems related to body image and self-concept because of the complex emotional reaction all adults experience as toddlers during the development of continence, a hard-learned task. Although body image (or the mental picture of one's appearance) is changing constantly, a time lag exists between the actual change in the body and the mental acceptance of it.[20] Lee[17] described four phases in the process of resolving alterations in body image after an illness or injury that are applicable to the patient having ostomy surgery. She terms the phases *impact, retreat, acknowledgment,* and *reconstruction.* Other authors have used different terms to describe similar phases; Busch, for example, uses the terms *shock and disbelief, development of awareness, restitution,* and *resolution.*[6] Lee's terms are used here.

**Impact.** The impact phase for the patient with an ostomy comprises loss of function (lifelong pattern of elimination and possibly sexual function), loss of a bodily part (rectum, bladder, colon, uterus, prostate), and loss of the mental image of the body (adding a surgical scar, stoma, and external pouching system). The patient may mentally compute these losses to determine whether he or she will be less of a person, less than whole. Each loss has an individual meaning and significance to each patient. Shame may be a component of the impact phase when elimination or sexual function is affected.

During the impact phase the patient may rely on denial for coping and may reject explanations about his or her condition or any attempts to teach self-care. The patient has no need to learn about a loss that is not yet "real" in his or her mind. The patient may appear uncooperative, whereas actually the problem is so anxiety-provoking that the patient cannot rely on his or her usual, rational problem-solving techniques. At this point the nurse should not try to remove the defense of denial by saying "Mr. Smith, this stoma is yours. You have to learn to take care of it!" Instead, support and acknowledgment of the patient's difficulty are indicated by a statement such as, "Mr. Smith, I know this is really a difficult time for you. Let me do your care for you today, and perhaps tomorrow you can start learning part of it." This response is supportive and caring; at the same time it plants the expectation that Mr. Smith will learn to care for himself.

**Retreat.** The second phase according to Lee is retreat. When patients discover they have not died as a result of the surgery, the reality of the ostomy becomes a problem. The patient's mental processes still hold on to the old body image, although the mirror and the patient's physical energy status reveal major changes. The nurse is reacting to this "new body" and wants to "teach care" to the patient who just wants to retreat.

Patients may find the reality ugly and disgusting. They may be angry or irritable, or they may ask, "Why me?" Their anger frequently is addressed to the person associated with the stoma, the nurse. The patient may complain about the nurse's tardiness, pouch leakages, or oversights, or the patient may address anger toward those with whom he or she feels the safest, family members. The spouse may be the target of emotional abuse and anger related not specifically to the person but to the situation.

Because the patient cannot physically leave, he or she may emotionally retreat. This action is not totally negative because it gives the patient some time to mourn the loss and reflect on the meaning of the stoma and its effect on his or her life. During this phase the nurse and staff members must not respond to the patient's anger with alienation and avoidance. Patients need to be allowed to express their anger without being abusive and need support in assessing their self-worth. Addressing the patient by name and encouraging the patient to comb his or her hair and to shave or apply makeup add to the patient's sense of personal worth. Stopping by to visit a patient when no direct physical task must be performed says, "I wanted to see you. I care about how you are feeling, not just whether your pouch is adhering."

**Acknowledgment.** The acknowledgment phase is the time when the patient puts aside anger and resistance and tries to find methods of coping. The patient realizes something is wrong or changed with his or her body, that this is stressful, and that he or she must face this reality to return to daily life. As the patient deals with changes in individuality and uniqueness, he or she may feel sad or cry. As the patient begins to adapt to a new image, he or she may spend considerable time going over memories of life before the loss.[6] He or she also may verbalize fears about the future—how he or she will deal with the ostomy on the job, while playing, or in social situations.

The family can help by acknowledging the illness and focusing on how the patient feels as a whole rather than concentrating on the stoma or bodily changes. When the spouse is to view the stoma for the first time, the nurse must support and prepare the spouse by describing how it looks, relating it to the pink, moist mucous membranes of the mouth, and explaining about the small sutures and mucus collection. The nurse should tell the spouse how important his or her reaction will be to the patient, who may interpret any negative response as rejection.

The nurse should be prepared to listen when the patient reminisces about the past and formulates visions of how he or she will manage in the future. This is a good time to bring in an ostomy visitor who has successfully recovered from a similar type of surgery. The nurse also can effectively support the family members and direct their support back to the patient.

**Reconstruction.** Lee's fourth stage is reconstruction. Reconstruction does not mean a return to perfection, but it is a process during which the patient realizes he or she has survived the physical loss and must adapt to the psychologic and social loss.[17] The patient may intellectualize that the ostomy surgery has saved his or her life and at the same time make derogatory remarks about his or her body such as, "I don't know why he (the surgeon) didn't just take that off; it doesn't work." The patient may give the stoma a name, in effect alienating it from his or her body in an effort to detach emotionally from the source of body change. The nurse who helps support the patient toward independence must be aware that the patient will vacillate between periods of dependence and independence. When pride in the accomplishments involved in learning self-care and adapting to body changes develops, the patient may find it helpful to serve as a role model to others who have just had the same type of surgery and still are having identity crises. Frequently patients returning to clinic for their first return appointments visit the inpatient care unit to see the staff members and, if appropriate, may be directed to rooms of patients who have had similar operations.

## Referral

If the patient who is grieving the losses is unable to find a balance in the effort to acknowledge his or her situation realistically, the patient's resources and coping mechanisms may be inadequate to avert a psychologic crisis. Physiologic responses such as anorexia, weight loss, hypertension, and tachycardia may combine with psychologic responses of anger, hostility, hopelessness, withdrawal, and depression.[20] Sometimes interventions designed to minimize the disturbance to the patient's body image are not effective. These patients may require a referral to the mental health care team to facilitate continued adaptation. The patient who feels hopeless and despairing about this situation may need a thorough psychologic evaluation and definitive treatment. The nurse can be alert to signs of despair and can help the patient deal with feelings of hopelessness and the sense that everything is impossible. To provide a positive effect on the patient's emotional status, the goals set for recovery should be immediate and achievable. Even in grave situations the patient can draw on the nurse's hopeful attitude and energy.

Watson, in her study of the effects of short-term counseling after ostomy surgery,[32] identified feelings that the participants in her study frequently reported: anger at the stoma and overall physical condition, feelings of ugliness because of the changed body image, fears regarding sexual function, grief over loss of continence, and worthlessness. These clinical patient responses support what could be predicted from theoretic models of adaptation and crisis.

## SEXUAL DYSFUNCTION

A specific and emotionally charged loss, which may be a result of several operations that necessitate an ostomy, is the loss of or alteration in sexual function. It is important for the nurse to have a basic understanding of the normal sexual-response cycle and how various types of surgery affect it. Interference in one function does not mean that all physical mechanisms are disrupted. Correct information is imperative so that myths and misinformation do not contribute to the patient's problems. Over the past decade much has been learned regarding sexual function itself and its preservation during pelvic surgery, yet there is still more to discover.

Incorporating sexual health in patient care is no longer disputed as a legitimate role for health care professionals.[13] It is a natural inclusion for the nurse, since so many of the patients receiving ostomy surgery have anxiety as a result of sexual alterations. The nurse can help the patient realize that although sexual function may be affected or sexual activity altered, sexuality cannot be destroyed. Sexuality is a physiologic and psychologic component of the person that is based on genes, hormones, and life experiences. Sexuality is not as simple as a single act of intercourse. It can be expressed physically through touch and acts of sexual intercourse, or it can be shared verbally or emotionally through intimacy and closeness. Sexuality is present throughout our lives and is constantly undergoing alteration. Any threat to sexual function creates complex emotional reactions.

### Causes

The patient with an ostomy is vulnerable to three categories of threats to sexual health: physical, psychologic, and social. Each is discussed here as it relates specifically to ostomy surgery.

**Physical.** An ostomy is the result of some degree of surgery, often pelvic. Pelvic surgery can physically disrupt important nerve and vascular supplies to the genitals. Other components of treatment that affect sexual function may include radiation therapy, chemotherapy, or medications that alter sexual function.

Each part of the sexual-response cycle can be disrupted physically. Desire is greatly influenced by hormones and the overall condition of the patient. In men the removal of the testicles or medically blocking the action of testosterone can decrease sexual desire, whereas removing the ovaries does not cause lowered desire in women. Certain pain medications and antiemetics can lower sexual desire, as can the symptoms they treat, pain and nausea. Generalized fatigue caused by the illness also can influence desire. Alcohol and opiates can be sexual depressants or desire decreasers. Desire, the first component of the sexual-response cycle, frequently is forgotten in sexual health education, which pays most attention to arousal and capabilities for erection or intercourse. If, however, a woman who has had a radical cystectomy requires chemotherapy as a follow-up treatment, the nurse should tell the patient and her spouse that a combination of factors—antiemetics, nausea, and fatigue—may cause her sexual desire to decrease. This knowledge helps the couple to prepare for this occurrence and to avoid interpreting it as a message of "I don't love you any-more." It also gives the couple an opportunity to plan sexual activity around the wife's medication schedule and energy levels.

Arousal depends on blood supply to the genitals and innervation. A man's arousal includes engorgement of the blood vessels in the penis, subjective excitement, and genital pleasure. It depends on the parasympathetic nerves that control blood flow to the penis, the vascular supply to the penis, and the pudendal nerves that transmit sensory responses from the genital area.[28] Because the parasympathetic nerve plexus lies behind and alongside the prostate, any pelvic surgery that removes the rectum, bladder, or prostate has the potential of damaging this plexus. Nerve-sparing surgical techniques have been developed and are used when possible.[28] For example, in a bowel resection performed for reasons unrelated to malignancy (such as total proctocolectomy in a patient with ulcerative colitis), nerve-sparing techniques are use to preserve sexual function.[11]

The role of pelvic surgery in damaging the vascular supply to the penis is not clear. Men with vascular disease before surgery may have difficulty in achieving full erections because of a reduction in blood vessel caliber resulting from atherosclerosis. Radiation therapy to the pelvis can further reduce blood vascularity to the penis by causing scarring in the small blood vessels, constricting them over time; erectile difficulties may not develop immediately but may occur several months after therapy.

A woman's arousal includes expansion and lubrication of the vagina, which usually is not affected by pelvic surgery unless part or all of the vagina is removed. (The top third of the vagina is excised during a cystectomy, and the entire vagina is resected in a total pelvic exenteration.) Radiation therapy can influence vaginal expansion and lubrication by affecting the small blood vessels and reducing available blood supply. The sensory nerves for both men and women remain intact, however, and genital sensation remains normal; this is important in the orgasm phase, which depends on both the pudendal nerve and the central nervous system.[28]

The genital pleasure and muscular contractions that occur during orgasm are not disrupted by pelvic surgery. The male mechanism of emission can be disrupted, however, if the sympathetic nerves in the presacral area that control emission are damaged. This damage can occur in any abdominoperineal resection. In addition, when a man has a radical cystectomy or a total pelvic exenteration, the prostate and seminal vesicles are removed, thereby removing the fluid from emission. Nevertheless, orgasm can occur in both men and women with ostomies, although other aspects of the response cycle are damaged. For example, a man who reports no erectile capabilities after cystectomy should still be able to have an orgasm from touch or friction of the genital area. The orgasm is dry, with no fluid ejaculated. Likewise women can have orgasms after a total pelvic exenteration and complete vaginal reconstruction.

**Psychologic.** The psychologic impact of an ostomy and how it affects a patient's body image and self-esteem have already been discussed in detail. The way a person feels about himself or herself also affects the person sexually. Sexuality is influenced by feelings of attractiveness and desirability. Each person needs to feel desirable, and the degree of impairment of his or her body image influences the person's recovery into a lovable partner.[28]

Emotional distress and emotional pain can be contributors to sexual problems. An illness that is threatening a person's life can rearrange his or her priorities; initially, concerns about survival override concerns about sexual function. Emotional responses to the crisis, such as anxiety, anger, and depression, also can influence sexual activity. Anxiety about the disease, the treatment, or the effect of the treatment on sexual function can convert each sexual act into a performance test. The patient's attention is more focused on the problems at hand than on the immediate sensual pleasure of the act. Prior episodes of failure of erection may come to the forefront of the patient's mind, contributing to the anxieties already present.

Anger, whether directed toward the disease, fate, or one's sexual partner, also can interfere with sexual function. Sometimes the "safest" person for the patient to be angry with is his or her sexual partner. The partner usually perceives this anger and for emotional safety backs away from the patient. This caution usually does not disappear in the presence of sexual approaches from the patient. The spouse also may have feelings of anger that must be resolved. Frustration, resentment, aggression, and tension render lovemaking difficult.

A multitude of factors can contribute to depression in medical patients: interruption of activities in their daily life, social rejection, loss of control over events surrounding the illness, pain and discomfort, loss of social and recreational benefits, effects of medications, odors, or even physiologic alterations as a result of the disease process. A depressed patient may feel loss of desire for sexual activity or a decrease in pleasure during sexual activity. The patient may not be able to generate enough energy or concentration to participate in sexual activities. Although a normal sadness accompanies serious illness, not all patients subsequently have clinical depression. The nurse can help the patient identify ways of coping with the dysphoria resulting from illness, surgery, and postsurgical consequences.

**Social.** The social impact of an ostomy intermingles with the psychologic, the physical, and the sexual aspects. Coe and Kluka[10] compiled a list of concerns expressed by ostomy patients and their spouses; included were concerns about being able to resume sexual activity, feeling alone, making changes in clothing styles, wondering how the ostomy will affect daily activities, trying to sleep while wearing a pouch, having an unpleasant odor, passing gas, deciding whom to tell, and cleanliness. The patient with an ostomy may fear rejection from his or her partner; if the patient does not have a partner, the patient may fear that no one will ever desire him or her as a sexual partner. Open communication about feelings and good sexual communication can help a couple. Most patients need time to adjust to their pouches and their body changes before they feel comfortable and secure in their sexual functioning.

## Sexual Rehabilitation

**The *PLISSIT* Model.** The nurse can make a major contribution to the health care team's function in sexual rehabilitation. Jack Annon's model, the PLISSIT mnemonic (*per*mission, *l*imited *i*nformation, *s*pecific *s*uggestion, and *i*ntensive *t*herapy),[2,3] is useful in defining levels of intervention for health professionals who provide sexual health care. The levels increase in complexity, knowledge, and communication skills, and the nurse should be able to respond to the needs of ostomy patients at the first three of the four levels (see the box on p. 18).

*Permission.* Permission gives the patient approval to express sexual concerns and anxieties. The nurse also gives professional "permission" to continue sexual behaviors the patient has been practicing provided that the practices are not harmful. This is the least complex of the intervention levels and requires the least preparation. It does, however,

---

### *PLISSIT* MODEL: AN EXAMPLE OF APPLICATION

**P   PERMISSION**
Introduction of sexual functioning information
   as part of preoperative education; patient
   questions encouraged and explored

**SS   SPECIFIC SUGGESTION**
Ideas regarding ostomy management during
   intercourse; positions, touching, and
   stimulating

**LI   *LIMITED INFORMATION***
Factual information regarding normal
   functioning, surgical alterations, teaching
   materials and models used

**IT   *INTENSIVE THERAPY***
Surgical implants, reconstruction, counseling
   by sex therapist or specialist

---

From Annon JS: *Behavioral treatment of sexual problems: brief therapy,* Hagerstown, Md, 1976, Harper & Row.

require the development of a relationship and a comfort zone in which the patient feels valued for himself or herself and safe in discussing personal and private issues with the nurse. The patient who senses that he or she will be judged or made to feel guilt or shame does not feel "permission." The nurse can give permission openly by overtly addressing sexual concerns. Questions such as, "Did your doctor discuss the sexual aspects of your surgery?" or "Do you or your spouse have any questions about the sexual effects of your surgery?" are open invitations, or permission, to ask questions and to discuss concerns. If the permission is not given openly, the patient may express sexual anxiety or test the safety of discussing sexual issues by trying to shock the nurse. For example, a man may expose himself or make such statements as, "I am a dead man now. I know she won't love me." Any sign of a negative response from the nurse makes the patient hesitant to bring up the subject again. By showing willingness to listen to the patient, the nurse is validating the importance of sexual health and providing an accepting environment in which the patient can express concerns.

*Limited information.* Limited information is the appropriate level of intervention during the preoperative teaching of patient and partner. On this level the ET nurse provides the patient with factual information that is directly related to the individual's condition and surgery. The nurse should use sensitivity and timing in discussing sexual information and should not take advantage of a time of personal vulnerability. Sexual information should be considered a part of the package of information given to the patient. Teaching aids help provide factual information, correct misinformation, and open the door for questions from the patient or partner. Pictures or three-dimensional models can show both normal sexual functioning and how the surgery will affect it. Most patients are not sure where the prostate is and what it does, why the uterus is removed with a radical cystectomy, or that the penis has three compartments. An information session for a man about to have a cystectomy may include an explanation of the mechanisms of erection and a description of the function and placement of penile prosthetic devices. A session for a woman requiring a cystectomy may include information concerning vaginal expansion and lubrication and the availability and use of suppositories or creams for vaginal lubrication. After the nurse has provided basic information, the patient or partner may raise questions that require further responses or the patient may dismiss the subject for the moment. The nurse should not force the matter on the patient. Rather, give correct information; the patient knows that he or she can return to this subject at any time. Providing information can relieve concerns and anxieties about sexuality. The nurse should help the patient to view sexuality as more than a single sexual activity and to realize that damaging one aspect of sexual functioning does not mean eliminating all aspects. Therefore those sexual functions that remain normal after surgery should be emphasized.

This level of intervention requires that the nurse have knowledge related to the sexual consequences of diseases and treatments. An increasing base of knowledge regarding sexuality is available through texts, journals, conferences, workshops, and the audiovisual media. This level also requires that the nurse have some degree of comfort in discussing a sensitive subject. Comfort increases with knowledge and practice. Discussing sexual issues with peers in unit patient care conferences or at clinical workshops provides gradual desensitization of the emotional charge associated with these topics. The nurse should recognize sexual health care as a component of professional nursing care and present it as such.

***Specific suggestions.*** The third level of the Annon model also is appropriate for the nurse, since specific suggestions for sexual activity can easily be combined with the specific suggestions for ostomy care. Many times assigning a patient specific behavioral tasks is sufficient to resolve the sexual problem. Helpful suggestions for the patient with an ostomy include practicing proper hygiene in ostomy care, making sure the pouch is empty and securely in place before starting sexual activity, using an attractive pouch cover or underwear, applying vaginal lubrication if appropriate, and drawing on a sense of humor to remind the couple that sexual activity should be fun and pleasurable, not stressful and disappointing.

Couples also may need some specific suggestions about their communication skills to ensure that each partner is aware of the other's needs and fears. For example, sexual miscommunication may lead a man to move to another bedroom to sleep alone when he is no longer able to have an erection, whereas the woman may be missing the snuggling, hugging, and kissing aspects of their shared bed. Such a couple may need some guidance in expressing what each would like from the other, which usually is not more than the partner is able to give. The nurse also may be able to suggest specific positions that are more comfortable (for example, the side-to-side position may be more comfortable for a patient whose stoma and abdominal incision are only a few weeks old) or specific touching activities to help a couple reach orgasm through noncoital stimulation. The offering of specific suggestions may encourage the couple and speed their return to sexual activity. This in turn may help reduce feelings of loss and can aid the rehabilitation process. The couple without sufficient information to deal with sexual recovery may attempt sexual activities before surgical discomfort or psychologic sensitivities have subsided and meet with disappointing failure. Failure may temper the next attempt at sexual activity, adding anxiety to a cycle of frustrations until eventually, to avoid emotional pain, the attempts cease. Some guidance and information from the nurse can smooth the transitional period of sexual recovery from surgery and eliminate potential problems.

***Intensive therapy.*** The fourth level of intervention involves reconstructive surgery, surgical implants, and psychosexual therapy. Intensive therapy requires the expertise of a sex therapist, psychologist, psychiatrist, or surgeon.

Sex therapy may consist of brief sex counseling or intensive sex therapy. Brief counseling can include education, guiding the patient to change maladaptive beliefs about sexuality and the illness, and teaching the patient to cope with the distractions of the ostomy.[28] Intensive sex therapy, on the other hand, involves behavioral treatment that employs techniques for desensitizing anxiety, for communication training, and for behavioral tasks that increase in difficulty over the course of the therapy. It is helpful for the sex therapist to have some knowledge of the disease processes and surgical treatments that persons with ostomies have so that individualized therapy can be structured.

Combining sex therapy or counseling with medical treatments may be necessary. An estrogen cream, if not contraindicated by the diagnosis, may be prescribed for a woman with dyspareunia or vaginal dryness. Otherwise a water-based vaginal lubricant such as K-Y jelly, Ortho Personal Lubricant, Lubrin, or Transi-Lube can be recommended.[27] A woman who has had split-thickness skin grafts for a vaginal reconstruction may need to use a vaginal dilator several times a week in addition to lubrication for intercourse. In contrast, a muscle-graft vaginal reconstruction usually does not require dilation because the vaginal caliber and depth are sufficient and not subject to stricturing; nevertheless, lubrication is recommended for this type of neovagina.[27]

A variety of penile prostheses are available as surgical treatment for erectile dysfunction. The assortment of models includes rigid and semirigid types (hinged and malleable) and inflatable types (self-contained and compartmental). The penile prosthesis is not a miracle cure for sexual difficulties. It can restore erectile function, but it cannot repair lowered desire or impaired sensation on penile skin. The semirigid models, although providing permanent penile rigidity, can be concealed under athletic briefs by folding the penis up against the abdomen or down toward the thigh. Although these models are the least complicated mechanically and the least expensive to insert, they are considered the least aesthetically satisfactory. Inflatable prostheses are more expensive and technically complicated because they contain a reservoir, inflatable cylinders, and pump and valve mechanisms; however, they are considered more aesthetically acceptable because the penis is not constantly erect.

Other mechanisms for penile erection include injecting the penis with drugs that cause priapism. Papaverine, sometimes combined with phentolamine, can produce a full and prolonged erection unless the man has serious penile vascular disease.[26] Even after orgasm the erection may remain for several hours. Patients employing this method should be supervised medically and taught to watch for unresolved priapism, which necessitates medical treatment. Scarring of the cavernous bodies and damage to the sensory nerves are other potential sequelae to the injections.

Another device that can assist a patient in achieving an erection is a suction apparatus that pulls blood into the penis and traps it there with an external elastic band.[19] This device is much less expensive than a penile prosthesis and requires no surgical procedure. Patients report anecdotally that they can achieve an erection sufficient for vaginal penetration. This device also requires patient education regarding proper and safe use. As with any type of sexual dysfunction, the technical restoration of a function should be accompanied by proper assessment, education, and response to the couple's overall situation.

Vaginal reconstructive surgery varies with the degree of vaginal disruption and type of primary surgery. In the 1970s physicians did not perform vaginal reconstructions at the time of the original surgery. Instead the reconstruction was offered months after the patient had recovered from the exenteration. Frequently patients had been so traumatized by the major exenterative procedure that they chose not to have another operation. For those who did choose vaginal reconstruction the possible procedures involved skin grafts, split-thickness grafts, or the Williams procedure in which the labia were sewn together to form a pouch.[1] The skin graft procedures caused problems of stricture and required frequent dilations. The neovaginas created were not soft or pliable, and intercourse was frequently painful. The Williams procedure resulted in a neovagina with a severe upright angle of entry and, in many instances, was not suitable for penile entry.

In the late 1970s and the 1980s the use of myocutaneous flaps for vaginal reconstruction became popular.[23] This procedure is combined with the original surgery, and the flaps serve to fill the huge pelvic defect and provide a soft, pliable, adequate neovagina that requires no dilation.

Not all patients who have an ostomy want or require intensive therapy for their sexual concerns. However, the nurse must be aware of the resources open to the patient and should be available as a supportive professional during the period of therapy. For example, when a man returns to the hospital for a penile prosthesis after receiving an abdominoperineal resection, the nurse can relieve embarrassment and offer support by stating, "I see you're coming back into the hospital for your prosthesis. Are there any questions I can answer for you? Do you need anything?" This conveys to the patient the nurse's understanding and acceptance of the problem and provides a familiar, supportive person on whom the patient and his partner can rely.

*Special circumstances.* Sexual rehabilitation is not limited to the married heterosexual patient of reproductive age; it should be a component of health care for all patients and all groups. For a young patient facing procedures that may affect sexual growth, development, and function, an overall plan of rehabilitation should be developed at the time of the initial treatment. For example, when a 3-year-old-girl requires a total pelvic exenteration for the treatment of sarcoma botryoides, the health care team should establish an overall growth and rehabilitation plan that includes learning independence in ostomy care, hormonal replacement at puberty, vaginal reconstruction after puberty, and sexual counseling throughout the process. An older, widowed man who requires a radical cystectomy should be afforded sexual information and offered options for recovering penile erections. The homosexual or lesbian patient should be acknowledged without judgment and offered counseling and information appropriate to his or her individual concerns. Information about the human immunodeficiency virus (HIV) and about measures of protection should be included for all patients. Likewise, nurses should employ precautions when dealing with a patient's bodily secretions. The extended relationship the nurse develops with an ostomy patient, beginning preoperatively and continuing through the acute care period and follow-up, can be used to effect progress toward sexual rehabilitation and to gain acceptance as the pivotal person in the health care team who discovers needs and provides needed referrals.

## FOLLOW-UP CARE

Planning for patient discharge and establishing goals for rehabilitation after ostomy surgery are components of nursing care that must be considered from the beginning of the nurse-patient relationship. Assessments of the patient's technical and emotional needs and identification of the community and home resources available for ongoing support must be coordinated.[21] The goal of the teaching-learning process is for the patient to transfer the information presented and the skills practiced in the hospital to the home situation.

Planning for discharge includes learning about the patient's home environment. How many bathrooms are in the home? How many people live in the dwelling? Are running water and indoor bath facilities available? Is there a mirror or counter available in the bathroom for use in ostomy care? Is the bathroom private? Discharge planning also should include evaluations of patients' economic resources. Will they be able to buy needed ostomy supplies? Is there a supplier in their area, or do they need information about mail-order equipment? Are community resources available for supplies? Other components of the discharge plan include available relationships for the family. With whom does the patient live? Who is available for assistance immediately after discharge? Who should be the backup person to learn ostomy care? Who is available for support to the spouse? What related support groups are available in the community? Does the patient need visits from a home-care nurse?

The patient and family should participate in making the discharge plans. They should have in hand, upon discharge, written instructions for the ostomy care, the address of an ostomy product supplier, a telephone number for the ET nurse, and addresses of appropriate community resources such as the United Ostomy Association, the American Cancer Society, or the Crohn's and Colitis Foundation of America, Inc. They also should have the date for a return appointment to see the ET nurse.

Each patient should have a follow-up visit with an ET nurse, which offers an opportunity to identify any problems that have developed and to see how the patient's recovery has progressed. At home the patient has had time to practice caring for the stoma, learning what works well and what questions still are unresolved. There has been a chance to see how care fits into the individual's routine and environment. At the follow-up visit the ET nurse should assess the patient's stoma, pouching system, and methods of care. Has the stoma size changed? Do adjustments need to be made in the equipment? What is the condition of the skin? Is the patient ready to learn more? What has been the person's emotional response to living with an ostomy? Has he or she resumed work, social, or sexual activities?

The follow-up visit should be a time to look for clues of any problems, emotional or physical. Frequently the problems are interrelated but not overtly presented. The patient who has had a colostomy for 9 months may profess to be having no problems; yet during the examination the ET nurse may find that this person is using a pin to prick a hole in the odor-proof pouch to release the gas, without realizing that this is the source of odor leaks. Another patient may demonstrate good methods of care and excellent hygiene but, when asked about her social life, reveal that she has not returned to her church and volunteer activities and refuses to visit her daughter in another town because she fears her pouch will leak.

The follow-up visit is an opportunity to identify such problems and find solutions. As a measure of recovery, the visit is a chance for the ET nurse to compare the patient's present activities with those before surgery and to evaluate the patient's progress in meeting the specified goals and objectives established earlier in the nursing plan. If necessary, the entire nursing management process remains in motion as assessment, planning, actions, and evaluation continue. Ultimately the goal in caring for the patient with an ostomy is rehabilitation, that is, return to the patient's optimal life-style. Because the patient's physical, psychosocial, and sexual adjustments may take months, the follow-up visits are important to provide needed guidance and support during the process of recovery.

## SUMMARY

Each aspect of the patient's care serves a function and is important to the overall program established by the ET nurse. The preoperative phase sets the stage for assessment, counseling, information giving, relationship building, and stoma site selection. The immediate postoperative period is the time to select the proper pouching system, to start lessons in care, and to provide acute care for incisional healing. The follow-up period allows the patient to develop independence and to assimilate the reality of the ostomy into his or her physical and emotional life. Each phase builds on the previous one as the patient copes, learns, and adapts.

# SELF-EVALUATION

## QUESTIONS

1. A primary reason for assessing a patient before the creation of a stoma is to:
   a. Determine which ostomy pouching system is appropriate
   b. Elicit the number of bathrooms in the home
   c. Discuss employment issues after discharge
   d. Identify patient ability and needs for learning self-care
2. Priority nursing activity(ies) with a patient who will have ostomy surgery include(s):
   a. Discussing the surgical procedure and stoma site selection
   b. Applying a pouch to validate the selected stoma site
   c. Stoma site selection and referral to a United Ostomy Association visitor
   d. Referral to a sex therapist and discharge planning
3. List four factors that influence the assessment process.
4. The patient with limited vision may best learn ostomy self-care by:
   a. Improved lighting and teaching by touch
   b. Enlarged size of print on resource materials
   c. Using audiovisual materials
   d. Selecting larger pieces of equipment
5. Asking questions about a patient's hobbies, work, and activities aids in the evaluation of:
   a. Hearing, dexterity, and sexual functioning
   b. Hearing, dexterity, and vision
   c. Dexterity, vision, and nutritional requirements
   d. None of the above
6. Preoperative patch testing of ostomy adhesives or dermatology referrals or both should be considered:
   a. In all preoperative ostomy situations
   b. Primarily with children because they have a thinner epidermis
   c. For patients with adhesive allergies and dermatologic disorders
   d. For patients with a history of radiation therapy
7. Including the patient in the decision-making process should enhance the patient's:
   a. Psychomotor skill
   b. Sense of control
   c. Quality of life
   d. Relationship with family members
8. When selecting ostomy equipment for an Islamic patient, what primary factor(s) should the nurse consider?
   a. Clothing selection
   b. Cultural and religious
   c. Sexual functioning and work environment
   d. Product availability
9. Examining the patient's abdomen before ostomy surgery is suggested for the following reason(s):
   a. To facilitate self-care and emotional adjustment
   b. To comply with physician's orders
   c. To identify potential stoma site(s)
   d. To order supplies and to patch test for allergies

10. Examining a patient's abdomen in different positions before ostomy surgery should be performed with the patient in what positions and why?

11. All of the following are principles of learning appropriate to the adult except:
    a. Adults are capable of self-direction.
    b. Adults have life experiences that influence learning.
    c. Adults learn in response to self-identified needs.
    d. Adults prefer to wait before applying their learning.

12. An example of the use of affective learning is:
    a. Planning a visit to the patient by an individual who has an ostomy and has returned to his or her preoperative life-style
    b. Visiting a patient who has physical disabilities to show that ostomy surgery is not so bad
    c. Frequent correction of the patient learning self-care
    d. None of the above

13. Name three factors that may interfere with early postoperative patient teaching and learning.

14. Small children who are learning self-care of an ostomy:
    a. Should participate in relation to normal developmental patterns
    b. May learn with the aid of a doll for practice
    c. Should be independent in self-care by the time they enter school
    d. All of the above

15. The correct sequence of the four phases in the process of resolving alterations in body image as described by Lee is:
    a. Retreat, acknowledgment, reconstruction, and impact
    b. Acknowledgment, impact, retreat, and reconstruction
    c. Impact, retreat, acknowledgment, and reconstruction
    d. Retreat, impact, reconstruction, and acknowledgment

16. A sexually active woman who requires a cystectomy may have difficulty with:
    a. Lubrication
    b. Arousal
    c. Climax
    d. Orgasm

17. Sexual functioning in individuals of either sex may be affected by:
    a. Radiation to the pelvis
    b. Chemotherapeutic agents
    c. Hormones
    d. All of the above

18. Sexual arousal in men depends on:
    a. The presence of the urethra
    b. Adequate blood and nerve supplies to the genitals
    c. A sexually creative partner
    d. Only an adequate nerve supply

19. List in order the levels of intervention in the PLISSIT model.

**20.** The use of a teaching model to explain normal sexual functioning is an example of which level of the PLISSIT model?
   **a.** Permission
   **b.** Limited information
   **c.** Specific suggestion
   **d.** Intensive therapy

**21.** Scarring of the cavernosa bodies and sensory nerve damage are potential side effects of:
   **a.** Inflatable penile prosthesis
   **b.** Injecting the penis with drugs that cause priapism
   **c.** Rigid penile prosthesis
   **d.** Semirigid penile prosthesis
   **e.** Suction device

**22.** A neovagina is created in the woman who has a:
   **a.** Cystectomy
   **b.** Abdominal perineal resection
   **c.** Hartmann's pouch
   **d.** Total pelvic exenteration

## SELF-EVALUATION

### ANSWERS

1. **d.** Identify ability and needs for learning self-care
2. **a.** Discussing the surgical procedure and stoma site selection
3. Factors that influence the assessment process:
   Physical, mental, and emotional statuses
   Cultural, social, and philosophic backgrounds
   Sensory abilities
   Past experiences
   Meaning of the event
   Interest, preoccupations, preconceptions, and motivational levels
   Knowledge of situation, environmental conditions, and distractions
   Attitudes and presence of others
4. **a.** Improved lighting and teaching by touch
5. **b.** Hearing, dexterity, and vision
6. **c.** For patients with adhesive allergies and dermatologic disorders
7. **b.** Sense of control
8. **b.** Cultural and religious
9. **c.** To identify potential stoma site(s)
10. The abdomen should be examined with the patient in the lying, standing, and sitting positions. As positions shift, changes occur in the abdominal contours and the pattern of scars, thus affecting the pouch adhesive surface.
11. **d.** Adults prefer to wait before applying their learning. (This is not true, since adults are more responsive when the need is present.)
12. **a.** Planning a visit to the patient by an individual who has an ostomy and has returned to his or her preoperative life-style
13. Factors that may interfere with early postoperative teaching and learning include pain, use of narcotics, nausea and vomiting, and the presence of tubes.
14. **d.** All the areas listed are appropriate for a child.
15. **c.** Impact, retreat, acknowledgment, and reconstruction
16. **a.** Lubrication inasmuch as the upper third of the vagina is excised
17. **d.** All the reasons listed may cause problems with sexual functioning.
18. **b.** Adequate blood and nerve supplies to the genitals
19. The PLISSIT model interventions are permission, limited information, specific suggestion, and intensive therapy.
20. **b.** Limited information
21. **b.** Injecting the penis with drugs that cause priapism
22. **d.** Total pelvic exenteration

# REFERENCES

1. Andersen BL, Turnquist DC: Psychological issues. In Berek JS, Hacker NF, editors: *Practical gynecologic oncology*, Baltimore, 1989, Williams & Wilkins.
2. Annon JS: The PLISSIT model: a proposed conceptual scheme for the behavioral treatment of sexual problems, *Sex Educ Ther* 2:1, 1972.
3. Annon JS: *Behavioral treatment of sexual problems: brief therapy*, New York, 1974, Harper & Row.
4. Billie DA: Patient/family teaching. In Dossey BM, Guzzetta CE, Kenner CV, editors: *Essentials of critical care nursing*, Philadelphia, 1990, JB Lippincott.
5. Bloom BS, ed: *Taxonomy of educational objectives. Handbook I: cognitive domain*, New York, 1956, David McKay.
5a. Boarini JH: Preoperative considerations. In Broadwell DC, Jackson BS: *Principles of ostomy care*, St Louis, 1982, Mosby–Year Book.
6. Busch KD: The concept of holism: the patient's experience with critical illness. In Hudak CM, Gallo BM, Benz JJ, editors: *Critical care nursing: a holistic approach*, ed 5, Philadelphia, 1990, JB Lippincott.
7. Busch KD: Patient and family teaching. In Hudak CM, Gallo BM, Benz JJ, editors: *Critical care nursing: a holistic approach*, ed 5, Philadelphia, 1990, JB Lippincott.
8. Carpenito LJ: Deriving nursing diagnosis: assessment and diagnosis. In Carpenito LJ, editor: *Nursing diagnosis: application to clinical practice*, ed 3, Philadelphia, 1989, JB Lippincott.
9. Christensen PJ: Assessment: overview of data collection. In Christensen PJ, Kenney JW, editors: *Nursing process: application of conceptual models*, ed 3, St Louis, 1990, Mosby–Year Book.
10. Coe M, Kluka S: Concerns of clients and spouses regarding ostomy surgery for cancer, *J Enterostom Ther* 15:232, 1988.
11. Corman ML: Nonspecific inflammatory bowel disease. In Corman ML, editor: *Colon and rectal surgery*, ed 2, Philadelphia, 1989, JB Lippincott.
12. Erwin-Toth P: Teaching ostomy care to the pediatric client: a developmental approach, *J Enterostom Ther* 15:126, 1988.
13. Fogel CI, Lauver D: *Sexual health promotion*, Philadelphia, 1990, WB Saunders.
14. Kenney JW: Overview of selected model. In Christensen PJ, Kenney JW, editors: *Nursing process: application of conceptual models*, ed 3, St Louis, 1990, Mosby–Year Book.
15. Knowles MS: *The modern practice of adult education*, New York, 1970, Association Press.
16. Krathwohl DR, Bloom BS, Masia BB: *Taxonomy of educational objectives. Handbook II: affective domain*, New York, 1964, David McKay.
17. Lee JM: Emotional reaction to trauma, *Nurs Clin North Am* 5:578, 1970.
18. Meleis A: The Arab American in the health care system, *Am J Nurs* 6:1180, 1981.
19. Nadig PW, Ware JC, Blumoff R: Noninvasive device to produce and maintain an erection-like state, *Urology* 27:126, 1986.
20. Roberts SL: Body image and self concept. In Roberts SL, editor: *Behavioral concepts and the critically ill patient*, ed 2, Englewood Cliffs, NJ, 1986, Prentice-Hall.
21. Rolstad BS: Facilitating psychosocial adaptation, *J Enterostom Ther* 14:28, 1987.
22. Roy SC: *Introduction to nursing: an adaption model*, ed 2, Englewood Cliffs, NJ, 1984, Prentice-Hall.
23. Rutledge FN: Pelvic exenteration. In Rutledge FN, Freedman RS, Gershenson DM, editors: *Gynecologic cancer: diagnosis and treatment strategies*, Austin, 1985, University of Texas Press.
24. Salvadalena GD: An enterostomal therapy nursing data base for use with ostomy surgery patients, *J Enterostom Ther* 18:100, 1991.
25. Scholz J: Cultural expressions affecting patient care, *Dimens Oncol Nurs* 4(1):16, 1990.
26. Schover LR: Sexual rehabilitation of the ostomy patient. In Smith DB, Johnson DE, editors: *Ostomy care and the cancer patient*, Orlando, Fla, 1986, Grune & Stratton.
27. Schover LR, Fife M: Sexual counseling and radical pelvic or genital cancer surgery, *J Psychosoc Oncol* 3:31, 1985.
28. Schover LR, Jensen SB: *Sexuality and chronic illness*, New York, 1988, The Guilford Press.
29. Shields M: Selected issues in treating Gypsy patients, *Hosp Physician* 2:85, 1981.

30. Smith DB, Johnson DE: Preoperative preparation. In Smith DB, Johnson DE, editors: *Ostomy care and the cancer patient,* Orlando, Fla, 1986, Grune & Stratton.
31. Walker A: Teaching the illiterate patient, *J Enterostom Ther* 14:83, 1987.
32. Watson PG: The effects of short-term post-operative counseling on cancer/ostomy patients, *Cancer Nurs* 6:21, 1983.
33. Watson PM: Patient education: the adult with cancer, *Nurs Clin North Am* 17:739, 1982.
34. Walsh PC, Lepor L, Eggleston J: Radical prostatectomy with preservation of sexual function: anatomical and pathological considerations, *Prostate* 4:473, 1983.
35. Watt R: Stoma site marking. In Broadwell DC, Jackson BS: *Principles of ostomy care,* St Louis, 1982, Mosby–Year Book.

# 2 Principles and Procedures of Stomal Management

PAULA ERWIN-TOTH
DOROTHY B. DOUGHTY

## OBJECTIVES

1. Identify assessment criteria and appropriate interventions for each of the following: ileus, intestinal obstruction, anastomotic leak, stomal ischemia and necrosis, and mucocutaneous separation.

2. Identify indications for lifelong replacement of vitamin $B_{12}$.

3. Identify factors to be included in postoperative assessment of the stoma and the peristomal skin.

4. Describe normal stomal color and turgor and the significance of deviations from normal.

5. Explain why a stoma that protrudes slightly usually is preferable to one that is flush, retracted, or excessively long.

6. Describe expected output for the following diversions: ureterostomy, intestinal conduit, jejunostomy, ileostomy, transverse colostomy, and descending or sigmoid colostomy.

7. Describe indications for use of the following products in pouching a fecal or urinary diversion:
   Sealants
   Solid skin barriers
   Skin barrier paste
   Skin barrier powder
   Adhesives
   Solvents

8. Identify factors to be considered in selecting a pouching system.

9. Compare and contrast the following:
   Fecal pouches and urinary pouches
   One-piece pouches and two-piece pouching systems
   Disposable and reusable pouching systems

10. Identify at least three effluent characteristics that the nurse must consider in providing peristomal skin protection.

11. Identify the most common cause of stomal damage and its nursing implications.

12. Identify measures that can be used to protect the skin from mechanical trauma and from chemical dermatitis.

13. Describe the procedure for accurately sizing the opening in the barrier or pouch for (a) a round stoma and (b) an irregularly shaped stoma.

14. Describe recommended procedures for cleansing the peristomal skin and for removal of peristomal hair.

15. Determine the amount of peristomal skin protection needed for each of the following:
    Ileostomy
    Transverse colostomy
    Descending or sigmoid colostomy
    Ileal conduit

16. Identify patients who may benefit from use of closed-end pouches with moderate capacity and those who may benefit from use of stoma caps.

17. Explain the purpose of external support devices for loop stomas, as well as the criteria and usual time frame for their removal.

18. Describe pouching options for the patient with a loop stoma stabilized with an external support.

19. Explain the purpose of antireflux valves in urinary pouches.

20. Describe two approaches that can be used to pouch a urinary stoma.

21. Identify factors to be assessed in managing the care of the patient with a difficult stoma.

22. Identify management options for each of the following:
    Stoma on a soft abdomen
    Flush or retracted stoma
    Deep peristomal creasing

23. For each of the following patients, patient with ileostomy, patient with transverse colostomy, patient with descending or sigmoid colostomy, and patient with urinary diversion, design a teaching plan that includes the following content areas:
    Normal stoma characteristics
    Normal output
    Self-care procedures
    Modifications in dietary or fluid intake
    Measures to promote normal function of urinary tract or intestinal tract
    Prevention and management of complications
    Resumption of activities of daily living

24. Identify self-care skills that the patient with an ostomy should acquire before discharge.

25. Identify factors that the nurse must consider in determining a colostomy patient's candidacy for regulation of fecal output by routine colostomy irrigation.

26. Describe the following procedures:
    Application of fecal pouch
    Application of urinary pouch
    Colostomy irrigation
    Ileostomy lavage
    Catheterization of urinary stoma

27. Identify problems that may occur with colostomy irrigation and appropriate intervention.

28. Describe measures for prevention and management of food blockage in the individual with an ileostomy.

29. Describe measures for prevention and management of fecal impaction in the person with a colostomy.

30. Describe measures for prevention and management of peristomal skin damage related to prolonged exposure to urine.

31. Identify factors to be considered in deciding whether the care of an infant or a toddler with an ostomy should be managed with diapering or by pouching.

32. Identify pouching modifications that may facilitate ostomy management for the preschooler and the school-aged child.

Successful adjustment to ostomy surgery begins during the preoperative phase and continues until patients have integrated changes in body image and function into their self-concepts and life-styles. Rehabilitation is significantly affected by the individual's ability to master ostomy care and to deal successfully with the change in body image. Therefore nursing care during the postoperative period is directed toward development of a secure pouching system, instruction in self-care, and counseling to facilitate emotional adjustment. Experiences during the immediate postoperative period have a critical bearing on how the individual adjusts to living with an ostomy, and initial impressions, either positive or negative, can promote or impede emotional adjustment and mastery of self-care.

## POSTOPERATIVE MANAGEMENT

Ideally the nurse providing ostomy care has met with the patient and family before surgery and has completed a comprehensive assessment of physical, psychologic, educational, and psychosocial status (see Chapter 1). If the patient was not seen preoperatively, this assessment must be conducted during the first few days after surgery.[22]

Care of the patient with an ostomy requires a multidisciplinary approach. After surgery the patient's general status should be fully assessed. Although the main responsibility for postoperative nursing care lies with staff nurses, the nurse providing ostomy care should be actively involved in the patient's care. The nurse should review the patient's medical record to determine the surgical procedure, operative findings, and types of incisions and drains. Pathology reports should be reviewed as soon as available because they provide data regarding prognosis. Pertinent laboratory data also should be reviewed by the nurse, including but not limited to complete blood cell count, prothrombin time, biochemical profile, and, if available, arterial blood gas values. The nurse providing ostomy care also should determine from the surgeon and staff nurse what information has been communicated to the patient and family and their level of understanding. The preceding information provides the basis for anticipatory care.

Nursing priorities during the immediate postoperative period are to maintain the patient's airway, to monitor fluid and electrolyte balance, and to assess and optimize the patient's cardiovascular and pulmonary status. The nurse also should monitor and promote wound healing, evaluate stoma condition and function, and maintain patency of catheters and drains. It is important to maximize patient comfort through pain control, positioning, and relaxation techniques and to provide emotional support for both the patient and family. Accurate and timely documentation and communication of assessment data are essential to promote optimum patient outcomes.

### Complications: Prevention and Management

As part of the health care team the nurse providing ostomy care should be cognizant of potential early and late postoperative complications. As with any major abdominal surgery, patients are at risk for myriad complications.

Common postoperative complications include the following: shock, hemorrhage, thrombophlebitis, pulmonary embolism, respiratory problems, genitourinary problems, gastrointestinal complications, wound and intraabdominal complications, sepsis, psychologic problems, and stoma complications.[4,9,11] (In-depth discussion of these complications is available in a medical-surgical text.[27]) In this chapter, discussion is limited to complications related specifically to the intestinal resection and anastomosis and to stoma construction: ileus, obstruction, loss of absorptive capacity, anastomotic leak, stomal ischemia and necrosis, and mucocutaneous separation.

**Paralytic Ileus.** Gastrointestinal complications after abdominal surgery may take the form of paralytic (adynamic) ileus, intestinal obstruction, or compromised absorption. Paralytic ileus refers to loss of intestinal motility, which is a normal response to bowel manipulation and anesthesia.[2] Peristalsis usually resumes in the small bowel within about 48 hours and in the colon within about 72 hours; ileus may be prolonged in the presence of intraabdominal abscess, hypokalemia, or heavy sedation or after lengthy surgical procedures or extensive bowel manipulation. Paralytic ileus manifests by absence of bowel sounds and failure to pass flatus or stool.[1,16] Distention of the proximal bowel commonly results and may necessitate placement of a nasogastric or gastrostomy tube to relieve distention and to prevent nausea and vomiting.

**Intestinal Obstruction.** Intestinal obstruction most commonly occurs as a result of adhesion formation; other causes include strictures, fecal impaction, and intussusception. Obstruction may be partial or complete. Specific symptoms produced by obstruction depend on the completeness of the obstruction and the level of the obstruction (e.g., proximal obstruction causes more severe nausea and vomiting, whereas distal obstruction causes more distention).[2] Bowel sounds initially are hyperactive and may be heard as high-pitched and tinkling; bowel sounds later become hypoactive.[1]

Obstruction usually is managed initially with conservative treatment, that is, proximal decompression (nasogastric or small bowel tube to suction) and bowel rest. Surgical intervention is required for persistent obstruction or to prevent necrosis or perforation associated with a closed-loop obstruction.[2]

**Altered Intestinal Absorption.** Surgery that involves construction of an ostomy also commonly involves resection or bypass of intestinal segments. The absorptive capacity of the bowel is of course affected by the segment and length of intestine resected or bypassed. Resection of significant lengths of small bowel affects absorption of nutrients, fluids, and electrolytes; colon resection or bypass affects fluid and electrolyte absorption but has no impact on absorption of nutrients inasmuch as nutrient absorption occurs only in the small bowel.

Specific absorptive sites also may be lost; for example, the patient who has a significant amount of the terminal ileum resected or bypassed may require lifelong vitamin $B_{12}$ supplementation because vitamin $B_{12}$ absorption occurs only in the terminal ileum. Depletion of this vitamin results in pernicious anemia and symptoms of vitamin $B_{12}$ deficiency, which are the same as those resulting from pernicious anemia (e.g., peripheral neuropathy). Inasmuch as the liver "stores" vitamin $B_{12}$, deficits may not occur until several years after resection or bypass; thus monitoring for declining serum $B_{12}$ levels is necessary so that replacement is begun when indicated to prevent vitamin $B_{12}$ deficiency.[2]

**Anastomotic Leaks.** Intestinal anastomotic leaks may occur and are associated with a significant increase in morbidity and mortality. Early signs of anastomotic breakdown include abdominal distention, signs of peritoneal irritation, and drainage of feces or urine through drains or incisions.[19] Any indications of anastomotic breakdown must be promptly reported; a thorough evaluation is indicated, and reoperation frequently is required. Abscesses must be drained, and aggressive antibiotic therapy is initiated.[4,11] Some patients require systemic antifungal therapy because peritoneal candidiasis can result from leakage of bowel contents or conduit urine after bowel preparation.

**Stomal Necrosis.** Stomal necrosis is most common during the first 3 to 5 days after surgery. Common causes include excessive dissection of the mesentery, resulting in inadequate blood flow to the distal bowel or stoma; traction on the mesentery as a result of abdominal distention or obesity; and edema of the bowel wall, caused by manipulation of the bowel or exposure of the bowel to air (edema can close off mucosal vessels). Ischemia commonly manifests by a dark red or purplish tint or a cyanotic hue; necrosis is evidenced as brown or black discoloration of the stoma, which usually is associated with loss of the normal tissue turgor and hydration.[26] The stoma may appear dry and firm, or flaccid (see Plate 12).

Necrosis may involve only the distal stoma or may extend proximally. The extent of necrosis must be assessed clinically and documented. To assess the extent of necrosis, a well-lubricated, clear test tube should be gently inserted into the stoma; the beam of a flashlight is then directed downward through the center of the test tube to determine the viability of the proximal bowel mucosa.[25] (A lubricated thermometer may be substituted for the test tube when stoma viability in the infant is checked.) If the proximal bowel is viable, the stoma and proximal bowel must be routinely reevaluated to assess for progression. Necrosis limited to the stoma itself does not present a surgical emergency; the stoma will slough, leaving a flush or slightly retracted stoma.[13] If, on the other hand, the necrosis extends to

---

### CONSERVATIVE MANAGEMENT OF MUCOCUTANEOUS SEPARATION

1. Flush separated area with normal saline.
2. Fill area of separation with absorptive powder or granules (e.g., skin barrier powder or hydroactive granules) to absorb drainage and maintain a moist wound surface.
3. Apply SteriStrips or microporous tape over absorptive powder or granules to provide a pouching surface.
4. Size pouch or barrier opening to fit closely around the stoma.
5. Apply skin barrier paste directly around the stoma.
6. Apply pouch.*

---

*Pouch with convexity may reduce the risk of stool migration.

fascia level, the physician should be notified immediately; emergency surgical intervention is indicated to prevent perforation and peritonitis.

**Mucocutaneous Separation.** Another early complication is mucocutaneous separation, that is, breakdown of the suture line securing the stoma to the abdominal surface[19,25] (see Plates 14 and 15). Any condition that interferes with wound healing can cause predisposition to mucocutaneous separation (e.g., malnutrition, corticosteroid administration, infection, or abdominal radiation). Mucocutaneous separation may in turn cause stomal retraction as a result of loss of support for the stoma at the abdominal surface. Although the surgeon may elect to administer local anesthesia and resuture wounds, it is more common to manage the separation conservatively, focusing on measures to support wound healing.[19] (Conservative management is described in the box above.)

Surgical intervention is required when the retraction is so severe that peritoneal contamination is a concern. In this case the patient is returned to the operating room for a formal laparotomy and stoma repair.

### Assessment Criteria

**Stoma Assessment.** Postoperative assessment of the stoma or stomas should include the following factors: (1) type, that is, segment of bowel, (2) viability, (3) stomal height, or degree of protrusion, (4) construction, (5) abdominal location, and (6) size.

*Stomal type.* The type of stoma cannot always be determined by inspection alone; all intestinal stomas are similar in color and appearance, and any segment of bowel may be brought out as a stoma in various abdominal locations. For example, an ileostomy may be located in the lower left quadrant of the abdomen and could be mistaken for a sigmoid colostomy. The nurse should always review the operative report to determine the procedure performed and the specific type of stoma constructed.

*Stomal viability.* Stomal viability is determined by assessing stomal color and turgor. Stomas constructed from intestinal mucosa normally are moist and beefy red in color. Urinary tract stomas, that is, ureterostomies and vesicostomies, often appear pale pink. Edema, which is a normal postoperative event, may give the stoma a taut, shiny, or translucent appearance.[13] A pale intestinal stoma may indicate a low hemoglobin level. A dark red or purplish tint to the mucosa may indicate bruising, early ischemia, effects of cortico-

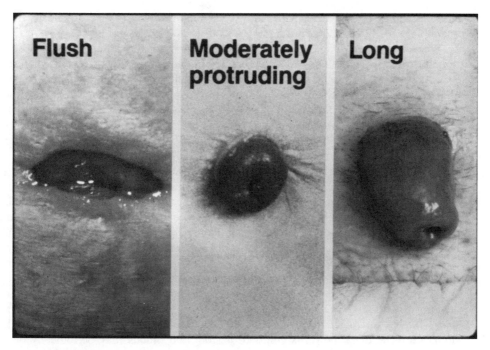

**Fig. 2-1**    Protruding stoma, flush stoma, and excessively long stoma. (Courtesy Hollister, Inc., Libertyville, Ill.)

steroid therapy, or signs of the disease process (e.g., Crohn's disease). A brownish cast to a colostomy may indicate a condition known as melanosis coli, the discoloration of the bowel mucosa resulting from long-term laxative use[5] (see Plate 13). A dark-brown to black stoma indicates ischemia, as does a loss of normal tissue turgor as evidenced by a flaccid or floppy appearance to the stoma.[13]

   *Stomal height.* The stoma also is assessed for degree of protrusion. Most stomas are matured (that is, everted and sutured to the abdominal surface) in the operating room. Interrupted sutures are placed through the mucosa and the subcutaneous tissue; this prevents implantation of the bowel mucosa onto the skin, which may occur if the sutures are placed through the mucosa and the epidermal layers.[9] Although the length of the stoma can range from flush to protruding, the ideal stoma should protrude slightly (Fig. 2-1). The small spout of a protruding stoma makes it easier to obtain a secure seal around the base of the stoma and promotes the drainage of the effluent into the pouch rather than around the base of the stoma and underneath the seal. A flush stoma (Fig. 2-1) or a stoma that is below skin level can make it difficult to obtain a secure seal, especially if there are creases adjacent to the stoma that become accentuated with position changes. When the effluent empties at or below skin level, there is a marked tendency for it to migrate underneath the seal of the pouch, resulting in leakage and skin irritation. Conversely, a stoma with excessive length (Fig. 2-1) can cause difficulty when the pouching system is being centered or when the pouch of a two-piece system is being attached. A stoma with excessive length is more vulnerable to trauma such as being pinched or lacerated by the pouching system or clothing. Finally, some patients find an especially long stoma to be aesthetically displeasing and to have phallic connotations.[9]

***Stomal construction.*** The stoma should be described according to the type of construction, for example, end, loop, or double barrel. An end stoma is constructed when the bowel is divided (with or without resection) and the proximal end of the bowel is brought to the abdominal surface as a single stoma that represents the end of the proximal functioning bowel (see Fig. 11-1); the distal bowel may be resected or may be closed and left in the abdominal cavity (Hartmann's pouch) (see Fig. 11-3). A loop stoma is constructed by making an abdominal incision, bringing a loop of bowel to the abdominal surface, and stabilizing the loop to prevent retraction of the bowel back into the abdominal cavity (see Figs. 11-9 and 11-15). Stabilization most commonly is accomplished with the use of an external support such as a plastic bridge or rod; loop stomas also can be secured by surgical construction of a fascial bridge. A stoma is said to be double barrel when both ends of the divided bowel are brought to the abdominal surface as stomas; the proximal stoma eliminates stool, whereas the distal stoma drains only mucus (see Figs. 11-4 and 11-16). This type of procedure also is referred to as a proximal ostomy and distal mucous fistula. Type of stomal construction is important because it provides information about permanence of the stoma and presence of bowel distal to the stoma. For example, when the rectum and anus remain intact in the patient with a fecal diversion, the potential exists for later takedown of the ostomy. The nurse also should be aware that the patient with a fecal diversion who has an intact distal bowel may expel stool through the rectum as well as the stoma until the distal bowel is emptied of stool and mucus may periodically be expelled per rectum on a long-term basis. (See Chapter 11 for further discussion of surgical procedures and implications.)

Additional factors relevant to construction of a gastrointestinal stoma that should be documented include the presence of a supporting rod or bridge, the method by which the supporting device is secured, and the amount of tension on the bowel. Construction of a urinary stoma may include the placement of ureteral stents or catheters; therefore their presence and patency should be described.

***Abdominal location.*** Abdominal location of the stoma should be documented, that is, right or left side of the abdomen, upper or lower quadrant. Furthermore, the nurse should describe the peristomal contours and should document the proximity of the stoma to any of the following: incision, waistline, abdominal skin fold or crease, or bony prominences.

***Size.*** The size of the stoma should be accurately assessed in either inches or millimeters with use of a stoma-measuring guide. Disposable measuring guides generally are included with all types of pouching equipment. Because most pouching systems are labeled in inches, it may be more convenient to measure in a like manner. The stoma should be measured at its base, precisely where the mucosa meets the skin (that is, from mucosa to mucosa). Oval stomas should be measured at both the widest and narrowest points, and the skin barrier or pouch opening shaped accordingly.

The characteristics of an ideal stoma are summarized in Table 2-1.

**Mucocutaneous Suture Line.** The peristomal sutures at the mucocutaneous junction should be examined and assessed for any evidence of mucosal separation, allergic reaction to the suture material, or infection. Ideally the mucosa of the stoma should be well approximated to the subcuticular layer, without evidence of tension or exposure of the dermis.

**Table 2-1**    Characteristics of an ideal stoma

| Characteristic | Ideal | Rationale | Variances |
|---|---|---|---|
| Height | Approximatey 2.5 cm | Easier for patient to see and facilitates drainage of effluent | Excessively long stomas may be cosmetically undesirable and difficult to conceal under clothing; stomas flush with skin may require additional convexity in appliance |
| Location of lumen | At apex of stoma | Facilitates drainage of effluent into pouch | If the lumen is at skin level, patient may have problems with leakage and pouch adherence. |
| Color | Red | Indicates good circulation | Temporary color changes may occur (e.g., anemia, when baby cries) and are normal. |
| Shape | Round | All presized appliances are round; makes procedure easier for client | If stoma is irregularly shaped, patient may need to cut appliances if total skin protection is required. |
| Location on body | Smooth surface below the belt line | Creases, bony prominences, suture lines, or umbilicus may interfere with pouch adherence; easier to conceal under clothing | |

From Thelan LA, Davie JK, Urden LD: *Textbook of critical care nursing: diagnosis and management*, St. Louis, 1990, Mosby–Year Book.

**Peristomal Skin.** Optimally the peristomal skin appears healthy and intact, with no differences between the peristomal skin and the adjacent skin surface. Peristomal skin damage is evidenced by erythema, maceration, denudation, rash, ulceration, or blister formation. In persons with dark skin, the damaged skin may appear lighter or darker than the surrounding skin, as opposed to erythematous. Table 2-2 presents common causes of peristomal skin damage, identifying characteristics, and principles of management.

**Genitourinary Function.** A urinary diversion stoma functions immediately upon construction. The urine is blood-tinged initially but progresses to amber or straw-colored. Because mucus is produced by the goblet cells in the intestinal mucosa, mucous shreds are normal in intestinal conduits; care should be taken to maintain the patency of the continuous drainage system. The pouch should be connected to gravity drainage to accurately monitor urinary output and to prevent overdistention of the pouch with resultant leakage. The source of urinary output, that is, the stoma, ureteral stents, or conduit catheter, should be documented. Output from abdominal drains also should be observed to determine

**Table 2-2**   Peristomal skin damage

| Type or cause of damage | Appearance | Treatment principles |
|---|---|---|
| **CHEMICAL DAMAGE**<br>Effluent in contact with skin<br>Incorrect use of adhesives or solvents | Erythematous and denuded areas corresponding to leakage of effluent *or* areas of product use (adhesives, solvents) | Eliminate effluent contact with skin; allow adhesives to dry and remove solvents from skin<br>*Topical:* Skin barrier powder; sealants if needed |
| **MECHANICAL DAMAGE**<br>Inappropriate skin care (scrubbing or "picking")<br>Incorrect tape removal or fragile skin, resulting in "stripping" of epidermis | Patchy areas of erythema or denudation corresponding with areas subjected to trauma or "taped" areas | Eliminate cause; teach atraumatic skin care, appropriate tape removal, and use of sealants when indicated<br>*Topical:* Skin barriers (powder; with sealant as indicated; solid barriers until area has healed) |
| **FUNGAL RASH** *(CANDIDA)*<br>Antibiotics resulting in fungal overgrowth<br>Persistent skin moisture | Maculopapular rash with satellite lesions | Keep skin dry: eliminate pooled urine; restore normal flora<br>*Topical:* Antifungal powder and sealant as indicated |
| **ALLERGIC REACTION**<br>Can be caused by any product | Areas of erythema, pruritis corresponding to area of skin exposed to allergen | Use patch test if needed to determine allergen; eliminate contact with allergen<br>*Topical:* Corticosteroid agent if needed for control of pruritis (cream or spray, not ointment, which would interfere with pouch adherence) |

whether the drainage is serosanguineous fluid or urine; urine output through abdominal drains is an ominous sign that may indicate an anastomotic leak at the site of the stents or the end of the conduit itself.[19]

### Gastrointestinal Function

*Jejunostomy.* Jejunostomy function usually begins within the first 48 hours after surgery, and the effluent initially is watery, clear, and dark green. Because the volume of output may approach 2400 ml in 24 hours, the patient should be closely monitored for signs of electrolyte imbalance. In addition, the absorption of nutrients, fluids, and electrolytes may be radically reduced in the patient with a jejunostomy; absorptive capacity depends on the length and function of the proximal bowel.[9] Therefore nutritional maintenance with hyperalimentation is not uncommon.[13]

*Ileostomy.* An ileostomy (see Fig. 11-6) generally begins to function within the first 48 to 72 hours after surgery. The initial effluent is viscous, green, and shiny. This output does not necessarily indicate return of peristalsis; rather, this initial drainage may be the elimination of fluid that has been collected in the distal small bowel. Once peristalsis returns, the patient may enter a period of high-volume output known as the adaptation phase. Output during this period exceeds 1000 ml per day and frequently is around 1500 to 1800 ml per day. The physiologic basis for this high-output phase is the loss of the colon's absorptive surface coupled with loss of the delay factor normally provided by the ileocecal valve.[18] During this period the patient must be monitored closely for signs and symptoms of fluid and electrolyte imbalance; replacement is critical. Replacement may be managed by the intravenous route or with oral electrolyte replacement solutions, depending on the status of bowel function.

Over a period of days to weeks the proximal small bowel increases fluid absorption and the bowel "adapts"[2]; there is a gradual reduction in the volume of output and a thickening of stool to a "toothpaste" consistency that is light to medium brown. Initially the amount of output from an ileostomy can vary from 500 to 1500 ml in a 24-hour period. After adaptation the average amount produced by most ileostomies decreases to between 500 and 800 ml daily.[9]

*Colostomy.* The initial output from a colostomy varies depending on the location of the stoma within the colon. Because the colon absorbs all but about 100 ml of the 1000 ml passed through the ileocecal valve daily,[5] distal colonic stomas produce stool of thicker consistency and lower volume output than do proximal colonic stomas, which produce higher volume and more fluid output.

*Cecostomy.* A cecostomy is located within the cecum, just distal to the ileocecal valve. This stoma usually begins to function by about the third postoperative day; output may be projectile (because of the close proximity of the ileocecal valve) and initially is watery. A cecostomy can be either a skin-level or a "tube" diversion and is located low in the right lower quadrant; location, output characteristics, and construction may combine to make this a difficult stoma to manage. This is particularly true of the tube cecostomy because stool tends to flow both through and around the tube. Tube cecostomies also are associated with a greater risk of intraabdominal spillage.

*Transverse colostomy.* A transverse colostomy usually begins to function on the third to fourth day after surgery. Output usually is pasty to soft and occurs after meals and at intervals throughout the day. Transverse colostomies frequently are located near or in the patient's waistline, and they often are constructed as loop stomas (see Fig. 11-14). In loop transverse colostomies a support device (e.g., rod or bridge) may be placed during surgery and removed 5 to 7 days later. The alternative is to construct a fascial bridge at the time of surgery, which obviates the need for a commercial stomal support device.

*Descending or sigmoid colostomy.* A descending or sigmoid colostomy takes the longest to regain normal peristalsis and may not begin to function until the fifth postoperative day (see Figs. 11-12 and 11-13). On occasion some liquid output and flatus may be seen by the third or fourth postoperative day. Patients with active bowel sounds who have not passed flatus or stool by the fifth day after surgery should be assessed for the presence of factors that would contribute to the delay in return of function (e.g., administration of nar-

**Table 2-3**   Characteristic output of gastrointestinal stomas

| Type | Amount (ml) | Consistency | pH |
|---|---|---|---|
| Esophagostomy | 1000-1500 | Saliva | Slightly alkaline |
| Gastrostomy | 2000-2500 | Liquid | 0.5-1.5 |
| Jejunostomy | 1000-3000 | Liquid | Slightly acid |
| Ileostomy | 750-1000 | Toothpaste | Alkaline |
| Cecostomy and ascending colostomy | 500-750 | Toothpaste | Alkaline |
| Transvere colostomy | | Mushy to semiformed | Alkaline |
| Descending and sigmoid colostomy | | Semiformed to formed | Alkaline |

Thelan LA, Davie JK, Urden LD: *Textbook of critical care nursing: diagnosis and management,* St Louis, 1990, Mosby–Year Book.

cotics). Such patients may benefit from a gentle, low-volume colostomy irrigation to stimulate bowel function. The routine colostomy irrigation procedure should be followed, as discussed later in this chapter.

Once normal function has resumed, the output from a descending or sigmoid colostomy usually is soft-formed stool, and elimination patterns generally are similar to preoperative patterns.

The amount and consistency of stool from any gastrointestinal stoma is influenced by the amount of bowel resected, the length and condition of the proximal bowel, medications, and diet. Over a period of several months the remaining bowel increases its absorption capacity,[5] and output decreases in volume and becomes thicker. Table 2-3 provides a description of the characteristic output of gastrointestinal stomas.

## POUCHING PRODUCTS

The primary goal in pouching an ostomy is to provide the patient with an odor-proof, secure seal. Secondary goals include promotion of self-care and provision of a cost-effective management system.

### Commonly Used Products

Many products are available that can be used to provide an appropriate and secure pouching system. The nurse must be familiar with available products and must select and integrate them appropriately to establish an effective pouching system for the individual patient. The most commonly used products, which are discussed briefly here, are listed in Table 2-4.

**Sealants.** Skin sealants contain a plasticizing agent (usually a copolymer) as the primary ingredient, along with variable amounts of isopropyl alcohol. These products are used to provide a thin protective film to the skin surface; this protective film helps prevent stripping of the epidermis during adhesive removal and also acts as a moisture barrier. Sealants may not be recommended for use under skin barriers because the protective film may reduce the adherence of the barrier. For selected patients (e.g., the patient with dry skin), however, the film actually improves barrier adhesion.

**Table 2-4**    Commonly used ostomy products

| Product | Forms | Composition |
|---------|-------|-------------|
| Skin sealants | Wipes, sprays, gels, liquids, and roll-on | Plasticizing agent such as copolymer; variable amounts of isopropyl alcohol |
| Skin barriers | Wafers, rings or washers, pastes, strips, and powders | May be made from karaya gum, pectin, gelatin, carboxymethylcellulose, and copolymers |
| Skin cleansers | Liquids, wipes, sprays, and foams | May contain water, lanolin, urea, propylene glycol, fragrance, and artificial colors; rinsing may be required to remove residue before pouch application |
| Skin adhesives | Liquids and sprays | May be silicone based or latex based; must allow solvents to evaporate to prevent skin damage |

Sealants are produced in the form of wipes, sprays, and liquids. Because of the alcohol content in the sealant, burning and stinging occur during application in patients with denuded skin. Therefore sealants should not be used on denuded skin unless a skin barrier powder is applied first; the skin barrier powder provides an absorptive and protective layer and helps minimize the burning and discomfort.

**Barriers.** Skin barriers in the form of wafers, rings, pastes, and powders are used to protect the peristomal skin from effluent, to create a level pouching surface, and to treat peristomal skin loss.

Many one-piece and two-piece pouching systems are now available with an attached skin barrier ring or wafer. Separate barrier wafers and rings also are available and can be used with adhesive-only pouches to produce pouching systems. Skin barriers can be composed of karaya gum, pectin, gelatin, and synthetic materials. Barriers vary in their resistance to breakdown by feces and urine; for example, karaya and pectin-based barriers dissolve with urine, whereas the newer synthetic barriers are more resistant. Karaya-based products may cause a temporary burning sensation on denuded skin as a result of the release of acetic acid during contact with moisture; this sensation does not occur with pectin, gelatin, and synthetic barriers.

Skin barrier pastes are used to create a level pouching surface, to prevent migration of drainage under the pouch seal, and to enhance the resistance of the solid skin barrier. All commercial skin barrier pastes contain alcohol, which causes a burning sensation if used on denuded skin.

Skin barrier powders are commonly dusted onto denuded skin to provide an absorptive, protective layer; if needed, the powder can then be "sealed" by lightly blotting the area with a damp finger or a sealant to ensure a dry, nonpowdery pouching surface. Skin barrier powders also can be mixed with glycerin to form a noncommercial paste that does not contain alcohol and is not painful to denuded skin.

**Adhesives.** Application of a silicone-based or latex-based skin adhesive may be used to increase the adhesion of an adhesive pouching system or to provide adhesion for a reusable (nonadhesive) system. It is important to teach the patient, family, and staff members to allow the adhesive to dry adequately before the pouch is applied; this prevents chemical damage to the skin resulting from trapped solvents.

**Solvents.** Adhesive removers are solvents that aid in the removal of tape, skin adhesives, and residue from skin barrier products. They may be helpful to the patient with sensitive skin (to reduce trauma from pouch removal) and also may be used in the care of reusable equipment. The patient and family are taught to rinse the skin after use of a solvent to prevent a chemical dermatitis.

**Pouching Systems.** Pouching systems are commonly classified as fecal or urinary, one-piece or two-piece, and disposable or reusable. Although most pouching systems are adhesive, several nonadhesive pouches are now available.

*Fecal versus urinary.* Urinary pouches have small spouts attached to the pouch, which facilitate drainage; these systems also have adapters to permit connection of the pouch to bedside drainage. Each company manufactures an adapter that fits its pouches. Most urinary pouches also are equipped with antireflux valves, which serve to reduce backflow of urine onto the skin, thus providing skin protection. Urinary pouches usually are odor-resistant.

Fecal pouches can be further categorized as drainable or closed-end (Fig. 2-2). Drainable pouches have an opening in the bottom of the pouch that permits emptying; commercial clips or rubber bands are used to maintain pouch closure. Closed-end pouches have no spout and cannot be emptied; they vary in size, capacity, and ability to vent flatus. Some are moderately sized and intended to accommodate a moderate amount of fecal output; these may be used for patients who want to change their pouches once or twice daily. Others have minimal or no capacity and should be used only for patients with descending or sigmoid colostomies that are well regulated by irrigation. Many are equipped with integrated flatus filters; these are beneficial in that they force the flatus through a charcoal layer and thus both vent and deodorize the flatus. Fecal pouches generally are odorproof.

*One-piece versus two-piece.* Pouches also are available as both one-piece and two-piece systems. The one-piece pouch incorporates the pouch with an adhesive surface used to attach the pouch to the body; many disposable pouches also have an attached skin barrier. Advantages of one-piece pouches include simplicity of application and low profile.

The two-piece pouching system has a separate faceplate (or wafer with flange) that is attached to the body and a pouch that is snapped onto or stretched over the flange (Fig. 2-3). Advantages of two-piece systems include increased accessibility to the stoma for care or monitoring, the ability to change the pouch without disrupting the adhesive, and enhanced ability to visualize the stoma and center the wafer or faceplate during pouch changes.

Most two-piece systems are rigid or semirigid (because of the flange); therefore they require relatively flat pouching surfaces. Another consideration in use of two-piece systems is whether the flange is stationary or floating; floating flanges are advantageous during the

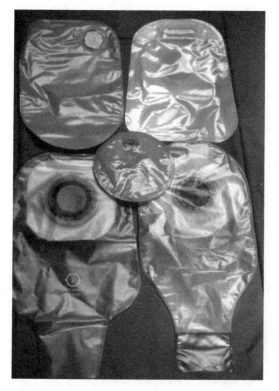

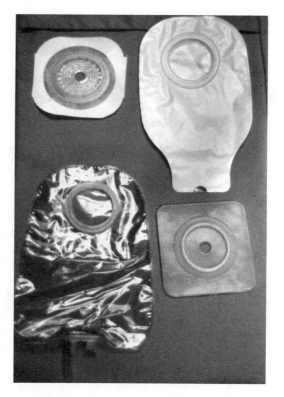

**Fig. 2-2** Fecal pouches: drainable and closed-end.

**Fig. 2-3** Two-piece disposable pouches.

early postoperative period because the nurse or patient can slide the fingers under the flange for pouch application (which prevents pressure on the sensitive abdominal wall).

*Precut versus cut-to-fit.* Many pouches are available that are presized, that is, the center opening has already been created. Since these pouches do not require cutting, they are simpler to apply; they are particularly beneficial for patients with reduced manual dexterity or visual acuity and for patients with learning disabilities. However, these pouches are not appropriate for patients who have irregularly shaped stomas; these patients require pouches with starter holes that can be custom cut to fit the stoma. Starter holes are small openings in the center of the pouch, which serve as starting points for creating an appropriate pouch opening. Most institutions find it advantageous to stock these "custom cut" pouches because less stock is required to meet a variety of patient needs.

*Disposable versus reusable.* Pouches are available in both disposable and reusable forms. Disposable pouches generally are constructed of lightweight, odorproof materials and may be one piece or two piece. The obvious advantage is that the disposable pouch requires no maintenance; it is simply discarded after use.

Reusable pouches are heavier pouches constructed of more durable materials such as rubber, heavy plastic, or vinyl. The plastic and vinyl products are intended for short-term use (weeks to months), whereas the heavy rubber products are intended for long-term use

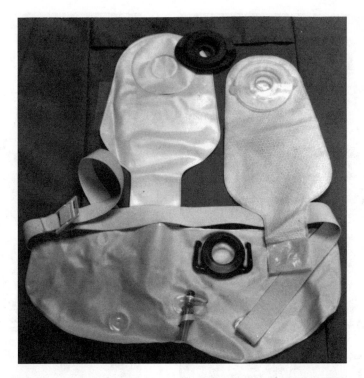

**Fig. 2-4**   One-piece and two-piece reusable pouching systems.

(months to years). Reusable products may be advantageous for the patient with financial constraints who requires frequent pouch changes or for the patient who needs more support and convexity than can be provided by disposable pouching equipment. Some patients simply may prefer reusable equipment.

Reusable products are presized and are available as both one- or two-piece systems (Fig. 2-4). One-piece systems have a faceplate already attached to a pouch. In contrast, reusable two-piece systems require assembly of the pouch and faceplate; the pouch is stretched around the flange, or gasket, of the faceplate and is secured in place with a commercial elastic ring or a rubber band.

One-piece systems offer some advantages in that they require less assembly and eliminate the risk of leakage between the pouch and the faceplate. However, one-piece reusable products may be more difficult to center over the stoma, particularly if the pouch is opaque. Furthermore, one-piece reusable pouches do not provide as wide a range of options as do two-piece systems, for example, use of one company's faceplate with another company's pouch.

Two-piece reusable systems also have advantages and disadvantages. Reusable faceplates and pouches are interchangeable because the gasket on reusable faceplates is a standard size; therefore two-piece systems permit the use of one company's faceplate with another company's pouch. However, the assembly required for a two-piece system may be difficult for some elderly patients or patients with arthritis. Two-piece systems also present a risk of leakage between the pouch and faceplate; this is more likely to occur with repeated stretching of the pouch.

Most reusable systems require the addition of adhesives to secure the pouch to the skin; pouches secured with a silicone ring and a belt are the exception. Contact cement or double-faced adhesive disks (sized to fit the faceplate) may be used to provide adhesion. Selected skin barriers that have tack on both sides also may be used.

Reusable systems require maintenance. The patient must be taught how to clean the pouch and how to appropriately use and remove adhesives or cements. For example, the cement does not have to be removed from the faceplate at each pouch change, but it should be removed whenever cement buildup on the faceplate is sufficient to create grooves. Some patients find it helpful to attach a double-faced adhesive disk to the faceplate as a "base" for the cement; the adhesive disk is easily removed when it is time to clean the faceplate. Application of a skin sealant to the faceplate before application of adhesive disks or cement also may facilitate the removal of adhesive products.

The nurse should wait until stoma shrinkage is complete (about 6 to 8 weeks after surgery) before ordering reusable equipment.

**Accessory Products.** A number of accessory products are available to support stoma management (see the box on p. 46). Belts and binders are used to provide additional support for the patient with a soft abdomen and a flush or retracted stoma. Convex inserts may be used in selected situations to add convexity to two-piece disposable systems. Convex inserts add limited degrees of convexity, however, and they are difficult for many patients to manipulate.

## Pouch Selection

Pouch selection is a complex process that requires thorough assessment of both the stoma and the patient (see the box on p. 47). Stomal characteristics that affect pouch selection include type and consistency of effluent, stoma size and construction, abdominal contours, and degree of stomal protrusion.[6] Patient characteristics that must be assessed include manual dexterity and visual acuity; level of physical activity; financial resources; and preferences concerning pouch size, opacity, and one-piece or two-piece construction. Finally, the nurse must consider availability of the product.

**Type of Stoma.** An important consideration is choosing a system that is appropriate for the stoma. A pouching system with a spout to facilitate emptying is required for the patient with a urinary stoma. For an intestinal stoma a drainable pouch with a closure clamp usually is indicated. One exception is the patient with a descending or sigmoid colostomy who performs colostomy irrigation and has minimal spillage between irrigations; this patient may elect to use a closed-end pouch or a stoma cap or cover. Patients who regulate their colostomies by diet may choose to use closed-end pouches, and pediatric patients who find it awkward or difficult to empty pouches at school also may benefit from use of closed-end pouches.

**Stoma Construction.** Stoma construction can affect selection of a pouching system. For example, creative pouching techniques may be required for the loop stoma stabilized by

## ACCESSORY PRODUCTS

### BELTS
Company specific or interchangeable; available in several adult sizes and in pediatric sizes; provide support at the 9 o'clock and 3 o'clock positions

### BINDERS
Available in widths ranging from 2 to 6 inches; Velcro closures; can be ordered with prolapse overbelt; can be custom ordered in terms of placement for cutout to accommodate pouch, for example, pouch opening can be placed in center of binder or toward the top or bottom

### CONVEX INSERTS
Can be added to selected two-piece systems to provide convexity and additional support; some systems can accommodate two inserts; insert must be carefully sized to clear the stoma by one-eighth inch (internal diameter) and to fit the flange of the wafer (external diameter); *not* interchangeable among companies

### POUCH COVERS
Provide moisture barrier between pouch and skin; available in adult and pediatric sizes to fit various pouches; provide concealment for pouch, which may enhance body image

### BEDSIDE DRAINAGE SYSTEMS FOR URINARY STOMAS
Available as bags or bottles (plastic jugs) with drainage tubing attached; adapter required to attach urinary pouch to drainage tubing; drainage system may be secured to the bed frame or may be placed in a plastic wastebasket on the floor

### UNDERWEAR AND SWIMWEAR
Designed to conceal and support pouch; may enhance body image; available in various sizes

### TAIL CLOSURES FOR DRAINABLE POUCHES
Available from numerous ostomy manufacturers; interchangeable or company specific

### STOMA GUIDE STRIPS
Made from rice paper; can be inserted into opening of pouching system to assist patient in centering pouch; strip dissolves when it comes in contact with moisture

### TAPES
Available from a variety of manufacturers in many sizes and types; some are waterproof, which may be beneficial for the patient who participates in water sports

### SOLVENTS
Available in liquid and "wipe" forms; most are petroleum based; skin must be washed and rinsed after use of solvents to prevent chemical dermatitis

---

**FACTORS TO CONSIDER IN SELECTING A POUCHING SYSTEM**

| STOMA CHARACTERISTICS | PATIENT CHARACTERISTICS |
|---|---|
| Type and consistency of effluent | Manual dexterity and visual acuity |
| Stoma size and construction | Level of physical activity |
| Abdominal contours | Financial resources |
| Degree of stomal protrusion | Preferences regarding pouch size, opacity, one-piece versus two-piece construction |

---

a rod or bridge. Stomas located adjacent to or in incisions must be pouched with incisional care in mind; the incisions can be protected with SteriStrips or strips of nonadherent gauze before pouch application.

**Abdominal Contours and Stomal Height.** Among the most important considerations in providing a secure pouch seal are the patient's abdominal contours and the degree of stomal protrusion. Careful assessment of these factors enables the nurse to select a pouching system that most closely approximates the peristomal contours. Pouching systems may be flexible or rigid and flat or convex, with varying degrees of convexity. Greater degrees of rigidity and support are required for soft abdomens, and greater degrees of convexity are required for retracted stomas. Care of the patient with a flat, firm abdominal surface and a flush or protruding stoma usually can be managed with a flat pouching system, either flexible or semirigid. The patient with a soft abdomen and a flush or retracted stoma may require a pouching system with support (rigidity) or convexity, or both, to obtain a secure seal. The patient with a stoma located in a deep crease usually requires an all-flexible pouching system or deep convexity.

**Visual Acuity and Manual Dexterity.** The nurse must consider the patient's visual acuity and manual dexterity in the selection of a pouching system. The patient with limited visual acuity may benefit from a pouching system that facilitates application by touch (e.g., a two-piece system), and the patient with poor dexterity may find it easier to apply a semirigid one-piece system than to apply a flexible system or a two-piece system that must be snapped together. The patient with poor visual acuity or limited dexterity also benefits from a precut system. It is important to recognize that a precut system requires a regularly shaped stoma and a semirigid system requires a relatively flat pouching surface; pouching options may be limited for some patients because of soft abdomens, deep creases, or retracted stomas.

**Activity Level.** In selecting a pouching system, the nurse should consider the patient's activity level. The active patient may benefit from use of a belt or binder; the patient who participates in water sports may need waterproof tape. Pouch flexibility may affect comfort in the active patient; once again, this consideration must take second place to the critical need to match the pouching system to the patient's abdominal contours.

---

### PRINCIPLES OF POUCHING

1. The skin must be protected from damaging effluent.
2. The stoma must be protected from trauma.
3. The peristomal skin must be protected from mechanical trauma.

4. The skin must be protected from damage caused by products used for pouching and skin protection.

---

**Additional Considerations.** Additional considerations include cost factors and reimbursement issues, patient preference (assuming that several systems are appropriate), and product availability.

The preceding principles serve to guide the nurse in selection of an appropriate pouching system. Accurate matching of pouch to patient depends on an understanding of these principles coupled with astute assessment skills and an appreciation for the unique challenges presented by individual patients. Frequently the nurse must modify existing pouching systems or must try several approaches to determine the most effective one. As the patient's abdominal contours and activity levels change, pouching needs also change. Thus follow-up in an outpatient setting is an essential component of care for these patients.

## POUCHING PROCEDURES

Once an appropriate pouching system has been selected on the basis of assessment of stoma characteristics and individual patient needs, the system must be applied and maintained to protect the peristomal skin. Four principles provide the basis for pouching techniques (see the box above). These principles are based on an understanding of the types of damage that can result from exposure to effluent and repetitive removal or inappropriate use of barriers and adhesives.

### Principles

**Skin Protection from Effluent.** The skin must be protected from effluent, which can cause varying degrees of damage, depending on the effluent's enzymatic content, pH level, volume, and consistency. The nurse must consider these factors in determining the amount of protection required for an individual patient.

For example, the output from a small-bowel stoma contains proteolytic enzymes that can rapidly produce skin erosion; large-bowel drainage contains no enzymes or only residual enzymes (ascending colon effluent) and is therefore less irritating to the skin. Urine, which contains no enzymes, does not cause chemical erosion. Effluent that is alkaline or markedly acidic is more damaging to the skin than is neutral or slightly acidic effluent; therefore alkaline urine is more likely to damage the skin than is acidic urine (because the normal pH level of skin is slightly acidic). Large volumes of effluent are likely to damage the skin, and effluent that is liquid in consistency can cause maceration if allowed to pool on the skin.

To protect the skin from effluent damage, the nurse must select products that provide the appropriate resistance and must size the pouch opening appropriately to limit the amount of skin exposed to the effluent. For example, the patient with a small-bowel stoma needs a barrier that resists breakdown by proteolytic enzymes and a pouch carefully sized to minimize peristomal skin exposure; any exposed skin must be protected with a skin barrier paste. In contrast, care of a large-bowel stoma can be managed with a less resistant barrier because colon effluent contains few, if any, enzymes. The primary requirement for the patient with a urinary stoma is elimination of pooling, since urine contains no enzymes and normally is slightly acidic; use of skin barriers is optional for this patient.

**Stoma Protection.** The stoma itself must be protected from trauma. Because it lacks nerve endings, it is insensitive, and damage can occur without the patient's awareness. Stomal damage usually results from an improperly sized pouch opening. Thus pouch openings should be carefully sized to clear the stoma and minimize skin exposure. Pouches with rigid faceplates, that is, reusable faceplates, should be sized to clear the stoma by at least one-eighth inch to prevent damage that can result from stomal movement during peristaltic activity. If the stoma is edematous, the pouch or barrier may be sized slightly larger than the stoma or radial slits can be made around the aperture to prevent any stomal damage. (If the pouch or barrier is sized larger than the stoma, the nurse must remember to provide the needed amount of peristomal skin protection; for example, the patient with an ileostomy who is using a reusable faceplate also requires a barrier ring or paste, or both, for skin protection.)

**Skin Protection from Mechanical Trauma.** The peristomal skin must be protected from mechanical trauma. Mechanical damage can occur as a result of inappropriate adhesive removal, which causes epidermal stripping, or inappropriate cleansing, which causes epidermal abrasions. The patient must be taught to gently peel the pouching system away from the skin and to use atraumatic cleansing techniques. The use of sealants may reduce mechanical trauma because they provide a protective film over the epidermis. Solvents may benefit the patient with fragile skin inasmuch as they facilitate atraumatic removal of tapes, adhesives, and barriers.

**Protection from Product-Related Damage.** The nurse must be alert to damage related to products used for pouching and skin protection. Incorrect use of products that contain solvents, for example, can cause a chemical dermatitis; such products (e.g., latex adhesives and pastes or sealants that contain alcohol) must be allowed to dry before pouch application. Patients who use solvents for pouch removal must be instructed to clean the skin and remove the solvent before pouch application.

Products used in pouching can be allergens. The nurse caring for the patient with an ostomy must be alert to the development of any sensitivity to the products used; if there is a question of allergic reaction, the patient should be tested for sensitivity to products being used and the pouching system should be modified to eliminate the offending product (see Chapter 3 for further discussion).

## Procedures

**General Issues.** General issues that must be considered in establishing pouching procedures include the following: organizational measures; timing for pouch changes; optimal schedule for pouch changes; and accurate sizing of the barrier or pouch opening.

*Organization.* It is helpful to organize all the products required for pouch changes in one area and to assemble all needed supplies before the pouch changing procedure is begun. Needed supplies include a plastic trash bag for disposing of soiled items, a wet washcloth or disposable wipes, the pouch to be applied, and any products for skin protection, such as skin barrier powder, sealants, or paste. When a "cut-to-fit" pouch is used, a measuring guide or pattern, pencil, and scissors also are needed. An electric or a disposable razor may be needed if hair is present in the peristomal area. When pouching a urinary stoma or a high-output fecal stoma, it is advisable to have an ample supply of absorbent wicks such as folded and rolled squares of soft paper towel or nonsterile gauze, tampons, or dental wicks.

*Timing.* Optimally the pouch change is scheduled for a time when the stoma is less active. A fecal stoma usually is less active at least 2 hours after a meal; for a urinary stoma the best time usually is early in the morning before fluid consumption. Each patient learns his or her own "best time" for pouch changes.

*Schedule for pouch change.* There is no "correct" frequency for pouch changes; the goal is to establish a routine frequency for pouch change that prevents leakage and provides the individual with control. The stoma that is appropriately sited and well constructed usually can be managed with a pouch change frequency of every 5 to 7 days; with more durable products some individuals can maintain secure seals for 10 days or even longer. In contrast, the person with a poorly sited stoma or a retracted stoma may require a twice-weekly pouch change to prevent leakage; occasionally, daily or alternate-day changes may be required.

Establishment of the optimal frequency for pouch change requires individual adjustment and experimentation. In the immediate postoperative period the pouch usually is changed more frequently to permit stoma assessment and to provide instruction in self-care procedures. After discharge the patient should be encouraged to gradually extend the interval between pouch changes until optimal frequency is determined. This frequency then becomes the basis for routine pouch changes. The patient also is taught to recognize the signs of undermining and impending leakage (that is, itching or burning of the peristomal skin, odor occurring when the pouch is closed, or visible "melting down" of the skin barrier) and to change the pouch promptly whenever any of these indicators are present.

**Sizing the Pouch or Barrier Opening.** The nurse must be able to accurately size the opening in the skin barrier or pouch, or both. As noted earlier, most manufacturers of ostomy supplies include disposable stoma-measuring guides in each box of pouches; these are easily used to determine the size of a round stoma. The opening that clears the stoma and minimizes exposure of the peristomal skin should be selected. For irregularly shaped stomas it is necessary to make a pattern that can then be used to size the barrier or pouch opening. One simple way to make a pattern is to use a transparent piece of plastic and a felt-tip marker to trace the stomal contours. The pattern is then cut out and altered as needed until a good fit is obtained. The pattern should be labeled with arrows indicating the head and the foot, as well as "pouch side" and "skin side." The pouch side is the side facing the nurse when the pattern is placed on the patient, and the skin side is the side resting on the patient's skin. The pattern can be used to trace the desired opening on the "skin side" of the barrier or pouch (the side covered with protective paper); to prevent pattern reversal it is important to place the pattern with the "skin side" facing the nurse and the "pouch side" of the pattern against the barrier or pouch (Fig. 2-5). Another way to avoid pattern reversal is to place the pattern on the patient's skin so that it fits correctly, then place the barrier or

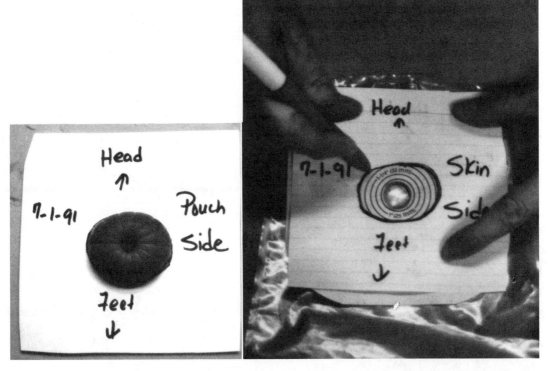

**Fig. 2-5** Pattern construction. **A,** Pattern is labeled "head" and "foot" and "pouch side" and "skin side." **B,** Pattern is traced onto skin side of barrier or pouch; pattern is placed with "pouch side" against barrier or pouch.

pouch "skin side" down against the pattern. Both are then picked up and turned over as a unit, and the pattern is traced onto the barrier or pouch.

When adding a barrier to an adhesive pouch, the barrier is sized to fit closely around the stoma (Fig. 2-6, *A*), whereas the pouch is sized to clear the stoma by at least one-eighth inch (Fig. 2-6, *B*). This method prevents the rigid pouch opening from causing damage to the stoma and also prevents tunneling of the effluent between the barrier and the pouch (see the box on p. 52.)

Because the stoma normally shrinks during the first 6 to 8 weeks after surgery, the barrier or pouch should be resized at each pouch change during this period. Once shrinkage is complete, further resizing is not indicated unless the stoma changes. The patient who is not able to measure his or her stoma or who has an irregularly shaped stoma must be reassessed closely during the first 6 to 8 weeks after surgery, either by a home-care nurse or in an outpatient clinic.

**Routine Peristomal Hygiene.** Routine cleansing of the peristomal skin is effectively accomplished with warm water; use of soap is discouraged because soap residue could cause a dermatitis and many soaps contain moisturizers that could interfere with pouch

## ADDING A SKIN BARRIER TO AN ADHESIVE POUCH

1. Use a commercial stoma-measuring guide to determine stoma size (if stoma is round), or make a pattern (if stoma is irregular).
2. Trace the pattern onto the "skin side" of the barrier (side covered with protective paper). Pattern should be placed with "pouch side" against the barrier (see Fig. 2-6, *A*). Cut the barrier out.
3. Trace the pattern onto the "skin side" of the pouch. Cut out a pouch opening at least one-eighth inch *larger* than the pattern (see Fig. 2-6, *B*).
4. Peel paper backing from the pouch to expose the adhesive surface, and attach the pouch to the barrier (see Fig. 2-6, *C*).

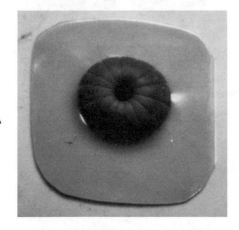

**A**

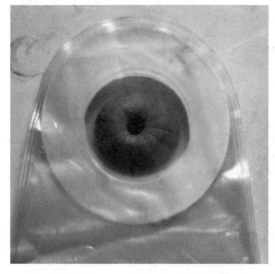

**B**

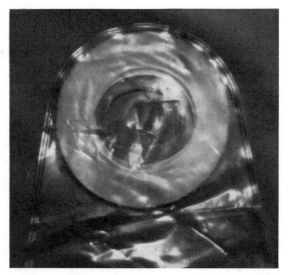

**C**

**Fig. 2-6** Adding barrier to adhesive pouch, as described in box above. **A,** Barrier sized to fit snugly around stoma. **B,** Pouch sized to clear stoma by one-eighth inch. **C,** Pouch attached to barrier.

adherence. If the patient wishes to use soap, the nurse must stress the importance of using a mild, nonoily soap and rinsing thoroughly. Patients occasionally may need to use commercial cleansing pads for peristomal skin care, for example, while camping or backpacking or when changing the pouch in a public restroom. In these situations a commercial cleansing pad that does not require rinsing and does not leave an oily residue is recommended. Most commonly available commercial wipes are intended for infant care and are lanolin based; these are not appropriate for peristomal skin care.

Peristomal hair removal is recommended for persons with hirsute abdomens; routine hair removal reduces the potential for folliculitis, which may occur when hair growth is impeded by the application of a pouching system. Specific procedures for hair removal differ; some patients are taught to shave, and others are taught to clip the peristomal hair. When the peristomal area is shaved, two guidelines should be followed. (1) Shave outward from the stoma to prevent inadvertent stomal damage. (2) When shaving with a safety razor, use either a "dry shave" technique (using a skin barrier powder) or a "wet shave" technique (using soap or shaving cream). If soap or shaving cream is used, rinse the peristomal area well before pouch application.

**Pouching a Fecal Stoma.** Issues that may affect the management of fecal diversions include protection of the peristomal skin from fecal contact; use of drainable versus closed-end pouches; and modifications required for effective pouching of loop stomas.

*Peristomal skin protection.* The degree of skin protection required for a fecal stoma is variable and depends on the enzymatic content, consistency, and volume of the effluent, which in turn depends on the location of the stoma within the gastrointestinal tract. The following is a general guideline in determining the degree of skin protection required for a fecal diversion: the more proximal the stoma, the more corrosive the drainage. For example, a jejunostomy or ileostomy requires protection of all peristomal skin[13]; most commonly a pectin, gelatin, or synthetic barrier is sized to fit closely around the stoma, and pectin-based paste is used as "caulk" to prevent undermining of the barrier and to protect the skin immediately adjacent to the stoma. Colostomy effluent usually is less corrosive than small-bowel effluent; although a barrier ring or wafer still is indicated to prevent fecal contact with the skin, karaya-based barrier rings and paste may be used effectively for these patients. The patient whose sigmoid colostomy is well regulated by irrigation has only small amounts of mucoid drainage and simply requires protection from maceration; a barrier ring or wafer usually is not needed.

In determining the amount of protection required for any patient, the nurse must consider the length and function of the proximal bowel. For example, the patient with Crohn's disease who has a colostomy and has had multiple small bowel resections may have corrosive ileostomy-type effluent and requires maximum skin protection, as do patients who have had previous radiation therapy that has damaged the bowel, resulting in a short-bowel syndrome.

Another consideration in determining the amount of peristomal protection required for an individual patient is the patient's self-care potential. Although an ileostomy is best managed with a pectin-based paste and a pectin, gelatin, or synthetic barrier sized to fit snugly around the stoma, not all patients are able to apply the paste; in these situations the nurse may omit the paste and focus on correctly sizing the barrier opening and on increased frequency of pouch changes. The ultimate goals are to protect the peristomal skin, to maintain a secure pouching system, and to promote self-care.

***Closed-end versus drainable pouches.*** Fecal pouches are available in both drainable and closed-end styles. The type of pouch selected depends on the volume and frequency of fecal output and the patient's ability and willingness to manipulate a drainable pouch.

Drainable pouches have an opening in the tail of the pouch, which permits drainage of fecal contents while the pouch remains in place. Drainable pouches usually are recommended for the patient who does not regulate fecal output (by colostomy irrigation or diet) and for the patient who has high-volume output. Use of drainable pouches reduces the frequency of pouch changes, which reduces cost and also reduces the risk of skin damage resulting from frequent pouch changes. Drainable pouches are closed with commercial tail closures, rubber bands, or binder clips. Although many individuals prefer the commercial clips, others find the rubber bands or binder clips easier to manipulate, at least initially.

Closed-end pouches are nondrainable and vary in construction and capacity. For example, closed pouches may be constructed with a simple adhesive faceplate, or they may have an attached skin barrier. Many closed pouches are constructed with flatus filters, which are particularly important features in one-piece closed pouches because they both vent and deodorize the flatus. The only other alternative for elimination of flatus from a closed pouch is to make a hole in the pouch; this is an undesirable option because there is no mechanism for odor control.

The capacity of closed-end pouches varies greatly; some contain a moderate amount of stool, whereas others may contain only small amounts of spillage between irrigations. The closed pouch with the least capacity is the stoma cap; it is intended primarily for mucus absorption and venting of flatus.

Closed-end pouches with moderate capacity may be beneficial for patients who have low-volume output and are unable or unwilling to empty the pouch. These patients may find closed pouches with two-piece systems preferable to one-piece closed pouches because the two-piece system permits exchange of pouches without the skin trauma and cost associated with removal of the adhesive one-piece pouch. Patients who use two-piece systems also may choose to use closed-end pouches, which are smaller, during sexual activity. Stoma caps and closed-end pouches with minimal capacity are appropriate only for patients with descending or sigmoid colostomies that are well regulated by irrigation or for the patient with a nonfunctioning mucous fistula.

***Stoma plugs.*** Disposable stoma plugs are available in both one-piece and two-piece forms; they are constructed of an inert material that conforms to the contour of the individual's colon and are designed for insertion *into* the stoma. Because they occlude the stomal opening, plugs prevent leakage of stool; an integrated flatus filter vents and deodorizes the flatus. Stomal plugs are intended for patients with descending or sigmoid colostomies who regulate fecal output with routine colostomy irrigations and who desire increased security against leakage between irrigations. They also may be used to provide short periods of continence (usually 4 to 6 hours) for the patient with a descending or sigmoid colostomy who does not irrigate. It is important to realize that these plugs are not suitable for all patients and that the patient must go through an adaptation phase during which wear time gradually is increased; guidelines for the adaptation phase are provided by the company (Coloplast, Tampa, Fla.). The patient using a stoma plug must be carefully monitored by an ET nurse throughout the adaptation phase.

***Pouching modifications for loop ostomies.*** Loop stomas may be stabilized on the abdominal surface by a fascial bridge or by an external rod or bridge; external supports are used to prevent stomal retraction and are left in place until the stoma has granulated to the abdominal wall. External supports usually are removed about 1 week after surgery; however, removal is delayed in patients with compromised healing resulting from infection, malnutrition, irradiation, or corticosteroids.

Pouching a stoma that is stabilized by a rod or bridge may require creative pouching techniques. If the support is small and flat, a flexible pouch and barrier can be placed directly over the support. If the stoma is stabilized by a small rod that can be manipulated, the stoma can be pouched with a one-piece pouch with attached skin barrier by means of the following approach:

1. The pouch is sized to fit around the stoma.
2. The rod is positioned so that the peristomal skin on one side of the stoma is exposed.
3. Half of the paper backing on the pouch is removed to expose half of the adhesive surface; this half of the pouch is pressed into place onto the exposed peristomal skin surface.
4. The rod is repositioned to expose the peristomal skin on the other side of the stoma. (The rod is now extending onto the pouch or barrier surface.)
5. The remaining paper backing is removed from the pouch, and the pouch is pressed into place.

With bulkier support devices such as a large rod it may be necessary to apply the skin barrier and the pouch separately. In this case the barrier is sized to fit around the stoma; a top slit is then cut down to the stoma opening. The barrier can then be fitted into place underneath the rod and the slit reinforced with skin barrier paste; a flexible, adhesive-only pouch is then applied over the barrier. (The opening in the pouch is cut about 1 inch larger than the stoma to permit manipulation of the pouch over the stoma and support device; this does not compromise skin protection because the skin is covered by the barrier [Fig. 2-7].) Regardless of the pouching technique used, it is important to indicate on the pouch that a rod is present. Such a notice serves as a caution to the individual who removes the pouch.

In some centers the nurse caring for the ostomy is asked to remove the support device. A physician's order should be obtained before removal of the support, and the nurse must ascertain satisfactory granulation of the stoma to the abdominal wall. Granulation is evidenced by absence of tension on the support device and adherence of the stoma to the abdominal wall.

Procedures for applying one-piece and two-piece fecal pouches are outlined in the boxes on p. 57.

**Pouching a Urinary Stoma.** Issues that must be addressed in pouching a urinary stoma include peristomal skin protection, pouching options, and modifications required for pouching a stoma with stents.

*Peristomal skin protection.* Urine contains no enzymes and normally is slightly acidic; therefore skin damage from urine usually is caused by pooling of the urine on the peristomal skin, which results in maceration. Alkaline urine can further damage the skin and can result in encrustations and crystal deposits.[13] Therefore skin protection for the patient with a urinary diversion focuses on prevention of pooling and maintenance of acidic urine.

Pooling is prevented by maintaining a tight seal between the skin and the pouch so that urine flows over the skin and into the pouch and is not trapped under the pouch adhesive. Pouches with antireflux valves further protect the peristomal skin by preventing or limiting

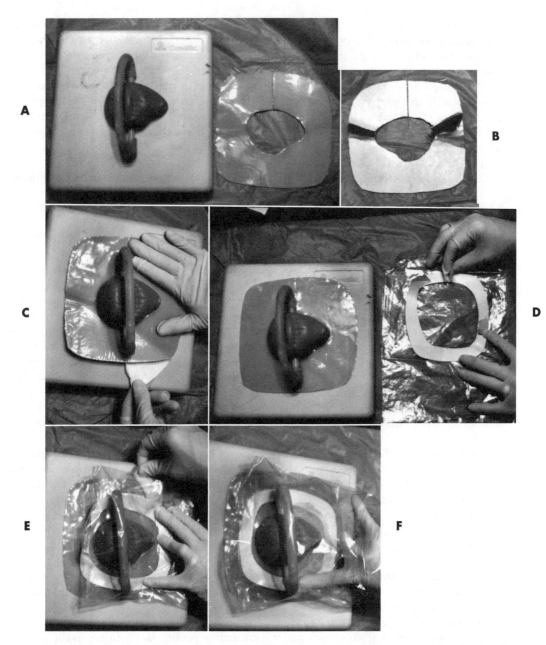

**Fig. 2-7**   Pouching loop ostomy stabilized by large support device. **A,** Barrier sized to fit stoma and top slit cut down to stomal opening. **B,** Protective paper on barrier torn but left in place. **C,** Protective paper strips removed and barrier pressed into place. **D,** Pouch sized to clear stoma by about 1 inch; protective paper strips torn but left in place. **E,** Pouch fitted into place and paper strips removed; pouch pressed securely against barrier. **F,** Barrier paste applied to skin-barrier junction and to barrier-pouch junction.

## APPLICATION OF ONE-PIECE FECAL POUCH*

1. Gather all supplies.
2. Gently remove soiled pouch by pushing down on skin while lifting up on pouch. Discard soiled pouch in odorproof plastic bag. *Save tail closure.*
3. Clean stoma and peristomal skin with water; pat dry. *If indicated,* shave or clip peristomal hair.
4. Use stoma-measuring guide or established pattern to determine size of stoma.
   *Presized pouch.* Check to be sure pouch opening is correct size. Order new supplies if indicated.
   *Cut-to-fit pouch.* Trace correctly sized pattern onto back of barrier or pouch surface, and cut stomal opening to match pattern.
   NOTE: Once stoma shrinkage is complete, this step may be omitted and preparation of clean pouch may be completed before soiled pouch is removed.
5. Apply skin barrier paste around stoma. (*Tip:* Wet finger to facilitate paste application.) An alternative approach is to apply skin barrier paste to aperture in prepared pouch or barrier. Allow paste to dry.
   *Optional:* Apply skin sealant to skin that will be covered by tape.
   Allow to dry.
6. Remove paper backing from pouch or barrier to expose adhesive surface; center pouch opening over stoma and press into place. Attach closure.
   *Optional:* Apply tape strips to "picture-frame" pouch-skin junction.

*Universal precautions* must be followed when this procedure is performed.

## APPLICATION OF TWO-PIECE FECAL POUCH*

1. Gather all supplies.
2. Gently remove soiled pouching system by pushing down on skin while lifting up on barrier wafer. Discard soiled pouch and wafer in odorproof plastic bag. *Save tail closure.*
3. Clean stoma and peristomal skin with water; pat dry. *If indicated,* shave or clip peristomal hair.
4. Use stoma-measuring guide or established pattern to determine size of stoma.
   *Cut-to-fit barrier wafer.* Trace correctly sized pattern onto back of wafer, and cut stomal opening to match pattern.
   *Presized barrier wafer.* Check to be sure pouch opening is correct size. Order new supplies if indicated.
   NOTE: Once stomal shrinkage is complete, this step may be omitted. If cut-to-fit wafer is being used, wafer may be cut out before soiled system is removed.
5. Apply skin barrier paste around stoma. (*Tip:* Wet finger to facilitate paste application.) An alternative approach is to apply skin barrier paste to aperture in barrier wafer. Allow to dry.
   *Optional:* Apply skin sealant to skin that will be covered by tape. Allow to dry.
6. Remove paper backing from barrier wafer; center wafer opening over stoma and press into place.
7. Snap pouch onto flange of barrier wafer. Attach closure.
   *Optional:* Apply tape strips to "picture-frame" wafer-skin junction.

*Universal precautions* must be followed when this procedure is performed.

backflow of urine onto the peristomal skin; most disposable pouches and selected reusable pouches are constructed with antireflux valves. Skin sealants also can reduce the potential for maceration of the peristomal skin, since sealants help "waterproof" the skin.

Encrustations and crystal formation are best prevented by maintaining an acidic and dilute urine.[13] Factors that affect urine acidity are further discussed later in this chapter.

*Pouching options.* In pouching the urinary stoma, the nurse may use one of two approaches. (1) A pouch with an attached skin barrier may be used. The skin barrier is sized to fit snugly around the stoma. (2) An adhesive-only system with an antireflux valve may be used. In this approach the pouch opening is sized to adhere to a flat abdominal surface, even if this requires cutting the pouch opening "wide" and leaving skin exposed. Either approach is valid because the intent of both is to protect the skin from pooled urine; it is not necessary to use a skin barrier wafer or ring to protect the skin from urine.

Pouches with barriers are sized to fit closely around the stoma because barriers are moldable and usually can adapt to peristomal contours. If the stoma is protruding (budded) and the pouch is equipped with an antireflux valve, any barrier that adheres well to the peristomal skin is appropriate. For example, karaya and pectin barriers are known to melt with exposure to urine; however, they may be effective with a budded stoma *if* the pouch is equipped with an antireflux valve (because the urine projects into the pouch and backflow is limited by the antireflux valve). With a flush or skin-level stoma, however, it is important to select a barrier resistant to breakdown by urine; urine from a flush stoma constantly washes over the barrier, and a barrier that is not resistant to urine quickly deteriorates. When changing a pouch with a barrier, the nurse should assess the barrier and the peristomal skin to ascertain that the barrier is not absorbing the urine, thererby *causing* peristomal maceration.

Some individuals with urinary stomas obtain longer pouch seals and improved skin protection by using adhesive-only pouching systems. In applying an adhesive-only pouch with an antireflux valve, the goal is to obtain a tight seal between the pouch and the peristomal skin so that pooling is prevented. Adhesive surfaces cannot adapt to changing peristomal contours and may lift and permit pooling if applied over irregular contours and deep creases; therefore the pouch opening should be sized to permit adherence to a flat abdominal pouching surface. It must be stressed that this approach requires use of a pouch with an antireflux valve; backflow of urine must be prevented because the peristomal skin is exposed. Use of sealants or cements usually is recommended to further protect the skin from maceration.

*Pouching the stoma with ureteral stents.* Ureteral stents frequently are placed at the time of surgery to stabilize the ureterointestinal anastomosis and to prevent stenosis and obstruction while healing occurs. In addition, a small catheter may be placed in the conduit to promote drainage from the conduit itself.[19] Ureteral stents usually remain in place for the first 7 to 14 days after surgery. Pouching during this period may be facilitated by use of a two-piece system. (The patient who is discharged with stents in place will need assistance with the pouch change procedure; a family member or significant other must be involved in discharge teaching, and a home-care referral frequently is warranted.)

Mucus accumulation around the stents is common and may be distressing to the patient and family. It is important for the nurse to reassure the patient and family that this is a normal occurrence and that stent removal eliminates the mucus accumulation at the stomal surface.

Finally, the nurse must realize that ureteral stents provide an ascending pathway for bacteria; therefore careful attention to clean technique is indicated when a stoma is pouched with ureteral stents in place.

Procedures for application of one-piece and two-piece urinary pouches are outlined in the boxes below.

---

## APPLICATION OF ONE-PIECE URINARY POUCH*

1. Gather all supplies.
2. Gently remove soiled pouch by pushing down on skin while lifting up on pouch. Discard soiled pouch.
3. Use stoma-measuring guide or established pattern to determine size of stoma.
   *Presized pouch.* Check to be sure pouch opening is correct size. Order new supplies if indicated.
   *Cut-to-fit pouch.* Trace correctly sized pattern onto back of pouch, and cut stomal opening to match pattern.
   NOTE: Once stomal shrinkage is complete, this step may be omitted. If a cut-to-fit pouch is used, pouch may be cut out before soiled pouch is removed.
4. Remove paper backing from pouch, and lay pouch to one side.
5. Clean stoma and peristomal skin with water; pat dry. *If indicated,* shave or clip peristomal hair.
   *Use wicks against stoma to absorb urine and to keep skin dry for steps 6 and 7.*
6. *Optional:* Apply skin sealant to skin that will be covered by tape. Allow to dry.
7. Remove paper backing from pouch; center pouch opening over stoma and press pouch into place.
8. *Optional:* Apply tape strips to "picture-frame" the pouch-skin junction.

*Universal precautions* must be followed when this procedure is performed.

---

## APPLICATION OF TWO-PIECE URINARY POUCH*

1. Gather all supplies.
2. Gently remove soiled pouching system by pushing down on skin while lifting up on barrier wafer. Discard soiled pouch and wafer.
3. Use stoma-measuring guide or established pattern to determine size of stoma:
   *Presized barrier wafer.* Check to be sure pouch opening is correct size. Order new supplies if indicated.
   *Cut-to-fit barrier wafer.* Trace correctly sized pattern onto back of wafer, and cut stomal opening to match pattern.
   NOTE: Once stomal shrinkage is complete, this step may be omitted. If a cut-to-fit pouch is used, pouch may be cut out before soiled pouch is removed.
4. Remove paper backing from barrier wafer, and lay wafer to one side.
5. Clean stoma and peristomal skin with water; pat dry. *If indicated;* shave or clip peristomal hair.
   *Use wicks to absorb urine and to keep skin dry for steps 6 and 7.*
6. *Optional:* Apply skin sealant to skin that will be covered by tape. Allow to dry.
7. Center wafer opening over stoma, and press into place.
8. Snap pouch onto barrier wafer. Close spout.
9. *Optional:* Apply tape strips to "picture-frame" the wafer-skin junction.

*Universal precautions* must be followed when this procedure is performed.

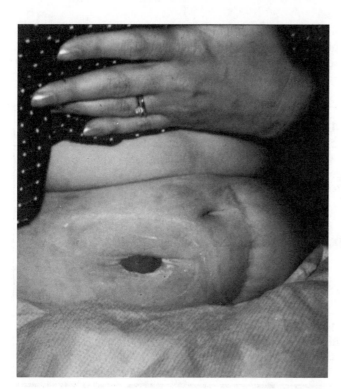

**Fig. 2-8** Stoma located on soft abdomen. Slight retraction of peristomal skin at muco-cutaneous junction from 3 o'clock to 9 o'clock position is evident.

**Pouching the Difficult Stoma.** Usually the preceding procedures provide the patient with a secure seal for a predictable period of time. The patient with a retracted stoma, irregular peristomal contours, or a soft abdomen may require modifications in either the pouching system or its application, to obtain a secure seal for even a limited period of time. In caring for the patient with a difficult stoma, the nurse must be skilled in assessment and pouch application and knowledgeable regarding options in pouching systems. The goals in pouching any stoma are to effectively match the patient's peristomal contours to the pouch surface or to modify the peristomal contours to conform to a pouch.

*Assessment.* Before modifying either the pouch or the application technique, the nurse must carefully assess the stoma and the peristomal contours. The patient should be observed in both the supine and the sitting positions to determine the degree of stomal protrusion, the point and angle at which the stoma empties, and the contours of the peristomal skin. It also is important to examine the adhesive surface any time the pouch is removed for leakage; this provides information regarding the point at which the pouch seal is being lost.

*Stoma on a soft abdomen.* The patient with a soft abdomen usually benefits from a more rigid pouching system; the addition of a belt or binder also may be indicated (Fig. 2-8). Some disposable pouching systems incorporate a plastic gasket and belt tabs into the pouch design; the gasket serves to increase the firmness or rigidity of the faceplate, and the belt tabs facilitate the use of a belt. Disposable pouches with built-in convexity have plastic rings incorporated into the pouch, which also provide support for a soft abdomen. However, the pouches that offer the greatest amount of rigidity are reusable systems; the faceplates for these systems are constructed of hard plastic or heavy rubber, and some have metal reinforcing rings.

Several factors should be considered in the decision to use either a belt or a binder. (1) A belt primarily adds support at the 9 o'clock and 3 o'clock positions, whereas a binder provides circumferential support. (2) If the stoma is not located in a belt plane, the standard belt may tend to "ride up," actually compromising the pouch seal; binders are much more likely to remain in place. (3) Binders are available in a variety of widths and can be custom designed to provide an adequate pouch opening and needed support; for example, a 6-inch binder can be constructed with the pouch opening in the center, toward the top, or toward the bottom, depending on stoma location and abdominal contours.

*Flush or retracted stoma.* The goal in managing a flush or retracted stoma is to maintain a secure seal between the pouch and the skin to prevent undermining (Fig. 2-8; see Plates 14 and 18), which may be accomplished through the addition of support and convexity and through measures that improve pouch adherence.

Successful management of the stoma that empties at or below skin level usually requires use of a pouching system with convexity. A convex faceplate presses into the tissue around the stoma, which increases the degree of stomal protrusion and reduces the risk of undermining. Pouches vary in the degree of convexity provided; pouch selection should be based on a careful assessment of the patient's stomal and peristomal contours so that the correct degree of convexity is chosen.

Disposable pouches are available with convexity that ranges from shallow to deep. One-piece systems usually are presized and available with standard round openings, although custom-cut pouches with oval convexity are now available (NuHope, Pacoima, Calif.). To obtain convexity with a two-piece disposable system the use of convex inserts usually is required, although two-piece wafers are available that are presized and convex. Convex inserts are plastic rings that fit within the flange of the wafer; they must be carefully sized so that the internal diameter clears the stoma by at least one-eighth inch and the external diameter fits the flange of the wafer. Convex inserts provide only slight convexity; two inserts can be used with selected wafers, but the degree of convexity provided still does not equal that of one-piece disposable systems with deep convexity. The use of convex inserts may not be feasible for many patients; considerable dexterity and strength are required to insert and remove the inserts. For this reason most patients desiring disposable pouches and needing convexity are best served with one-piece systems.

Patients who require greater convexity or support than can be provided by disposable pouching systems should be evaluated for a reusable pouching system. Reusable faceplates provide more support than do disposable faceplates because they are made of heavier, more durable materials; in addition, reusable systems offer more options in terms of convexity. For example, the Permatype Company (Farmington, Conn.) offers six different convexities, with custom-cut or standard stomal openings (Fig. 2-9). When the stoma is measured for a reusable faceplate, it is essential to allow one-eighth inch clearance to prevent stomal damage resulting from the rigid faceplate. When pouching a fecal stoma, especially an ileostomy, the nurse must remember to apply a barrier ring or paste, or both, immediately around the stoma to protect this exposed skin.

Binders or belts frequently are used with convex pouching systems to provide additional support, particularly when the patient has both a retracted or flush stoma and a soft abdomen. However, belts and binders may also be used for patients with firm abdomens because belts and binders enhance convexity by holding the faceplate securely against the

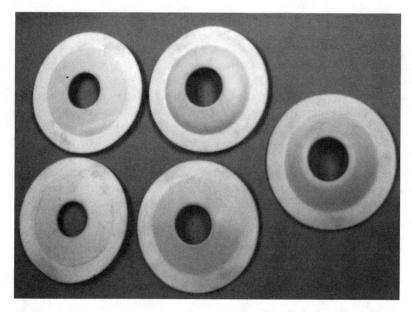

**Fig. 2-9**   Permatype reusable faceplates with convexity. (From Permatype Company, Farmington, Conn.)

abdominal wall. Convexity can also be added or enhanced by applying skin barrier rings or wafers around the stoma or by applying skin barrier wedges in peristomal creases.

Another approach to management of the flush or retracted stoma is to improve the adhesion between the skin and the pouching system, thus preventing undermining. Skin barrier paste commonly is used to reduce undermining with fecal stomas. When the stoma is flush or retracted, it is important to apply the paste in a thin, smooth layer that is even with the skin so that the effluent drains over the paste as opposed to tunneling under it. Skin barrier paste usually is not recommended for use on the skin adjacent to a urinary stoma because currently available pastes dissolve when in contact with urine. Paste *may* be used to create a level pouching surface around a urinary stoma, since the paste is covered by the barrier or pouch and is not exposed to the urine. Occasionally paste may be used adjacent to the stoma, then covered with contact cement to "waterproof" the paste. Another way to improve adhesion is to add contact cement to the faceplate and the skin; this approach can be used with both fecal and urinary systems.

***Deep peristomal creasing.*** Deep peristomal creasing usually is best managed with an all-flexible pouching system and measures to increase pouch adherence; this approach is based on matching the pouch to the patient's contours (Fig. 2-10). The alternative is to evaluate the patient for use of a reusable system that provides support and deep convexity; the intent is to support the peristomal tissues in a more normal configuration. If a reusable system is used in this case, the addition of a belt provides further support at the 9 o'clock and 3 o'clock positions, usually the areas of deepest creasing.

Use of all-flexible systems is usually the best choice for the patient with deep creasing and a firm abdomen; support and convexity may be more effective for the patient with deep

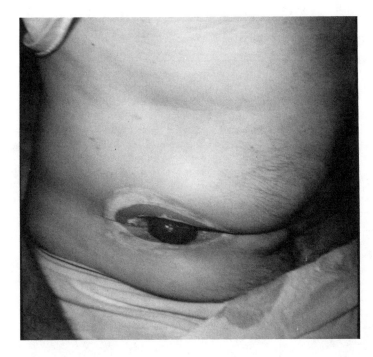

**Fig. 2-10**   Deep peristomal creasing at 9 o'clock and 3 o'clock positions. Stoma has good protrusion, and abdomen appears firm.

---

## APPLICATION OF ONE-PIECE REUSABLE POUCH*

1. Gather all supplies.
2. Prepare pouch for application by adding adhesive to faceplate.
   a. Apply double-faced adhesive disk sized to fit reusable pouch faceplate. Remove paper backing, and lay pouch to one side, *or*
   b. Apply thin layer of contact cement to one side of the reusable pouch faceplate. Lay pouch to one side.
3. Gently remove soiled pouch, and lay it to one side for cleaning.
4. Clean peristomal skin with water; pat dry. *If indicated,* shave or clip peristomal hair.
5. Prepare skin.
   *Fecal stoma.* Apply barrier ring or barrier paste, or both, to protect skin immediately adjacent to stoma.
   *Urinary stoma.* Use wicks to absorb urine and to keep peristomal skin dry for steps 6 and 7.

NOTE: Barrier ring is optional for patient with urinary diversion.

6. *If contact cement is used as adhesive,* apply thin layer of contact cement to peristomal skin surface, and allow it to dry.
7. Center pouch opening over stoma, and press it into place. *Tip:* Centering an opaque pouch over a flush stoma may be facilitated by use of stoma guide strips or by applying the inferior half of the pouch faceplate, then the superior half, which permits better visualization of the stoma.
8. *Optional:* Apply tape strips to "picture-frame" the pouch-skin junction, or add belt or binder for increased security. Both tape strips and belt or binder may be used.
9. Clean soiled pouch, and prepare for repeat use.

---

*Universal precautions* must be followed when this procedure is performed.

---

**APPLICATION OF TWO-PIECE REUSABLE POUCH***

1. Gather all supplies.
2. Prepare faceplate and pouch for application.
   a. Stretch pouch over flange of faceplate, and secure with commercial O ring or rubber band. Proceed as if applying a one-piece reusable system (see the box on p. 63), *or*
   b. Apply adhesive to faceplate. Apply thin coat of contact cement and put faceplate to one side to permit drying, *or* attach a double-faced adhesive disk sized to fit faceplate, remove the paper backing to expose the adhesive surface, and put faceplate to one side.
3. Gently remove soiled pouch, and put it to one side for later cleaning.
4. Clean peristomal skin with water; pat dry. *If indicated,* shave or clip peristomal hair.
5. Prepare skin.
   *Fecal stoma.* Apply barrier ring or

barrier paste, or both, to protect skin immediately adjacent to the stoma.
   *Urinary stoma.* Use wicks to absorb urine and to keep peristomal skin dry for steps 6 and 7.
   NOTE: Barrier ring is optional for patient with urinary diversion.
6. *If contact cement is used as adhesive,* apply thin coat of contact cement to peristomal skin, and allow it to dry.
7. Center faceplate opening over stoma, and press it into place. Further secure faceplate to faceplate-skin junction with tape strips or with application of belt or binder.
8. Stretch pouch over flange of faceplate, being careful not to disrupt seal between faceplate and skin; secure with O ring or rubber band.
9. Cleanse soiled pouch and faceplate; prepare for repeat use.

*\*Universal precautions* must be followed used when this procedure is performed.

---

creasing and a soft abdomen. Procedures for applying reusable systems are outlined in the boxes on pp. 63 and 64.

***Indications for surgical revision.*** The nurse should be aware that it is not always possible to compensate for a poorly sited or poorly constructed stoma with innovative pouching techniques. When all available options have been explored without satisfactory results (that is, a predictable pouch seal duration of at least 2 to 3 days), the patient should be referred to the surgeon for possible stoma revision. It is important to ascertain whether the conditions that resulted in a difficult stoma have been corrected; the patient should not be subjected to further surgery unless improvement is expected. For example, the patient who was not evaluated preoperatively and as a result has a poorly sited stoma *and* who has appropriate sites available is likely to benefit from surgical revision. On the other hand, the patient who has a retracted stoma because of marked obesity is unlikely to benefit from additional surgical intervention unless weight loss occurs first.

## EDUCATION FOR SELF-CARE

Adaptation to an ostomy depends in large part on mastery of self-care; thus instruction in ostomy management is a major component of postoperative nursing care. Because principles that underlie effective patient teaching have been discussed in Chapter 1, this section focuses on the content of patient teaching. In teaching the ostomy patient, the nurse must always remember that the patient is dealing with many issues other than self-care and must modify the teaching plan on the basis of the patient's physical and psychologic status and readiness to learn. The nurse also must remember that it usually is not possible or necessary to accomplish all teaching before discharge from the hospital. In most settings it is more realistic to identify critical content that must be taught before the patient is discharged, such as self-care procedures; additional instruction is then provided by the home-care nurse or in the outpatient clinic.[20,23,28]

Content to be included in the teaching plan for an individual with an ostomy includes general concepts relevant to anyone with an ostomy, as well as concepts specific to the type of ostomy, that is, fecal or urinary diversion. This section first addresses general concepts, then describes concepts specific to the type of ostomy.

## General Concepts

Instruction regarding normal stoma characteristics and function, self-care procedures, and peristomal skin care must be included in the teaching plan for any person with an ostomy. In addition, all patients must be provided with information regarding supplies used and supply sources.

**Stoma Characteristics and Function.** Instruction regarding normal stoma characteristics and function usually begins with preoperative teaching and is continued in the postoperative phase during ostomy care procedures.[8] The nurse caring for the patient with an ostomy should point out (1) that the stoma normally is pink or red and that it is moist, (2) that because the stoma has many small blood vessels, it may bleed slightly during cleansing, (3) that the stoma is edematous after surgery and gradually shrinks over the next 6 to 8 weeks, and (4) that because the stoma has no nerve endings, it is not sensitive to touch. Normal output should be described in terms of frequency, volume, and consistency. For example, the nurse explains to the patient with an intestinal conduit that urine drains from the stoma almost constantly and that it is normal for the urine to contain mucus strands; the urine itself should appear clear and dilute. In contrast, the patient with a ureterostomy or vesicostomy should be instructed that the urine should appear clear and dilute *without* strands of mucus. The patient with an ileostomy should be aware that fecal output during the first few weeks (adaptation phase) is likely to be fairly liquid and of high volume (up to 2 quarts per day) but that the stool gradually thickens to a mushy consistency and the volume decreases to less than a quart a day. The patient with a transverse colostomy is instructed to expect mushy or soft stool to drain several times a day, particularly after meals. The nurse should explain to the patient with a descending or sigmoid colostomy that the postoperative stool pattern probably will be similar to the preoperative, preillness pattern in terms of frequency and consistency.

The patient with a fecal diversion should be prepared for large volumes of flatus and noise when peristalsis resumes. It is important to reassure the patient that flatus is temporary and is related to the return of bowel function after an operation; large volumes of flatus are *not* likely to be a long-term problem.

**Self-Care Procedures.** Instruction in self-care procedures *must* be accomplished before discharge; these are survival skills for the person who plans to live independently with an ostomy. Minimal self-care procedures include pouch emptying (and rinsing, if desired) and pouch change procedures.

***Pouch emptying.*** Patients must be taught to empty the pouch, whether fecal or urinary, when it is one-third to one-half full; this prevents overfilling of the pouch and consequent disruption of the pouch seal. The nurse explains that by sitting on the toilet with spread legs, the patient can empty the pouch directly into the toilet. Toilet paper may be placed in the toilet before emptying to prevent splashing.

Individuals using two-piece systems may choose to snap off the pouch that must be emptied and snap a clean pouch onto the intact wafer. The soiled pouch can then be emptied and rinsed. Two pouches can be alternated in this way for 1 to 2 weeks.

***Pouch change procedure.*** Instruction in the pouch change procedure usually begins with the patient observing while the nurse demonstrates and explains each step of the procedure. During subsequent pouch changes the patient (or caregiver) assumes increasing responsibility until he or she demonstrates the ability to change the pouch independently. It may be helpful to use a stoma model to provide the needed number of practice sessions without frequent disruption of the pouch seal. The patient should *not* be discharged until independence in pouch changing has been demonstrated either by the patient or by a caregiver. It is not necessary for the patient or caregiver to demonstrate perfect technique; however, it *is* essential that the person demonstrate the basic steps of the procedure, including the ability to correctly center and apply the pouch.

The nurse bases the teaching plan on the pouching system and application techniques found to be effective for the individual patient. Although specific pouching techniques are individualized, the following outline can be used as a guide for teaching.

#### ROUTINE AND UNSCHEDULED CHANGES

Routine pouch change frequency and indications for unscheduled pouch changes are described. The patient is instructed to establish a routine for pouch changes and is assisted to determine an appropriate schedule (e.g., every Monday and Thursday, every 5 days, or once a week). The nurse also emphasizes that the pouch *must* be changed immediately for any indications of leakage such as itching or burning sensations in the peristomal skin.

#### OPTIMAL TIME FOR POUCH CHANGE

The patient is encouraged to schedule routine pouch changes during periods of reduced stomal activity, such as early morning before fluid intake for the patient with a urinary diversion.

#### ORGANIZATIONAL HINTS

The patient is encouraged to keep all supplies needed for a pouch change in one area; any written instructions should be kept in the same area. Before changing the pouch, the patient should gather all needed supplies to avoid unnecessary delay and possible frustration.

#### TECHNIQUES FOR REMOVING USED POUCH

The importance of atraumatic pouch removal must be stressed. The nurse also instructs the patient in options for pouch disposal or, in the case of reusable pouches, in appropriate cleansing procedures.

#### PERISTOMAL SKIN CARE AND INSPECTION

The patient is taught to gently cleanse the peristomal skin and to inspect the skin for evidence of irritation (red or broken areas, maceration, or rash). The patient with a hirsute abdomen also is taught an appropriate method for hair removal.

#### PERISTOMAL SKIN PROTECTION

The patient is taught the purpose and the application procedure for all products used on the skin (e.g., skin sealants, contact cements, and skin barrier paste). This teaching is individualized for the patient; for example, the patient who uses a skin barrier paste may be taught to use a damp finger to apply the paste directly to the peristomal skin adjacent to the stoma or may be taught to apply the paste to the opening of the prepared pouch, whichever is easier and provides the best protection. The patient who has a urinary stoma or a high-output fecal stoma must be taught how to use wicks so that the skin can be kept dry and a secure pouch seal obtained.

### POUCH PREPARATION AND APPLICATION

The patient is taught to remove all protective plastic and paper from the pouch before application and to carefully center the stomal opening when applying the pouch. The patient also is taught to size the stoma at each pouch change during the first 6 to 8 weeks; the patient with a round stoma may use a stoma measuring guide, whereas the patient with an irregularly shaped stoma uses the pattern that he or she was given at discharge. If the stoma is smaller than the presized pouch or the pattern, the patient is instructed to obtain pouches corresponding to the new stomal size or to construct a new pattern. Resizing also can be performed by the home-care nurse or by the nurse in the outpatient clinic. It is important to provide close outpatient follow-up for the patient with an ostomy during the first 6 to 8 weeks after surgery or until stomal shrinkage is complete.

### APPLICATION OF CLOSURE (OR CLOSURE OF URINARY SPOUT)

The patient is taught the procedure for applying a closure clip or a rubber band and is taught to check for security by gently tugging on the closure. The patient with a urinary diversion is taught to close the spout of the pouch.

**Skin Care.** Instruction in routine peristomal skin care is incorporated into the pouch change procedure and includes (1) gentle cleansing with water or with a mild soap, followed by thorough rinsing, (2) safe techniques for peristomal hair removal (i.e., with scissors, electric shaver, or safety razor directed away from the stoma and used in conjunction with shaving cream or skin barrier powder), and (3) appropriate use of products such as sealants, barrier pastes, adhesives, and solvents.

The patient is taught to inspect the peristomal skin at each pouch change and to recognize minor skin damage such as erythema, maceration, or denudation. The patient is instructed to treat the damaged skin with skin barrier powder and, when indicated, to use water or sealant over the powder to provide a suitable pouching surface. The patient also is taught to check the stoma and the pouch-barrier opening to ensure optimal skin protection.

Because of the large amount of information the patient must assimilate before discharge, the nurse may elect *not* to include treatment of skin breakdown in the teaching plan. This choice is particularly appropriate when the potential for skin damage is low, when close outpatient follow-up is available, and when the patient is overwhelmed. These patients are instructed to contact the ET nurse (or nurse providing ostomy care) for skin problems. All patients are taught to contact the ET nurse for any skin problems unresponsive to treatment and for any severe or "unusual" skin damage.

**Supply Information.** The patient or caregiver should be provided a list of necessary supplies that includes product numbers and suppliers. The patient is encouraged to contact the various suppliers and inquire about product availability, product cost, and payment policy. For example, some companies file an insurance claim and charge the patient only the deductible; others require that the patient pay the entire bill and then seek reimbursement from the insurance carrier.

The nurse may need to assist the patient in obtaining reimbursement. In some cases a letter of medical necessity or a prescription is required.

### General Instructions for the Patient with a Fecal Diversion

In addition to the general issues addressed in the previous section, some concerns are unique to the type of diversion. Patients with fecal diversions must be taught how to empty the pouch and how to keep the pouch tail clean and free of odor. Additional concerns common to patients with fecal diversions include dietary and fluid modifications, control of gas and odor, and management of diarrhea.

In addition, the patient with an ileostomy needs specific instruction related to fluid and electrolyte balance, food blockage, and guidelines for medications. The patient with a transverse colostomy may have concerns related to clothing and concealment of the stoma, whereas the patient with a descending or sigmoid colostomy needs instruction in prevention and management of constipation and may need guidance regarding management options and specific instruction in colostomy irrigation.

**Pouch Emptying Procedure.** Patients with fecal diversions are taught how to manipulate the clip (or alternate tail closure) and are usually instructed to "cuff" the bottom of the pouch before emptying. This cuff keeps the bottom of the pouch clean, which helps prevent odor; the cuff also helps the patient to keep his or her hands clean during the procedure. The patient is taught to empty the stool by gently squeezing, or "milking," the walls of the pouch and to clean the bottom of the pouch thoroughly with toilet paper, a disposable wipe, or a damp paper towel. The nurse should explain that rinsing the pouch is not necessary because the pouch is odorproof; however, patients who prefer to rinse the pouch are instructed to use a squeeze bottle with lukewarm water and to avoid vigorous rinsing of the stoma, which can rinse away the barrier paste and contribute to disruption of the pouch seal. After the pouch has been emptied and the tail cleaned, the patient is taught to "uncuff" the pouch and to reapply the closure.

**Dietary and Fluid Modifications.** The patient with an ostomy commonly has concerns and questions related to diet, and this is an important area in patient education. The box on p. 69 lists the effects of various foods on ostomy output. For most patients there are few if any restrictions; instruction focuses primarily on the importance of a well-balanced diet and adequate fluid intake. The nurse must always be cognizant of the patient's medical and surgical history and must individualize patient instruction accordingly; for example, the patient with Crohn's disease who has had multiple previous small-bowel resections may require significant dietary adjustments unrelated to the ostomy.

**Control of Gas and Odor.** The nurse explains to the patient that there are two major sources of intestinal gas: swallowed air and gas formed by bacterial action on undigested carbohydrates. Swallowed air gradually is absorbed in its transit through the intestinal tract; therefore swallowed air is more likely to affect the patient with a small-bowel stoma, especially a stoma located in the proximal small bowel. Swallowed air is increased by use of straws, talking while eating, chewing gum, and smoking; the patient who swallows large amounts of air may benefit from reduction or elimination of these practices. Gas formed by bacterial action on undigested carbohydrates is of greater significance to the patient with a large-bowel stoma because most intestinal bacteria are located in the colon (the small bowel has low bacterial counts). The nurse assists the patient to identify gas-forming foods (e.g., beans, cabbage, broccoli, brussels sprouts, and beer)[21] and explains the lag time between intake of gas-producing foods and actual flatulence, which usually is about 6 hours for the person with a colostomy (based on average transit time from mouth to colon). The

## EFFECTS OF FOOD ON STOMA OUTPUT

**FOODS THAT THICKEN STOOL**
Bananas
Rice
Bread
Potatoes
Creamy peanut butter
Applesauce
Cheese
Tapioca
Yogurt
Pasta
Pretzels
Marshmallows

**FOODS THAT LOOSEN STOOL**
Dried or string beans
Chocolate
Raw fruits
Raw vegetables
Highly spiced foods
Fried foods
Greasy foods
Prune or grape juice
Leafy green vegetables (lettuce, broccoli, and spinach)

**FOODS THAT CAUSE STOOL ODOR**
Fish
Eggs
Asparagus
Garlic
Some spices
Beans
Turnips
Cabbage family vegetables (onions, cabbage, brussel sprouts, broccoli, cauliflower)

**FOODS THAT CAUSE URINE ODOR**
Seafood
Asparagus

**FOODS THAT CAUSE GAS**
Dried and string beans
Beer
Carbonated beverages
Cucumbers
Cabbage family of vegetables (onions, brussel sprouts, cabbage, broccoli, and cauliflower)
Dairy products
Spinach
Corn
Radishes

**FOODS THAT COLOR STOOL**
Beets
Red jello

individual can then decide to omit these foods or to eat them selectively at times when flatulence will not cause embarrassment. The patient is reminded that pouches are odorproof and is taught measures for muffling flatus sounds, such as putting pressure against the stoma with the hand or elbow. (Patients with large amounts of flatus may benefit from pouches with deodorizing flatus filters; these filters vent the gas through a charcoal filter, thus eliminating flatus odor while keeping the pouch relatively flat.)

The most important odor-control measures are use of odorproof pouches and good hygiene, that is, keeping the bottom of the pouch clean. The patient who is using an odorproof pouch and who keeps the pouch spout clean should have fecal odor only when the pouch is emptied or changed. It often is helpful to remind the patient that fecal odor during elimination is normal. Additional options for odor control include pouch deodorants, room deodorants, and oral deodorizing agents; some individuals use dietary manipulation as well. Agents used as pouch deodorants include commercial deodorants, commercial per-

**Table 2-5**   Oral deodorants

| Type | Effects | Contraindications and guidelines for use |
| --- | --- | --- |
| Activated charcoal | Reduces fecal odor; darkens stool | Large doses can interfere with vitamin absorption |
| Chlorophyllin copper complex | Reduces fecal and urinary odor; turns stool dark green; may cause temporary slight diarrhea | Should not be used in children younger than 12 years old; effective dose usually 100 to 200 mg daily |
| Bismuth subgallate | Reduces fecal odor; reduces flatus; thickens stool; turns stool dark green-black | Excessively large doses may cause heavy metal toxicity; may cause shadows on abdominal films; may interfere with absorption of anticoagulants and antibiotics; contraindicated for patients with renal failure; recommended dose: 1 to 2 tablets 3 to 4 times daily initially, then titrated to lowest effective dose, e.g., 1 to 2 tablets daily |

ineal cleansers, and mouthwashes, all of which contain antibacterial agents. Deodorizing agents for use in the pouch are added to the pouch after it is emptied. Room sprays are intended for use when the pouch is emptied or changed. Room sprays are particularly beneficial when the patient must empty the pouch in a public restroom; they are available in purse or pocket size. Oral agents commonly used include bismuth subgallate (Devrom) and chlorophyllin copper complex; these over-the-counter agents significantly reduce fecal odor when taken consistently. Effects, contraindications, and guidelines for use are outlined in Table 2-5. Some individuals may choose to alter their diets to reduce fecal odor; foods that have been associated with reduced odor include yogurt, parsley, and orange juice. Again it must be emphasized that the best odor-control measures are a secure, odor-proof pouch and good hygiene.

**Management of Diarrhea.** The person with a fecal diversion is just as susceptible to episodes of diarrhea as the person whose bowel is intact; diarrhea may occur as a result of a viral or bacterial gastroenteritis, antibiotic therapy, radiation therapy, chemotherapy, some medications (e.g., antacids containing magnesium), or food intolerance. Management of diarrhea depends partially on the location of the fecal diversion within the gastrointestinal tract and on the length and function of the proximal bowel; however, the principles of management are the same for all patients and can be summarized as follows:

1. Eliminate the cause, if possible; for example, the patient who is taking antibiotics may benefit from a lactobacillus preparation to restore normal bowel flora.[10]
2. Maintain a bland, constipating diet; recommended foods include rice, pasta, cheese, bananas, and applesauce.
3. Replace fluid and electrolytes; the patient is instructed to replace both fluid volume and fluid components, that is, electrolytes. One approach is to drink a glass of

replacement fluid each time the pouch is emptied; suggested replacement fluids include sports drinks, fruit or vegetable juices, and broth.

4. Over-the-counter antidiarrheal medications usually are acceptable. One exception is for the patient receiving radiation therapy; this patient should not take over-the-counter antidiarrheal agents without physician approval because many of these preparations contain bismuth, which is a metallic agent.

The patient also should be instructed to notify the physician of signs and symptoms of fluid-electrolyte imbalance, such as weakness, lethargy, dry mouth and tongue, reduced urine output and increased urine concentration, abdominal cramps, and dizziness when standing.[12] Notifying the physician is particularly important for the patient with a small-bowel or proximal large-bowel stoma, since these patients are at greater risk than normal for fluid-electrolyte imbalance during episodes of increased fluid loss.[9]

## Specific Instruction for the Patient with an Ileostomy

The patient with an ileostomy has unique educational needs related to dietary and fluid modifications, recognition and management of food blockage, measures to prevent fluid-electrolyte imbalance, and guidelines for medication administration.

**Dietary and Fluid Modifications.** In teaching the patient with an ileostomy, the nurse emphasizes the importance of a balanced diet, adequate fluid intake, and measures to prevent food blockage. An ileostomy does not alter a person's ability to digest and absorb nutrients; thus dietary restrictions are minimal. Restrictions based on previous bowel resections or medical conditions are continued; however, it is important to give the patient with inflammatory bowel disease permission to slowly reintroduce foods that were problem foods before surgery.

Because an ileostomy causes the loss of 500 to 750 ml of fluid a day through the stool, the patient is counseled to increase fluid intake to 10 to 12 glasses daily.

Instruction should be given regarding the potential for food blockage and preventive measures. The nurse explains why a person with an ileostomy is at risk for food blockage: the ileum has a relatively narrow lumen (about 1 inch in diameter), which may be narrowed further if any scar tissue develops at the fascia-muscle layer. Undigested fibrous residue can then accumulate at this point of narrowing and can cause a partial or complete obstruction of the bowel lumen.[13] (The person with a colostomy is not at risk for food blockage because the colon has a wider lumen and any fibrous residue is mixed in with the solid stool.) The nurse identifies high-fiber foods that may contribute to a food blockage (see the box on p. 72, *top*) and emphasizes that this complication usually can be prevented by adherence to the following guidelines:

1. Omit high-fiber foods for the first 6 to 8 weeks after surgery; during this time the bowel is edematous and the bowel lumen is narrower than normal.

2. Add high-fiber foods one at a time in small amounts; this permits the individual to monitor tolerance and determine those foods that are not tolerated.

3. Chew food well, and drink plenty of fluids. Chewing breaks down the high-fiber foods into smaller units that are less likely to accumulate at a narrow point within the bowel. Adequate fluid intake also promotes elimination of fecal residue.

4. Monitor response to new foods; intolerance usually is indicated by cramping or diarrhea or both.

---

## HIGH-FIBER FOODS

| | |
|---|---|
| Foods that are stringy and fibrous (e.g., corn, raw celery, coconut, and Chinese vegetables) | Nuts |
| | Popcorn |
| Foods with nondigestible fibrous peels (e.g., potatoes with peels, apples with peels, and grapes) | Meats with casings (e.g., sausage, wieners, and bologna) |
| | Mushrooms |
| Raw cabbage, as in cole slaw | Large seeds (such as watermelon seeds) |
| Dried fruits (such as raisins, dried figs, and apricots) | |

---

## CONSERVATIVE MANAGEMENT OF FOOD BLOCKAGE

1. Warm tub bath to relax abdominal muscles
2. Peristomal massage and knee chest position to attempt dislodgement of fibrous mass
3. If stoma is swollen, remove pouch and replace with pouch that has larger stoma opening.
4. If able to tolerate fluids (not vomiting) and passing stool, avoid solid foods and increase intake of fluids to replace fluid and electrolytes. Drink one glass of liquid each time pouch is emptied. Juices such as grape juice exert a mild cathartic effect.
5. If vomiting or not passing stool, or both, do not take anything orally (liquids or solid food).

*Notify the physician or ET nurse* if any of the following develops:
  Stool output stops (complete blockage)
  Preceding conservative measures fail to resolve symptoms
  Signs of partial obstruction are persistent (high volume, odorous effluent, abdominal cramps, and nausea and vomiting)
  Inability to tolerate fluids or replace fluids and electrolytes
  Signs and symptoms of fluid and electrolyte imbalance

---

**Recognition and Management of Food Blockage.** Adherence to the guidelines for adding high-fiber foods to the diet usually prevents development of a food blockage. However, the person with an ileostomy should be taught the signs and symptoms of food blockage, appropriate home management, and indications for notifying the physician. Signs and symptoms of food blockage are the same as for any intestinal obstruction and vary depending on completeness of the obstruction. Partial obstruction usually manifests by cramping abdominal pain, watery output with a foul odor, and possible abdominal distention and stomal swelling. Nausea and vomiting may occur. Complete obstruction is evidenced by absence of output, severe cramping pain, abdominal distention, stomal swelling, nausea, and vomiting.[11,13] Home relief measures used in the treatment of partial and complete obstruction are outlined in the box above, *bottom*. The patient is taught to notify the physician (or ET nurse) promptly if signs of complete obstruction do not respond to the

---

### SIGNS AND SYMPTOMS OF FLUID-ELECTROLYTE IMBALANCE

**ADULT**
Dry mouth and mucous membranes
Orthostatic hypotension
Decreased urine volume
Increased urine concentration
Sunken eyes
Extreme weakness
Flaccid muscles
Diminished reflexes
Muscle cramps (abdominal or in legs)
Lethargy

Tingling or cramping in feet and hands
Confusion
Nausea and vomiting

**INFANT**
Depressed fontanelle
Lethargy
Sunken eyes
Weak cry
Decreased frequency of wet diaper

---

aforementioned measures or if signs of partial obstruction persist for more than 24 hours despite appropriate home management; these patients usually require ileal lavage as outlined in the section on long-term follow-up.[2]

**Prevention and Management of Fluid-Electrolyte Imbalance.** The person with an ileostomy has lost the absorptive functions provided by the colon, as well as the delay feature provided by the ileocecal valve. This individual loses about 500 to 750 ml of fluid daily through the stoma, compared with 100 to 200 ml lost by the average person with an intact colon. Thus these patients are at much greater risk for fluid-electrolyte imbalance during periods of increased loss, for example, gastroenteritis that causes diarrhea and vomiting. Self-care instruction for these patients must include the importance of vigorous replacement of fluid and electrolytes during periods of increased loss, recognition and prompt response to signs and symptoms of fluid-electrolyte imbalance, and the importance of notifying the physician promptly should they be unable to replace fluids during periods of increased loss.[12] (See the box above for signs and symptoms of fluid-electrolyte imbalance that necessitate physician notification.)

Fluid-electrolyte balance in the infant with an ileostomy can be particularly problematic. Close, accurate monitoring of stool output and all intake is essential. Gauze and diapers are weighed to calculate output; if a pouch is in place, the stool output is measured. Daily weights are obtained and should be examined to determine whether the infant's trend in daily weights reflects a slow gain or a loss. The infant who fails to demonstrate a trend in weight gain may be described as having "failure to thrive."

To determine whether the infant's output is normal or high, the following guide can be used: Normal stool output equals 1 mg per kilogram of body weight per 24 hours (see the box on p. 74). When the infant's stool output is high, the following interventions should be considered by the neonatologist, surgeon, nurse, and dietitian: (1) reevaluate the type of infant feeding solution being used, (2) implement or adjust antidiarrheals or bulking agents, and (3) supplement oral feedings with total parenteral nutrition. Occasionally the surgeon may elect to close the ileostomy once it is determined safe to do so, despite the typical preference to wait until the infant is 1 to 2 years of age.

---

### GUIDE TO EVALUATING VOLUME OF FECAL OUTPUT IN INFANTS

**NORMAL OUTPUT RANGE IN AN INFANT**

One milliliter per hour per kilogram of body weight

**EXAMPLES**

1. A 10-pound infant weighs 4.55 kg. The equation used to calculate normal stool output per 24 hours follows:

   4.55 kg × 24 hr = 109.2 ml
2. A preterm infant weighing 2.2 kg has an ileostomy because of necrotizing enterocolitis. Oral feedings are being introduced slowly, and the stool output increases to 8 ml per 2 hours. Normal stool volumes are estimated as follows:

   2.2 kg × 24 hr = 52.8 ml

At the current rate, 96 ml of stool will be produced in 24 hours, which is interpreted as high output. The neonatologist, surgeon, gastroenterologist, and nurse must collaborate to identify measures to control stool volume (type of oral solution, administration of immodium and bulking agents, or supplemental parenteral nutrition).

From Boarini JH: Principles of stoma care for infants, *J Enterostom Ther* 16(1):21, 1989.

**Guidelines for Medication Administration.** Some forms of medication are designed for gradual absorption along the full length of the bowel, including the colon; because of decreased bowel length and transit time, these medications are incompletely and unpredictably absorbed in the person with an ileostomy. Medications that may be incompletely absorbed include enteric-coated tablets, large tablets, and time-released capsules and spansules.[24] Tablets may be evaluated for breakdown by the following home test: the individual places the tablet in a glass of water and evaluates the rate of dissolution in 30 minutes. If the tablet has begun to dissolve, it usually can be adequately absorbed. The individual is instructed *never* to crush medications unless instructed to do so by the pharmacist; this results in exposure of the drug to the gastric fluids, which may inactivate the drug or cause severe gastric distress.[12] Instead, patients are counseled to inform their physicians, dentists, and pharmacists of the ileostomy and the possible need for alternate forms of medication. This is especially important for the patient taking antidiarrheal medication or antibiotics; liquid forms of these drugs may be recommended to ensure full intended effects. The liquid form of medications is particularly helpful during the first 6 to 12 months after ileostomy and for the patient with rapid transit resulting from multiple small-bowel resections, inflammatory disease, or radiation enteritis.

The patient with an ileostomy also must be counseled *never* to take a laxative because this could result in severe fluid-electrolyte imbalance. The patient should know that adequate preparation of the small bowel for diagnostic studies or for surgery can be achieved by restricting oral intake to clear liquids for 24 hours.[11] This is an extremely important point; because many patients see a variety of health care providers in years subsequent to surgery, it is imperative that all patients be knowledgeable and able to act in their own behalf.

## Specific Instruction for the Patient with a Transverse Colostomy

Issues specific to the patient with a transverse colostomy include dietary and fluid modifications and concealment of the stoma. Transverse colostomies most commonly are performed for temporary diversion; therefore an additional issue for many patients is incorporation of the colostomy into their life-styles on a temporary basis.

**Dietary and Fluid Modifications.** The nurse explains to the person with a transverse colostomy that nutrients are digested and absorbed in the small intestine and that the small intestine is not affected by a transverse colostomy.[5] Therefore this individual has *no* absolute restrictions imposed by the colostomy. The person with a transverse colostomy loses additional fluid through the stoma and should be instructed to increase fluid intake to 10 glasses of liquid per day. (Dietary modifications for control of gas were discussed in the section, General Instruction for the Patient with a Fecal Diversion.)

**Concealment of the Stoma.** The patient with a transverse colostomy often has a stoma located in the upper abdominal quadrants, above the beltline. These patients frequently have concerns related to clothing and concealment of the stoma. Although suggestions must be individualized for the particular patient, general guidelines include use of a knit layer of clothing next to the body to keep the pouch secure and smooth and use of a loose outer layer for concealment. The patient also may find vests, sweaters, scarves, and jackets helpful in concealing the stoma.

## Specific Instruction for the Patient with a Descending or Sigmoid Colostomy

The patient with a descending or sigmoid colostomy needs information regarding prevention, recognition, and management of constipation. These patients also need to be evaluated regarding candidacy for routine irrigation as a means of regulating bowel function. Patients who are candidates must be counseled regarding their management options, and those who elect to try colostomy irrigations must be instructed in the procedure.

**Prevention and Management of Constipation.** The nurse providing ostomy care must assess the patient's previous bowel habits, including history of constipation, past management of constipation, and life-style factors affecting bowel function, such as activity level and intake of fiber and fluid. The nurse should explain to the patient that a colostomy does not prevent constipation and should make specific recommendations for maintenance of healthy bowel function and prevention of constipation. Routine preventive measures include daily exercise and adequate intake of fluids and fiber. The nurse makes individual recommendations based on usual fluid and fiber intake, past bowel patterns, and activity tolerance. For example, the sedentary patient with a history of constipation and usual intake of fluids and fiber limited to six glasses of fluid a day and one serving of fiber (less than 5 gm) may be instructed to begin a simple, graduated walking program, to add two glasses of fluid a day, and to take a bulk laxative twice daily. (An alternative suggestion would be to increase dietary intake of bulk or to add bran to the diet.) The patient also is instructed in recognition of constipation: failure to pass stool for more than 24 hours, hard stools, or liquid stools associated with cramping and abdominal swelling. The patient is instructed to increase fiber and fluid intake and to notify the physician or ET nurse promptly in the event of constipation.

**Colostomy Irrigation.** Patient education for the person with a descending or sigmoid colostomy may include instruction in colostomy irrigation. The nurse first must assess the appropriateness of routine irrigation as a method of management and must then counsel the patient regarding management options. The patient who is determined to be a candidate for routine irrigation and elects this management approach is then instructed in the irrigation procedure.

*Criteria for irrigation.* The patient who meets the following criteria is a good candidate for management with routine irrigations:

1. Descending or sigmoid colostomy. Routine irrigation is a management option only for the patient with a descending or sigmoid colostomy. It is an inappropriate approach for the patient with a more proximal stoma because these stomas produce a more fluid, higher-volume output; thus these patients are unable to regulate fecal output with irrigation, and routine irrigations may induce fluid-electrolyte imbalance.

2. Normal bowel function. Routine irrigation is most appropriate for the person with a history of regular, formed bowel movements; it is least likely to be effective in the individual with frequent episodes of diarrhea or irregular bowel elimination patterns.[5]

3. Ability to learn and perform the procedure. The patient must be capable of learning and performing the irrigation procedure and must have access to adequate toilet facilities (running water and indoor plumbing).

4. Patient preference. Irrigation is the patient's preferred method of management. Irrigation is a management *option* and is not required to maintain normal bowel function. The decision to use this management approach should be made by the patient, not by the health care team.

There are some conditions and situations in which routine irrigation is contraindicated or at least not recommended. These include the following:

1. Stomal prolapse or peristomal hernia. Routine irrigation is contraindicated in these patients because of the potential for increased prolapse or bowel perforation and poor evacuation results.

2. Children and young adults. Routine irrigation usually is not appropriate for younger patients because of the potential for creation of bowel dependency.

3. Pelvic or abdominal radiation. Irrigation is contraindicated in the patient receiving pelvic or abdominal radiation, because of the extreme risk of bowel perforation. Irrigations should not be initiated or resumed until bowel friability has resolved, as indicated by restoration of normal bowel function and healthy stomal mucosa.

4. Temporary colostomy. Routine irrigation usually is not recommended for patients with temporary colostomies, because of the potential for creating bowel dependency and the time required to master the procedure; however, the nurse must use his or her judgment in determining appropriateness for an individual patient. For example, a young woman with a temporary colostomy for a rectovaginal fistula is unlikely to develop bowel dependency with short-term irrigation and the woman may benefit from this management approach if she has concerns about gas and emptying her pouch in public restrooms.

5. Poor prognosis. Routine irrigation usually is not recommended for patients who have a poor prognosis, because of the time and energy required for the procedure. Again, however, the nurse must determine candidacy based on the individual's status and priorities.

*Patient counseling regarding management options.* Once the nurse has determined the patient's candidacy for irrigation as a method of management, the nurse should counsel the patient regarding available options.

The nurse explains that irrigation acts to stimulate bowel emptying and that routine irrigations establish regular bowel elimination in response to the irrigation stimulus; the advantage is that the patient regains control of fecal elimination.[5] Disadvantages include the time required for the procedure and the risk of bowel dependency over time. It is important to stress that irrigation is *one approach* to colostomy management and that irrigation is not required to maintain normal bowel function. It also is important to explain to the patient that irrigation does not provide effective bowel regulation in all cases, that the time required for bowel regulation varies from about 3 to 6 weeks, and that the choice to discontinue irrigation is always available if the process becomes incompatible with the patient's life-style. However, the person who discontinues irrigation after many months or years may need to routinely use a bulk laxative or stimulant, or both, to maintain bowel function.

The nurse assists the patient to determine the method of management most compatible with both life-style and preferences. For the patient who chooses to try irrigation, the nurse provides instruction in the procedure.

***Potential problems with initial colostomy irrigation.*** When colostomy irrigations are initiated, the nurse should be aware of the following potential problems: unresolved postoperative ileus, vasovagal reaction, and anastomotic complications.

### POSTOPERATIVE ILEUS

Colostomy irrigations usually are delayed until normal bowel function has resumed, as evidenced by elimination of stool and flatus through the stoma and the patient's ability to tolerate oral intake. As noted earlier in this chapter, low-volume irrigations occasionally are performed to stimulate peristalsis in the presence of hypoactive bowel sounds. If some degree of ileus is thought to persist, irrigations should be performed with saline and the volume limited to 500 ml or less.

### VASOVAGAL REACTION

Colon distention occasionally causes excessive vagal stimulation, resulting in bradycardia, hypotension, and possibly loss of consciousness. The patient should be promptly placed in the supine position, which helps restore cerebral blood flow; fluid resuscitation also may be necessary. Vasovagal reaction is more likely to occur with initial irrigations and in the patient with a history of vagal stimulation or bradycardia. For this reason it may be advisable to perform the first irrigation with the patient in bed.

### ANASTOMOTIC COMPLICATIONS

Most descending or sigmoid colostomies are constructed as end colostomies, and there is no proximal bowel anastomosis; occasionally, however, additional resections result in bowel anastomoses proximal to the stoma. In this situation, colostomy irrigations should be delayed until the anastomoses are well healed, usually about 4 to 6 weeks after surgery.[5]

***Instruction in irrigation procedure.*** After the nurse has assessed the patient's readiness for colostomy irrigations, the patient is instructed in the procedure (see the box on p. 78). Key concepts to include in patient teaching follow.

### PRINCIPLES OF COLOSTOMY IRRIGATION

The nurse explains that the irrigating fluid distends the bowel, which causes the bowel to contract and empty. Routine irrigation causes the bowel to empty on a regular basis, which reduces the chance of fecal elimination between irrigations.

### SCHEDULE

Most individuals irrigate the colostomy daily or every other day, depending on the preoperative bowel pattern. Time of day is selected on the basis of the individual's life-style and preference. However, for optimum results irrigation should be regularly scheduled procedure.

## COLOSTOMY IRRIGATION*

1. Gather supplies. Explain procedure to patient, and provide for privacy and comfort.
2. Remove pouch or stomal covering.
3. Attach irrigation sleeve; place bottom of sleeve into toilet to direct returns, *or* close bottom of sleeve with rubber band, binder clip, or commercial tail closure.
   NOTE:Irrigation sleeves for two-piece systems are snapped onto the two-piece wafer with flange; other reusable sleeves are belted into place. Disposable adhesive sleeves also are available.
4. Prepare irrigating solution. Volume to be given is titrated for the patient and is based on the patient's tolerance and feelings of colonic distention ("fullness"). Initial irrigations usually are performed with 500 ml of solution or less to prevent overdistention and cramping. Routine irrigation for the average adult is performed using approximately 1000 ml of solution.
   Close clamp on irrigating bag, and fill bag with desired amount of tepid water or prescribed irrigant.

Open clamp, and allow irrigating solution to flow to clear tubing of air. Suspend irrigating bag at approximately shoulder height.
5. Lubricate the cone tip; insert cone tip gently into stoma, and hold tip securely in place to prevent backflow.
6. Open clamp, and allow irrigation solution to flow in steadily; the desired time frame for instillation of fluid is 5 to 10 minutes.
7. When desired amount of irrigant has been delivered *or* when the patient senses colonic distention, close the clamp and remove the cone.
8. Wait approximately 30 to 45 minutes for returns. After initial returns are complete (usually 10 to 15 minutes), the individual has the option to close the bottom of the sleeve and move around.
9. When returns are complete, rinse and remove the irrigation sleeve.
10. Clean peristomal skin, and apply pouch or desired stomal covering.
11. Prepare equipment for repeat use.

*Universal precautions* must be followed when this procedure is performed.

### TYPE AND VOLUME OF IRRIGATING SOLUTION

Most individuals use lukewarm tap water; the alternative is saline, which can be made by adding 2 teaspoons of salt to 1 quart of water. Volume is titrated for the individual; the goal is to use enough irrigant to distend the bowel but not enough to cause cramping pain. Most adults use between 600 and 1000 ml of water; the patient is instructed to instill the irrigant at a steady rate until a feeling of fullness is achieved.

### EQUIPMENT

The patient is instructed to use a cone tip rather than a catheter (Fig. 2-11); the cone tip prevents bowel perforation[9,13] and also prevents backflow of the irrigating solution, thereby promoting bowel distention and effective elimination. (The cone tip should be held securely against the stoma to prevent backflow.) An irrigation sleeve is snapped onto a two-piece wafer or belted into place around the stoma; disposable adhesive irrigation sleeves also may be used. The end of the sleeve can be closed with a clip or placed into the toilet to direct the flow of returns.

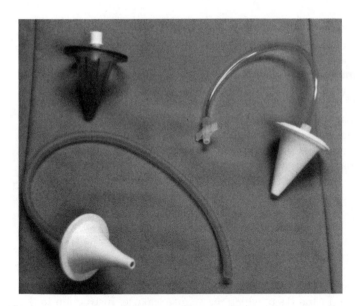

**Fig. 2-11** Cone tip for colostomy irrigation.

*TIME FRAME*

The time required for the entire irrigation procedure is usually about 1 hour: approximately 10 minutes for setup and instillation of irrigant, 30 to 40 minutes for returns, and 10 minutes for cleanup. (While waiting for returns, the individual is free to pursue other activities with the irrigation sleeve in place.)

*PROBLEM SOLVING*

The nurse instructs the patient in management of commonly encountered difficulties with irrigation and also reminds the patient that any questions can be directed to the ET nurse or physician. Commonly encountered problems include difficulty instilling the irrigant, failure of the irrigant to return, or cramping.

1. Difficulty in instillation of the irrigant usually is related to malposition of the cone tip, hard stool obstructing the cone tip, or a peristaltic wave. The patient is instructed to redirect the cone tip to make sure it is not against the bowel wall; if this does not resolve the problem, the patient should clamp the tubing, remove the cone tip, and check for hard stool obstructing the cone tip. Temporary removal of the cone tip also permits elimination of any stool in the distal bowel (if active peristalsis is the impeding factor). The patient may then resume the procedure.
2. Failure of the irrigant to return is most commonly related to inadequate fluid intake, resulting in a fluid volume deficit. (Postoperative ileus is another common cause, but this problem should be resolved before irrigations are initiated). The nurse explains to the patient that the large bowel absorbs fluid when the individual is dehydrated; the patient is instructed to wear a drainable pouch until the next irrigation and to increase oral fluid intake.
3. Cramping pain usually is due to overly rapid instillation of the irrigant or to instillation of irrigant that is too cool. The individual is instructed to instill only lukewarm fluid and to instill the fluid at a steady rate over a 5- to 10-minute period. If cramping occurs, the individual is instructed to stop the flow of irrigant until the cramping resolves.

### Specific Instruction for the Patient with a Urinary Diversion

General instruction is provided to any patient with an ostomy; in addition, the patient with a urinary diversion must be instructed in dietary and fluid modifications, use of night drainage, measures for prevention of urinary tract infection and stone formation, and measures to maintain dilute acidic urine.

**Dietary and Fluid Modifications.** In teaching the person with a urinary diversion, the nurse emphasizes the importance of fluid intake; adequate fluid intake usually is considered to be 1800 to 2400 ml per day and is the single most important factor in prevention of complications such as urinary tract infection and stone formation.[3,10] Usually no dietary modifications are required for this patient, although the patient should be informed of foods that may increase urine odor, such as asparagus, fish, and spices.

**Pouch Emptying and Use of Night Drainage.** Patients with urinary diversions are taught how to manipulate the spout on the urinary pouch and how to dry the spout after emptying; they may stand in front of the toilet or sit on the toilet to empty the pouch, whichever they prefer.

The patient with a urinary stoma is encouraged to use a night-drainage system to prevent overdistention of the pouch during sleep, which may cause leakage. Instruction in the use and maintenance of night drainage systems includes the following:

1. Use of an adapter to connect the pouch to the drainage tubing
2. Measures to stabilize the drainage tubing (e.g., running the tubing down a pajama leg or use of a catheter strap)
3. Measures to promote drainage and prevent vacuum formation (e.g., connecting the tubing to the pouch with some urine remaining in the pouch, coiling the tubing so there are no kinks, and using a night-drainage jug with a swivel top to maintain patency of the tubing)
4. Routine maintenance (emptying and rinsing the night-drainage system daily, capping the tubing when not in use to prevent contamination of tubing, and routine cleansing of the entire drainage system with a vinegar solution or a commercial cleanser)

The patient who does not wish to use a night-drainage system must be taught to waken during the night to empty the pouch.

**Prevention of Urinary Tract Infection.** Ureterostomies and small-bowel conduits are, in general, freely refluxing systems; therefore patients with urinary diversions are at risk for chronic urinary tract infections.[19] Chronic infections increase the patient's risk of calculi formation and eventual renal compromise.[3] Thus it is essential to teach the patient measures for prevention of infection and early recognition and prompt response to signs of infection. Prevention includes the following measures:

1. Adequate fluid intake. Adequate fluid intake is the single most important approach to prevention of urinary tract infections; it provides continual flushing of the urinary system, dilutes any bacteria present in the urine, and fosters an acidic pH, which inhibits bacterial growth. Patients are encouraged to drink 1800 to 2400 ml of fluid daily unless there is medical contraindication.
2. Reduction of bacterial proliferation around the stoma. Bacterial proliferation around the stoma can increase bacterial migration through the stoma and into the conduit, resulting in an ascending infection. Measures that reduce bacterial proliferation around the stoma include use of pouches with antireflux valves, regular emptying of

the pouch to prevent urinary stasis, and use of night drainage systems (or regular emptying of the pouch during the night). Thus patients are encouraged to use pouches with antireflux valves and to empty their pouches on a regular basis. Good hygiene in caring for reusable equipment and night-drainage systems also is important in reducing bacterial proliferation.

3. Elimination of urinary stasis. Urinary stasis promotes bacterial proliferation, which in turn can lead to ascending infection. Patients with urinary diversions should be monitored for urinary stasis by means of intravenous pyelograms or retrograde radiologic examinations (called "conduit-o-grams" or "loop-o-grams"), or both, on a regular basis; stasis may result from an overly long conduit, angulation of the conduit or of the ureters, or stenosis occurring at the ureteroileal junction or along the conduit. Significant stasis may require surgical correction.

Patients also must be taught the signs and symptoms of urinary tract infection: cloudy, malodorous urine; change in urine pH from acidic to alkaline; flank pain; fever; malaise; and anorexia, nausea, and vomiting. The patient is taught to report signs of infection promptly so that diagnostic studies can be performed and treatment can be initiated. The nurse stresses that early treatment of any infections helps prevent kidney damage. The nurse also should explain to the patient that a sterile urine specimen usually is needed to determine the presence of infection and the organism causing the infection; this specimen is obtained by inserting a sterile catheter through the stoma and into the conduit or ureterostomy.[10] The nurse reminds the patient that since the stoma has no nerve endings, this procedure is painless.

**Prevention of Stone Formation.** Stone formation is known to be promoted by the following factors: concentrated urine, chronic urinary tract infection, and alterations in urinary pH. Calculi are more likely to form in concentrated urine because the minerals eliminated through the urine are more likely to reach the "supersaturation" point, at which time precipitation occurs.[10] Chronic urinary tract infections with urea-splitting organisms create an alkaline urine and contribute to struvite stone formation. An alkaline urine pH also contributes to formation of stones that contain calcium, phosphate, and oxalate because these substances are more soluble in an acidic urine. In contrast, uric acid stones are more likely to form in an acidic urine because uric acid is less soluble and more prone to precipitation in an acid environment.[3,10]

*All* patients therefore must be instructed regarding the importance of adequate fluid intake and prevention or prompt treatment of urinary tract infections.

For the patient with a history of calculi formation it also is important to determine the type of stone and to implement measures to modify urine pH accordingly. For example, the patient with a history of calcium oxalate, calcium phosphate, or struvite calculi should strive to maintain an acidic urine pH, whereas the patient with uric acid stones should maintain an alkaline urine. Urine pH can be altered by medications; for example, sodium bicarbonate may be used to maintain an alkaline pH, and ascorbic acid commonly is used to help acidify the urine.[3,10] Dietary modifications also may be indicated for the patient with a history of calculi formation: the patient with calcium oxalate stones may be instructed to limit foods and fluids high in calcium and oxalate (e.g., dairy products, citrus juices, and tea), whereas the patient with uric acid calculi is instructed to limit foods high in purine (e.g., lean meats, organ meats, and whole grains).[3,10]

**Maintenance of Dilute and Acidic Urine.** As already noted, acidic urine can help prevent urinary tract infections because an acidic environment is hostile to bacterial growth.

In addition, acidic urine has less odor and is less damaging to the skin. For these reasons maintenance of acidic urine usually is encouraged for the person with a urinary diversion.

As previously discussed, urine pH may be altered by diet, fluid intake, presence or absence of infection, and medications. The urine of a healthy person with adequate fluid intake usually is acidic; average urine pH is about 6.0. On the basis of these facts, the patient with a urinary diversion is instructed to drink at least 1800 to 2400 ml of fluid per day, primarily water. Patients may be taught to monitor urine pH with nitrazine paper on a weekly or "as needed" basis. Persons who are to monitor their urine pH are taught the following guidelines. (1) The test strip should be dipped into *fresh* urine to achieve accurate results. (2) The test strip should not contact the stoma or the skin because these structures give different pH readings. (3) The test strip should be promptly compared with the color chart. (An easy way to check urine pH is to incorporate the testing into the pouch change procedure; after the clean pouch is applied, a small amount of urine is drained into a cup for testing.) Persons who are taught to monitor pH also must be taught how to interpret the results, for example, what to do if the urine pH is alkaline. The patient should know to evaluate fluid intake, increase water consumption, and be alert to other signs of infection. Any signs of infection should be reported.

The nurse must always remember that acidic urine is *contraindicated* for some patients: patients with a history of uric acid stones, patients with gout, and patients taking sulfa antibiotics or selected chemotherapeutic agents.[10,24] Therefore it is important for the nurse to review the patient's history before providing instruction in urine acidification; any questions regarding appropriate measures for the individual patient should prompt consultation with the patient's physician. finally, it is important to remember that the *most important factor* in prevention of infection and stone formation is *volume of fluid intake*.

## Specific Instruction for the Pediatric Patient with an Ostomy

Principles of growth and development and guidelines for teaching children and parents are presented in Chapter 1. Children with ostomies have unique management issues that are discussed in this section; these include management options, that is, diapering versus pouching; measures to increase pouch security; and measures to facilitate self-care by the school-aged child. The box on p. 83 summarizes special considerations for the parent of an infant with a stoma.

**Management Options.** Infants and toddlers normally are incontinent; the decision to manage by pouching as opposed to diapering is based primarily on the need for skin protection. For example, an ileostomy in the infant or toddler must be managed by pouching because the output is enzymatic and can rapidly cause severe skin breakdown. Care of the infant with a colostomy is also commonly managed with pouching, particularly when the colostomy is of high output.

Care of the infant with a colostomy can also be managed with skin protection and diapers. This option is chosen when it is either preferred by the parents or easier to maintain, that is, when the stoma is difficult to pouch. Occasionally, skin protection is the preferred option for a premature neonate who has an ileostomy but has not yet begun oral feedings. During this interim, pouching may not be desirable because of the infant's small size (typically less than 2 kg), immature skin, limited pouching surface, and minimal stool production. Pouching must be instituted once stool volume increases. Table 2-6 presents characteristics of the preterm infant's skin and nursing implications to be considered in ostomy management.

## SPECIAL CONSIDERATIONS WHEN CARING FOR THE INFANT WITH A STOMA

1. Use one-piece outfits so that the pouch is accessible for easy emptying and to prevent inadvertent dislodging of the pouch as the infant begins to explore body parts.
2. Encourage parents to instruct the grandparents and a babysitter in pouch change and emptying procedures so that the parents can resume a normal life-style and "go out" periodically.
3. Encourage parents to treat the infant as normally as possible; the presence of the stoma does not delay the infant's physical or cognitive development.
4. Encourage parents to discuss the infant's dietary advancement and immunization schedule with their pediatrician.
5. Use an electrolyte solution such as Pedialyte to supplement fluid-electrolyte intake if needed (instead of diluted Jello, for example).
6. Reassure parents that the stoma may discolor temporarily (white or purple) when infant is crying; normal color returns when infant stops crying.

**Table 2-6**   Characteristics of preterm infant's skin

| Characteristic | Consequence | Nursing implication |
|---|---|---|
| Skin more permeable | Increased absorption through skin | Minimize use of skin products containing chemicals that may be absorbed through the skin |
| Greater ratio of surface area to body weight | Chemicals contained in skin-care products can be absorbed systemically through the skin at higher than desired doses | Minimize use of skin-care products such as skin sealants and adhesives because of potential absorption through the skin |
| Diminished cohesion between epidermis and dermis | Epidermis can be easily traumatized | Minimize use of tapes or adhesives on skin; consider and evaluate appropriateness of using skin sealants and solvents on the skin; use solid-wafer skin barrier under tapes; peel adhesives away slowly and gently |
| Decreased thickness of stratum corneum | Stratum corneum only partially effective as a barrier and is easily damaged | Monitor skin for erythema or denudement, and reduce or eliminate causative factors; avoid use of harsh soaps or chemicals on skin; dab skin gently: do not rub or use a rough cloth |

NOTE: As the infant's gestational age increases, the preterm infant's skin becomes more similar to adult skin. For example, the skin of the infant born 2 months prematurely should become more characteristic of the newborn's skin by 2 months of age.

Modified from Kuller JM: Skin development and function. I. *Neonatal Network* 3:18, 1984, and Boarini JH: Principles of stoma care for infants, *J Enterostom Ther* 16(1):21, 1989.

For the infant whose care is managed with diapers, skin protection can be provided through use of sealants, skin barrier wafers or washers, or ointments. Parents and nurses must be aware that this management option is appropriate as long as peristomal skin integrity is maintained. If the peristomal skin becomes consistently denuded, however, pouching must be instituted.

Care of the infant with a urinary diversion usually is managed by diapering; pouching is indicated only if this is the parents' preference, if the skin is damaged, or when fecal contamination causes urinary tract infections. Pouching also may be required on an "as needed" basis for the toddler with a vesicostomy or ureterostomy, for example, to allow the child to swim without risk of urinary tract infection or to contain the urine during operative procedures.

**Measures to Increase Pouch Security.** The infant or toddler with an ostomy may require clothing alterations to promote pouch security and to reduce the frequency of pouch changes. As children begin to explore their bodies, they may, out of curiosity, inadvertently pull the pouch off; parents are encouraged to use one-piece sleepers and playsuits to avoid such inconveniences.[7]

As the infant becomes more active, the parent may find a two-piece pouching system to be preferable. To empty the pouch the parent needs only to snap off the soiled pouch and snap on a clean pouch; the infant does not have to lie quietly while the pouch is emptied. Once the infant is redressed and content, the parent can empty the pouch and clean it for repeat use. The box below lists pouching tips for the infant with a stoma.

**Measures to Facilitate Self-Care.** The school-aged child may require modifications in the pouching system to promote independence; for example, the child may find it easier to change a closed-end pouch than to manipulate the clip and empty a drainable pouch. The child also may require assistance in obtaining support for ostomy care at school; it may be

---

### POUCHING TIPS FOR CARE OF THE INFANT WITH A STOMA

1. Encourage that the pouch change procedure be a planned event with two people and the baby. One person is in charge of changing the pouch; the other person is responsible for entertaining the infant.
2. Change the pouch at a planned, convenient time; do not wait for the pouch to leak at a less than optimal time. Try to use the infant's usual quiet time.
3. Assemble all pouching equipment before changing the pouch, and place items within easy reach.
4. Empty the pouch off to the infant's side into a second diaper or into a container.
5. When the infant becomes more active (around 3 months of age), it may be convenient to use a two-piece pouch to facilate pouch emptying. In this way the pouch can be snapped off, a clean pouch snapped on, and the infant redressed. After the infant is redressed, the soiled pouch can be rinsed out and is reused later.
6. Use a gas filter to vent the pouch; infants produce considerable flatus as a result of the air swallowed while sucking.

necessary for the physician or ET nurse to write a letter explaining the child's ostomy, the child's need to go to the bathroom as needed, and the child's need for privacy when emptying or changing the pouch.[7] In some situations the ET nurse or the child's primary nurse can make a visit to the school to familiarize the teachers with the child's needs. The school nurse is a valuable resource and should be included in the education process.

## Teaching and Counseling for Resumption of Life-Style

The initial focus in patient teaching is on self-care skills and daily management issues such as dietary alterations; once these basic skills are mastered, the focus shifts to ways in which to incorporate the ostomy into the person's life-style. Common concerns include bathing; clothing; management of the ostomy at work; management of the ostomy during exercise, recreational activities, and travel; management of the ostomy during sexual activity; and disclosure issues.

**Bathing.** The nurse explains that the patient may take a tub bath or shower with the pouch on or off. The patient is encouraged to bathe with the pouch on unless it is time to change the pouch; routinely bathing with the pouch off may result in inadvertent removal of the skin barrier paste or washing of the skin barrier wafer or ring, which in turn contributes to premature disruption of the pouch seal. The patient may choose to "picture-frame" the edges of the pouch with waterproof tape to increase the resistance; the alternative is to pat the taped edges dry or to dry them with a hair dryer.

**Clothing.** The nurse encourages the patient to wear snug undergarments, with the pouch inside the undergarment; the nurse also informs the patient of the availability of pouch covers, soft cloth covers that protect the skin from the plastic of the pouch and also serve to conceal the pouch contents. For the patient with a flush or slightly protruding stoma located in the lower abdominal quadrants these measures usually are sufficient to conceal the stoma, and these patients may continue to wear their preoperative clothing. Clothing modifications usually are minimal for these patients; for example, the patient may wear slacks or skirts that have front pleats or are a little looser than normal. Women are instructed that panty hose are permissible, as are stretch panty girdles; regular girdles also may be worn provided that the stays do not cross the stoma. Bathing suits are available that effectively conceal the stoma; women are counseled to look for patterned suits with front shirring or draping. Patients also should be aware of specialty underclothing designed for the person with an ostomy (e.g., Options, Chicago, Ill.).

The patient with a large or protruding stoma and the patient with a stoma located in the upper quadrants of the abdomen may need to significantly modify clothing choices. These modifications are discussed in the section, Specific Instructions for the Patient with a Transverse Colostomy.

**Management of the Ostomy at Work.** The patient is counseled to keep an "emergency kit" available at all times (at work, when traveling, and the like); this kit should contain all supplies needed for an emergency pouch change. The nurse also helps the patient to solve problems regarding emptying the pouch in public restrooms; helpful hints include use of a room deodorizer and placement of toilet paper in the commode before emptying to prevent splashing. If the patient's occupation involves rigorous activity or heavy lifting, the physician must be consulted regarding any restrictions.

**Management of the Ostomy During Exercise and Recreational Activities.** The nurse explores with the patient usual activities and any modifications necessitated by the ostomy. For example, the patient who engages in vigorous exercise may benefit from use of a belt or binder to secure and support the pouch; the patient who enjoys water sports should be counseled to use pouches without fabric backing and may wish to reinforce the pouch edges with waterproof tape; the patient who enjoys backpacking may need information regarding commercial wipes that can be used as alternatives to water for cleansing the stoma and peristomal skin.

**Management of the Ostomy During Travel.** In discussing travel for the person with an ostomy, there are two areas of concern. The first is ostomy supplies. In determining the amount of supplies needed, the patient is counseled to take enough pouching supplies to last the entire trip and to factor in unexpected pouch changes, that is, to take enough additional supplies to cover problems with pouch failure, seal disruption, or, in the patient with a fecal diversion, diarrhea. It is important to instruct patients to keep their supplies with them at all times; ostomy supplies should not be packed in luggage that is to be "checked" and should not be kept in areas of extreme heat or cold. Finally, patients are advised to contact the ET nurse or the company that manufactures their ostomy supplies to obtain information regarding supply sources at their travel destination.

The second area of concern is the potential for gastroenteritis caused by food or water consumption in another country; this is of particular concern to the person with a fecal diversion. Patients are counseled to drink bottled water if there is any doubt as to the safety of the water; the person with a colostomy managed by routine irrigation should also use bottled water for irrigation.

**Management of the Ostomy During Sexual Activity.** The nurse counsels the patient to empty the pouch and to check the pouch seal before engaging in sexual activity. The nurse also may suggest options for securing or concealing the ostomy pouch, as described in Chapter 1. Finally, the nurse encourages the patient and partner to be open in discussing feelings and concerns regarding the ostomy and to accept negative feelings as a normal part of the adaptation process.

**Disclosure Issues.** One issue confronting the ostomy patient is "whom to tell, how to tell, when to tell" about the ostomy. The nurse may help patients deal with these issues by assisting them to identify their priorities and concerns, as well as by role-playing various approaches to disclosure.

**Support Groups.** The nurse should inform the patient of the availability of support groups and should provide contact information. Support groups that may be beneficial to the person with an ostomy include the United Ostomy Association (UOA), the Crohn's and Colitis Foundation of America (CCFA), various cancer support groups (e.g., Can Surmount and I Can Cope), ileoanal reservoir support groups, and parents' support groups.[14]

## DISCHARGE PLANNING

Discharge planning is a critical concern for the patient with an ostomy. As length of stay after ostomy surgery has declined, the time available for teaching and counseling also has declined. In today's environment the teaching focus during the postoperative phase must be

---

**RECOMMENDED FREQUENCY OF OUTPATIENT FOLLOW-UP AFTER OSTOMY SURGERY**

| | |
|---|---|
| Two weeks after discharge from hospital | Six months later (1 year after surgery) |
| Four weeks later (6 weeks out of hospital) | Yearly and for problems as needed |
| Six weeks later (3 months out of hospital) | |
| Three months later (6 months out of hospital) | |

---

**DISCHARGE CHECKLIST FOR THE OSTOMY PATIENT**

| | |
|---|---|
| Written pouch-change instructions (procedure and frequency of change) | Referral to support groups as indicated (UOA, CCFA, and the like) |
| Patient teaching booklet | Follow-up outpatient appointment with ET nurse |
| List of pouching equipment (product names and numbers) | Follow-up outpatient appointment with surgeon |
| List of ostomy equipment retailers (including telephone numbers) | Work telephone number for ET nurse |
| Referral to home-care nurse | |

---

on survival skills, that is, pouch emptying and pouch change procedures. Much additional teaching and counseling are required to support integration of the ostomy into the patient's life-style.[15,17] Thus all patients should have access to outpatient follow-up on a regular basis. A suggested regimen for outpatient follow-up is given in the box above, *top*.

In addition to outpatient follow-up, many patients need home health care after discharge; the home-care nurse can provide reinforcement and support for self-care, as well as additional instruction regarding ostomy management and counseling regarding psychosocial issues.[15,17] The nurse providing instruction should evaluate the ostomy patient's potential need for home-care follow-up and should initiate or contribute to the referral. Clear documentation regarding care and teaching provided in the acute care facility is essential, as is a current care plan for ostomy management. It frequently is beneficial for the ET nurse or nurse providing ostomy care to contact the home-care nurse and provide the nurse with additional information regarding the patient's care.

The box above, *bottom*, provides a sample discharge checklist for the patient with an ostomy.

## LONG-TERM FOLLOW-UP

The person with an ostomy should receive follow-up care on a long-term basis in an outpatient setting. Major concerns in outpatient follow-up include rehabilitation issues, supply information, and detection and management of complications.

## Rehabilitation Issues

The nurse should never assume that a patient is "comfortable" with the ostomy simply because he or she has had it for a period of time and is independent in self-care. Even if the patient has been "rehabilitated" and "well-adjusted," changes in life status may change his or her feelings about the ostomy. For example, the patient who goes through a divorce and is again single may suffer new fears and anxieties regarding acceptance by a sexual partner and may need to deal with disclosure issues once again.

## Technical Care Issues

As noted earlier, patients' pouching needs frequently change over time, as their abdominal contours, degree of stomal protrusion, and activity levels change; weight gain, weight loss, and pregnancy are common causes of changing abdominal contours. In addition, new products are constantly being developed. One reason for outpatient follow-up is to keep patients up-to-date regarding their options and to provide ongoing problem-solving for any pouching difficulties.

## Detection and Management of Complications

Common stomal and peristomal complications are discussed in Chapter 3; the ET nurse, must be alert to signs of these complications when providing outpatient follow-up. Issues and complications specific to various diversions are discussed in this section, along with appropriate nursing intervention.

## Fecal Diversions: Intact Distal Bowel Segment

As discussed earlier in this chapter, ostomies can be constructed as end, loop, or double-barrel stomas; end stomas may be constructed in conjunction with removal of the distal bowel, or the distal bowel may be oversewn and left in place (Hartmann's pouch). When the distal bowel segment remains intact, as occurs with a loop stoma, a double-barrel stoma, or an end stoma with Hartmann's pouch, the patient must be prepared for temporary output of stool per rectum once peristalsis returns. The nurse also explains that the distal bowel continues to produce mucus and that the patient periodically may feel rectal fullness and the need to expel the accumulated mucus.[26] Patients who sense rectal distention but are unable to expel the mucus may benefit from a low-volume rectal enema to flush out the mucus.

The patient who has a double-barrel ostomy must be taught how to manage the nonfunctioning mucous fistula stoma. If the distal mucous fistula stoma is immediately adjacent to the proximal functioning stoma, it should be included in the pouch. If the nonfunctioning stoma is located at a distance from the proximal stoma, it can be managed with a light dressing that the patient changes daily or as needed, or with a stoma cap or cover.

## Ileostomy: Food Blockage

As stated earlier, the patient with an ileostomy is at risk for food blockage. The ET nurse must be prepared to provide ileostomy lavage when the patient with an ileostomy develops a food blockage unresponsive to conservative management (e.g., peristomal massage or a warm bath). The purpose of ileostomy lavage is to gradually dislodge the fibrous mass by repetitive saline irrigations[2] (see the box on p. 89 for the suggested procedure). In performing ileostomy lavage, the nurse must be aware that the obstruction may be caused by factors other than a food blockage, for example, adhesions or a volvulus producing a small-

---

**ILEOSTOMY LAVAGE***

1. Gather supplies.
2. Explain procedure to patient, and provide for privacy and comfort.
3. Remove pouch and attach disposable adhesive irrigation sleeve. Close bottom of irrigation sleeve with tail closure, rubber band, or binder clip, *or* place bottom of sleeve in toilet or bedpan.
4. Perform gentle digital examination to determine the direction of the bowel and to break up any fibrous mass just proximal to stoma.
5. Lubricate a No. 14F or No. 16F catheter, and insert until blockage is reached.
   NOTE: If catheter can be inserted to a depth of 8 to 10 cm without reaching blockage, notify physician; this

situation usually indicates a more proximal obstruction resulting from adhesion formation, volvulus, or the like.
6. Instill 30 to 50 ml normal saline solution.
7. Remove catheter and wait for returns.
8. Repeat steps 5 through 7 until mass is removed. Then advance catheter to check for proximal blockage; perform additional irrigations as indicated.
9. When blockage is resolved, remove irrigation sleeve.
10. Clean peristomal skin and apply pouch.
11. Document procedure, patient tolerance, amount of solution instilled, and volume and consistency of returns.

*Universal precautions* must be followed when this procedure is performed.

---

bowel obstruction.[11] (Food blockage usually occurs at fascial level and frequently can be identified by digital examination[2]; the ability to insert the catheter further than 8 to 10 cm without difficulty usually indicates a more proximal obstruction, which probably is caused by factors other than a food blockage.) The nurse also must be alert to signs and symptoms of fluid-electrolyte imbalance, which commonly occurs with food blockage (as a result of high-volume fluid output or vomiting); the patient with fluid-electrolyte imbalance usually requires intravenous replacement. Finally, the nurse must be aware that food blockage requires dietary reevaluation and a review of the patient's understanding of preventive measures.

## Colostomy: Fecal Impaction

Constipation may develop in the patient with a descending or sigmoid colostomy; if uncorrected, this condition can progress to impaction. Mild to moderate constipation can be managed by increasing fluids and fiber, administering a mild laxative, or performing a colostomy irrigation. If the patient's history suggests a fecal impaction, that is, the patient has had no stool or only liquid stool for several days associated with abdominal distention and cramping pain, a digital examination should be performed to confirm the impaction.

Guidelines for disimpaction parallel those for rectal disimpaction and can be summarized as follows:

1. Digital breakup is attempted; if successful, breakup is followed by a cleansing irrigation. When attempting digital breakup, it is helpful to place one hand against the

abdominal wall under the stoma to stabilize the bowel; the other hand is then used to digitalize the stoma and to attempt breakup of the fecal mass by pressing the stool between the examining finger and the supporting hand.

2. If digital breakup is unsuccessful, a retention irrigation may be given. In administering retention irrigations the nurse must remember that the intent is to instill an emulsifying solution against the fecal mass, not to stimulate peristalsis. Thus retention irrigations are low in volume, usually 100 to 200 ml, and are given slowly; the cone tip or other antibackflow device may be held in place for a brief period after instillation to discourage premature evacuation of the solution. Solutions used vary according to institution protocols and practitioner preference; commonly used solutions include oil preparations[13] and stool softener solutions (e.g., docusate sodium sulfosuccinate and water). The solution should be left in the colon for several hours, and digital breakup is again attempted.

Once the impaction is broken up, a cleansing irrigation is performed, and the patient also may be given a laxative. Laxatives should *not* be given until the impaction has been at least partially resolved; in the presence of partial or complete bowel obstruction, laxatives can cause severe cramping pain. Repetitive instillation of small volumes of solutions that dissolve stool (e.g., milk and molasses) sometimes is used to eliminate resistant fecal impactions. Once the impaction is resolved, the nurse teaches the patient or caregiver appropriate measures for prevention of constipation and impaction.

## Loss of Bowel Regulation with Irrigation

Loss of bowel control may develop in the patient with a descending or sigmoid colostomy who is using routine irrigation as a management approach. Specifically, the patient may state that returns take longer and are less complete than usual and that spillage between irrigations occurs more frequently. In managing this problem, the nurse must perform a careful assessment of factors that affect peristaltic activity and peristaltic response to irrigation, such as changing activity levels, reduced amounts of dietary bulk, and the aging process itself.

Management involves correction of causative factors and incorporation of the following measures, which are known to increase peristalsis:

1. Increased bulk, either through dietary changes or the addition of a bulk laxative, and increased activity levels
2. Increased mechanical stretch of the bowel during the irrigation procedure, either by increasing the volume of irrigant by 100 to 200 ml or by correction of faulty irrigating technique (e.g., replacing a catheter tip that allows backflow with a cone tip that prevents backflow, as well as teaching the patient to hold the cone tip securely against the stoma)
3. Addition of a mild peristaltic stimulant such as casanthranol with administration timed so that maximum effect occurs at the time of irrigation (e.g., administration at bedtime for increased peristalsis during an early morning irrigation).

If these measures do not restore normal bowel function and control, the patient may be counseled to discontinue irrigations and to manage the colostomy with continuous pouching. The patient who has been irrigating for a number of years may have a dependent bowel and may need to take a bulk laxative or a mild peristaltic stimulant on a routine basis to prevent constipation and impaction.

## Colostomy: Bowel Preparation

The individual with a colostomy may require a bowel preparation before diagnostic studies or intestinal surgery. The following principles should guide the nurse in providing an appropriate preparation:

1. If the distal bowel is intact, as is true with a loop colostomy, a double-barrel colostomy, or a colostomy with Hartmann's pouch, the nurse first must determine whether the preparation is for the proximal bowel, the distal bowel, or both bowel segments. The proximal bowel can be cleansed by use of liquid diets, oral laxatives, and colostomy irrigations; the distal segment must be cleansed by rectal enemas or, in the case of a loop or double-barrel colostomy, by an irrigation through the distal stoma or the distal limb of a loop colostomy. (Returns from an irrigation of the distal bowel segment should be from the rectum.) If a rectal enema is administered to a patient with a Hartmann's pouch, the nurse must base the volume of solution administered on the length of the retained distal segment. For example, the patient with a Hartmann's pouch involving only the rectosigmoid colon should receive a low-volume enema to prevent perforation.

2. Standard bowel preparation procedures can be used for the person with a colostomy, with only minor modifications: oral agents can be given as prescribed, irrigations are substituted for enemas designed to prepare the proximal bowel, and suppositories usually are omitted (because they are likely to be expelled before they have completely dissolved, thus likely to be ineffective). Suppositories are most beneficial when administered rectally to prepare the distal bowel segment.

3. To prevent fluid-electrolyte imbalance, repetitive irrigations should be performed with saline solution rather than tap water.

4. To determine an appropriate preparatory course for an individual patient, the nurse must consider the reason for the bowel preparation, the usual consistency and volume of the stool, and the length and function of the proximal bowel.

## Urinary Diversion: Stomal Catheterization

Stomal catheterization is indicated when a sterile specimen is needed, for example, in the diagnosis of urinary tract infection; occasionally catheterization is used to determine the volume of residual urine in the conduit.

In obtaining a urine specimen for culture, the goal is to accurately reflect bacterial colony counts in the kidneys and the conduit.[29] Thus the nurse must incorporate measures to prevent a false-positive or a false-negative test result. Specific guidelines for stomal catheterization include the following:

1. The nurse explains the procedure and rationale to the patient and clarifies that the procedure is not painful. The urinary pouch is removed.

2. After handwashing, the nurse dons sterile gloves and sets up the sterile field.

3. The stoma is "prepped" with three swabs or cotton balls soaked in an antiseptic solution (e.g., povidone-iodine); each swab is used to deliver one cleansing stroke directly across the stoma. An adequate preparation helps reduce the risk of a false-positive test result, that is, a bacterial colony count indicative of infection that results from contamination of the specimen by surface organisms. An adequate preparation also reduces the risk of introducing bacteria into the conduit during the catheterization procedure, which could *cause* infection.

4. The preparation solution is removed by wiping the stoma with sterile gauze or cotton balls, by rinsing the stoma with sterile saline, or by allowing urine to run over the stoma. Failure to remove the preparation solution may result in a false-negative test result, that is, a bacterial colony count indicating the absence of infection that results because the preparation solution eradicated the organisms in the specimen.

5. The catheter is lubricated and inserted gently into the stoma to just below fascial level. The drainage end of the catheter is placed into a sterile container and held below the level of the conduit to facilitate drainage. Because the conduit does not serve as a reservoir, it frequently is necessary to wait for urine to drain into the sterile container. Urinary elimination sometimes can be stimulated by measures that increase intraabdominal pressure (e.g., having the patient cough or laugh) or measures that enhance gravity drainage (e.g., having the patient turn to the side).

Catheterization may be performed with either a single-lumen or a double-lumen catheter. The single-lumen catheter is a standard straight catheter; the double-lumen catheter has a fenestrated latex sheath that covers the catheter. The double-lumen catheter is inserted through the stoma into the conduit lumen to just past fascial level with the latex sheath intact; the inner catheter is then advanced through the latex sheath, and the urine specimen is collected. On a theoretic basis, the double-lumen catheter reduces the potential for false-positive or false-negative test results because the collection catheter does not contact the stoma. Limited studies seem to support this hypothesis, although there have been no reports of controlled and conclusive studies.[29]

Modifications in the aforementioned technique are required when ureteral stents are in place and for the patient with a ureterostomy. To obtain a sterile specimen from ureteral stents, the nurse should prepare the ends of the stents, allow urine to drip from the stents to flush away the preparation solution, then collect a drip specimen in a sterile container. (Before beginning the procedure, the nurse dons sterile gloves and sets up a sterile field. In obtaining a catheterized specimen from a ureterostomy, the nurse may need to use a sterile 5F or 8F catheter or feeding tube; stomal preparation and the catheterization procedure are performed as described for a conduit catheterization.

### Urinary Diversion: Peristomal Skin Damage Resulting from Prolonged Exposure to Urine

As noted earlier in this chapter, urine contains no enzymes and is not inherently harmful to the skin; however, prolonged exposure, as occurs when urine is allowed to pool on the skin, may cause maceration, "hyperplasia" of the involved epidermis, and encrustation, that is, accumulation of mineral deposits on the stoma and peristomal skin[13] (see Plate 6). Alkaline urine is particularly damaging to the skin, which normally is acidic in pH.

The first step in correcting the skin problem is to identify and eliminate the causative factors, including factors that make the urine more damaging to the skin (e.g., alkalinity, increased urine concentration, or urinary tract infection) and factors that increase exposure of the peristomal skin to urine (e.g., barrier meltdown, incorrect sizing of the pouch or barrier opening, use of a pouch without an antireflux valve, or an ineffective pouching system that results in frequent leakage).

The nurse educates the patient or caregiver, or both, regarding the causes of the skin damage and appropriate preventive measures: adequate fluid intake, prompt treatment of any infection, sizing of the barrier opening to minimize exposed skin, use of a pouch with an antireflux valve, and problem-solving regarding any pouching problems.

# COLOSTOMY TEACHING RECORD

| | | | Materials given: | | | | | | |
|---|---|---|---|---|---|---|---|---|---|
| | | | Pertinent data: | | | | | | |

Assessment guidelines code:
1. Needs complete Instruction
2. Needs further Instruction
3. Needs reinforcement
4. Comprehends
5. NA (not applicable)

| | OBJECTIVES | Assessment code | Instructions (date and initial) | | | | | PROGRESS |
|---|---|---|---|---|---|---|---|---|
| | | | 1st | 2nd | 3rd | Family | Complete | |
| **AFFECTIVE** | 1. Verbalizes feelings about disease process and surgery | | | | | | | |
| | 2. Verbalizes feelings about colostomy | | | | | | | |
| **COGNITIVE** | 3. Explains how bowel function has changed | | | | | | | |
| | 4. Explains three methods of colostomy management | | | | | | | |
| | 5. Explains one method for preventing and managing gas | | | | | | | |
| | 6. Explains one method for preventing and managing odor | | | | | | | |
| | 7. Explains one method for preventing and managing skin irritation | | | | | | | |
| | 8. Explains one method for preventing and managing diarrhea | | | | | | | |
| | 9. Explains two possible causes of constipation | | | | | | | |
| | 10. Discussion of method for cleaning irrigation equipment | | | | | | | |
| | 11. Identifies when ET nurse or physician should be called | | | | | | | |
| | 12. States type of equipment being used and where it can be purchased | | | | | | | |
| | 13. States community resources available | | | | | | | |
| **PSYCHOMOTOR** | 14. Demonstration of how to empty pouch | | | | | | | |
| | 15. Demonstration of how to clean peristo-mal skin | | | | | | | |
| | 16. Demonstration of how to perform colostomy irrigation | | | | | | | |
| | 17. Demonstration of how to apply pouch | | | | | | | |

**Fig. 2-12** Sample flowsheet for patient teaching documentation. (From Bishop Clarkson Memorial Hospital, Omaha, Nebr.)

The second focus in management of urine-induced skin damage is eliminating urine contact with the skin. The patient's pouching system is modified as indicated to provide a secure seal and to minimize urine contact with the skin. Specific measures that may be used include use of skin barrier powders and sealants to provide a dry pouching surface, addition of a urine-resistant barrier or adhesive, or both, to the pouching system, and addition of convexity and support devices to improve the pouch seal.

Stomal encrustations may be treated with vinegar soaks applied to the stoma at each pouch change; if the patient is wearing a two-piece system, the pouch may be removed and vinegar soaks may be applied to the stoma at regular intervals (e.g., three to four times a day).[10] Vinegar soaks are beneficial because the acetic acid dissolves the encrustations resulting from alkaline urine. It is important to caution the patient that the vinegar may temporarily cause the stoma to blanch and that this does not indicate any damage to the stoma.

## SUMMARY

Nursing care of the patient with an ostomy should be consistently focused on supporting the adaptation process. Nursing interventions include development of an appropriate and secure pouching system, instruction in self-care and ostomy management, and counseling to support positive integration of the ostomy into the patient's self-concept and lifestyle. The nurse providing ostomy care must be knowledgeable regarding ostomy management, astute in assessing patients' physical and psychologic status, and skilled in the areas of technical care, patient teaching, and counseling. Fig. 2-12 provides a sample flowsheet for patient teaching documentation, which can be initiated at the preoperative outpatient visit, used throughout the hospital stay, and continued in the outpatient follow-up clinic. Nursing management does not end with the patient's discharge from the hospital but should be available for as long as the patient has the ostomy.

# SELF-EVALUATION

## QUESTIONS

1. Which of the following is a normal occurrence during the first 48 to 72 hours after surgery for construction of a stoma?
   a. Mucocutaneous separation
   b. Stomal ischemia
   c. Ileus
   d. Anastomotic breakdown

2. Which of the following patients is most likely to require lifelong vitamin $B_{12}$ replacement?
   a. Patient who has had total colectomy
   b. Patient with a permanent ileostomy
   c. Patient who has had the terminal ileum resected or bypassed
   d. Patient who has an ileal conduit

3. Identify common causes of stomal necrosis and appropriate nursing response.

4. Describe one approach to management of mucocutaneous separation.

5. Identify factors to be included in postoperative assessment of the stoma and peristomal skin.

6. Describe normal output for each of the following diversions:
   a. Ureterostomy or vesicostomy
   b. Intestinal conduit
   c. Ileostomy
   d. Transverse colostomy
   e. Descending or sigmoid colostomy

7. Skin sealants are effective for which of the following?
   a. To protect the skin from enzymatic drainage
   b. To provide a moisture barrier and protection against epidermal "stripping" with adhesive removal
   c. To increase the adhesion between the skin and the adhesive pouch surface
   d. All of the above

8. Identify the three major forms of skin barriers and appropriate uses for each form.

9. Identify factors to be considered in selecting a pouching system.

10. Explain the benefit of antireflux valves in urinary pouches.

11. Which of the following patients is a candidate for a closed-end pouch?
    a. Patient with an ileostomy
    b. Patient with a sigmoid colostomy
    c. Patient with an ileal conduit
    d. Patient with a transverse colostomy

12. Identify at least one advantage of using reusable pouching systems.

13. The nurse should wait until stoma shrinkage is complete to order reusable equipment. Stoma shrinkage usually is complete by:
    a. 7 to 10 days after surgery
    b. 6 to 8 weeks after surgery
    c. 3 to 6 months after surgery
    d. 1 year after surgery

14. Which of the following is *most likely* to provide an effective seal for the patient with a retracted stoma?
   a. All-flexible pouching system
   b. Rigid pouching system
   c. Convex pouching system
   d. Any pouch used with a belt

15. Which of the following diversions produces the most damaging effluent and therefore requires the most peristomal skin protection?
   a. Ileostomy
   b. Ileal conduit
   c. Transverse colostomy
   d. Sigmoid colostomy

16. Removal of peristomal hair generally is recommended to prevent folliculitis.
   a. True
   b. False

17. Loop stomas initially are stabilized on the abdominal surface by either a fascial bridge or an external support. The purpose of this support is:
   a. To prevent stomal retraction
   b. To prevent stomal obstruction
   c. To prevent stomal prolapse
   d. To prevent peristomal hernia formation

18. Use of skin barriers is *optional* in pouching a urinary diversion because urine is not inherently damaging to the skin.
   a. True
   b. False

19. Identify key content to be included in the teaching plan for each of the following patients:
   a. Patient with an ileostomy
   b. Patient with a transverse colostomy
   c. Patient with a descending or sigmoid colostomy
   d. Patient with an ileal conduit

20. In teaching the patient with a new ostomy, which of the following represents "critical content," that is, content that must be taught before discharge?
   a. Dietary and fluid modifications
   b. Explanation of surgical procedure and rationale
   c. Pouch emptying and pouch change procedures
   d. Adaptation and sexual issues

21. Describe one approach for management of minor peristomal skin irritation that patients may be taught.

22. The lag time between ingestion of gas-forming foods and actual flatulence in the patient with a colostomy usually is:
   a. 1 to 2 hours
   b. 6 to 8 hours
   c. 8 to 12 hours
   d. 12 to 24 hours

23. Identify common gas-forming foods that the patient with a fecal diversion may wish to avoid or to eat selectively.
24. Describe measures the patient with a fecal diversion can use for odor control.
25. The individual with a fecal diversion is just as susceptible to episodes of diarrhea as is the person with an intact bowel.
    a. True
    b. False
26. Which of the following patients is at greatest risk for fluid-electrolyte imbalance during episodes of diarrhea?
    a. Patient with an ileostomy
    b. Patient with a transverse colostomy
    c. Patient with a descending colostomy
    d. Patient with a jejunostomy
27. Identify at least three replacement fluids that the patient with a fecal diversion can drink to help prevent fluid-electrolyte imbalance during periods of increased fluid loss.
28. List three measures that the patient with an ileostomy should be taught to prevent food blockage.
29. Identify criteria for use of routine colostomy irrigation as a method of management.
30. Colostomy irrigation is *contraindicated* for which of the following patients?
    a. Patient with a descending colostomy
    b. Patient with a peristomal fungal rash
    c. Patient receiving pelvic radiation
    d. Patient with a retracted stoma
31. You are performing the initial colostomy irrigation for Grace Hester 7 days after abdominoperineal resection and sigmoid colostomy. She suddenly complains of feeling faint and hot, and then she becomes unresponsive. This condition *most* likely is due to:
    a. Hysterical reaction to first irrigation
    b. Fluid-electrolyte imbalance resulting from irrigation
    c. Early bowel obstruction
    d. Vasovagal reaction
32. Mrs. Jones calls the outpatient clinic to report that the water she used to irrigate her colostomy has not returned. In talking with Mrs. Jones, the nurse should be aware that failure of irrigating solution to return *most* commonly is due to:
    a. Fluid volume deficit
    b. Fecal impaction
    c. Intestinal obstruction
    d. Peritonitis
33. The care of infants and toddlers with ostomies frequently is managed by diapering instead of pouching. Identify at least one contraindication to management by diapering.
34. The patient with a double-barrel or loop colostomy may periodically experience rectal fullness as a result of mucus accumulation.
    a. True
    b. False

35. John Williams is a 26-year old man with an ileostomy. He calls the ET outpatient clinic and states, "I think I have a food blockage." Questioning reveals that John is having no output, has stomal swelling and abdominal distention, and is having nausea, vomiting, and cramping pain. Which of the following is an *inappropriate* recommendation for John at this time?
   a. Try sitting in a warm tub of water
   b. Try peristomal massage
   c. Force fluids to prevent fluid-electrolyte imbalance
   d. Change your pouch to one with a larger stomal opening
36. Home relief measures are ineffective in relieving John's obstruction, and he comes to the outpatient clinic for evaluation and management. Which of the following represents appropriate management?
   a. Repetitive lavage with 30 to 50 ml normal saline
   b. Administration of laxative such as magnesium citrate
   c. Ileostomy irrigation with 1000 ml tap water
   d. Manual disimpaction
37. List at least two factors that may contribute to loss of bowel regulation in the patient who has managed his or her colostomy with routine irrigations.
38. You are asked to recommend an appropriate bowel preparation for the patient with a descending colostomy and Hartmann's pouch who is to have a proctoscopic examination of the rectum. Which of the following is the most appropriate recommendation?
   a. Oral laxatives followed by cleansing enema
   b. Oral laxatives followed by colostomy irrigations until clear
   c. Colostomy irrigations for both proximal and distal bowel until returns are clear
   d. Low-volume rectal enema
39. To obtain a urine specimen for culture and sensitivity testing from a patient with a urinary diversion, the nurse should:
   a. Apply a sterile pouch and collect freshly drained urine
   b. Cleanse the spout of the pouch before collecting the specimen
   c. Clean the stoma and catch a "drip" specimen from the stoma
   d. Catheterize the stoma using sterile technique
40. Urine acidification is contraindicated for which of the following patients?
   a. Patient with a history of calcium oxalate stones
   b. Patient with a history of struvite stones
   c. Patient with a history of uric acid stones

112566

# SELF-EVALUATION

## ANSWERS

1. **c.** Ileus
2. **c.** Patient who has had the terminal ileum resected or bypassed
3. Common causes of stomal necrosis include:

    Excessive dissection of the mesentery

    Traction on the mesentery

    Edema of the bowel wall

    Nursing response includes frequent assessment of the extent of necrosis and prompt physician notification for necrosis extending to the fascial level. The extent of necrosis can be assessed by inserting a well-lubricated, clear test tube into the stoma and directing the beam of a flashlight down through the test tube to illuminate the mucosa of the proximal bowel.
4. Management of mucocutaneous separation:

    Flush the separated area thoroughly with normal saline.

    Lightly pack the area of separation with an absorptive agent (e.g., hydroactive granules or powder or skin barrier powder).

    Cover the absorptive agent with skin barrier paste, SteriStrips, or microporous tape to provide a pouching surface.

    Size the pouch opening to fit closely around the stoma.

    Apply a thin layer of skin barrier paste directly around the stoma to prevent migration of stool under the pouch surface.

    Center the pouch and press into place.
5. Postoperative assessment:

    Stoma type (e.g., colostomy, ileostomy, or ileal conduit)

    Stoma viability

    Stomal height, or degree of protrusion

    Stomal construction (e.g., end, loop, or double-barrel)

    Stoma location on abdomen

    Stoma size

    Presence and status of stomal supports, ureteral stents, or conduit catheter

    Mucocutaneous suture line

    Peristomal skin status
6. Normal output:

    **a.** Clear dilute urine

    **b.** Clear urine with strands of mucus

    **c.** Ileostomy

    Initial output: usually viscous, green, and low volume

    Adaptation phase: high-volume liquid output (more than 1000 ml per day)

    Long-term: "toothpaste" consistency; 500 to 800 ml daily

    **d.** Pasty to soft stool occurring after meals and at unpredictable intervals throughout the day

    **e.** Soft, formed stool, with elimination patterns similar to preoperative patterns
7. **b.** To provide a moisture barrier and protection against epidermal "stripping" with adhesive removal

8. Forms of skin barriers:
   a. Solid barriers (rings or wafers) are used to protect the peristomal skin from effluent and to improve the adhesion of the pouch to the abdominal wall.
   b. Skin barrier pastes are used to create a level pouching surface, to prevent the migration of effluent under the pouch seal, and to enhance the resistance of the solid wafer skin barrier.
   c. Skin barrier powders are used to protect and treat peristomal skin damage. They also can be mixed with glycerin to produce a homemade paste that contains no alcohol and does not burn denuded skin.
9. Factors in selection of a pouching system:
   a. *Stoma assessment factors*
      Type and consistency of effluent
      Stoma size and construction
      Abdominal contours and degree of stomal protrusion
   b. *Patient assessment factors*
      Manual dexterity and visual acuity
      Level of physical activity
      Financial resources
      Preference (e.g., pouch size, opacity, and construction)
   c. *Product availability*
10. Antireflux valves reduce backflow of urine onto the peristomal skin and thus provide peristomal skin protection.
11. **b.** Patient with a sigmoid colostomy
12. Advantages of reusable pouching systems:
    a. Reusable systems generally provide more support than do disposable systems.
    b. Reusable systems are available in six levels of convexity.
    c. Reusable systems represent a more cost-effective option for the patient whose pouch requires frequent changing.
13. **b.** 6 to 8 weeks after surgery
14. **c.** Convex pouching system
15. **a.** Ileostomy
16. **a.** True
17. **a.** To prevent stomal retraction
18. **a.** True
19. **a.** *Patient with an ileostomy:*
    Stoma characteristics and function
    Self-care procedures: pouch emptying, pouch change
    Peristomal skin care
    Dietary and fluid modifications: need for increased fluid on daily basis, measures to prevent food blockage, and measures to control gas
    Measures to control odor
    Recognition and management of food blockage
    Prevention and management of fluid-electrolyte imbalance
    Guidelines for medication administration
    Life-style issues (bathing; clothing; management of ileostomy at work, when traveling, during exercise and recreational activity, and during sexual activity; and disclosure issues)
    If applicable, potential alteration in sexual function

    **b.** *Patient with a transverse colostomy*

        Stoma characteristics and function

        Self-care procedures: pouch emptying and pouch change

        Peristomal skin care

        Dietary and fluid modifications: measures to control gas

        Prevention and management of diarrhea

        Measures to control odor

        Life-style issues (bathing; clothing; management of colostomy at work, when traveling, during exercise and recreational activity, and during sexual activity; and disclosure issues)

    **c.** *Patient with a descending or sigmoid colostomy*

        Stoma characteristics and function

        Self-care procedures: pouch emptying, pouch change

        Peristomal skin care

        Dietary and fluid modifications: fluid and fiber to prevent constipation; measures to control gas

        Measures to control odor

        If patient meets criteria for management by routine irrigation, instruction in irrigation procedure and principles

        Management of diarrhea and constipation

        Life-style issues (bathing; clothing; management of colostomy at work, during exercise and recreational activity, during travel, and during sexual activity; and disclosure issues)

        If applicable, potential alterations in sexual function

    **d.** *Patient with a urinary diversion*

        Stoma characteristics and function

        Self-care procedures: pouch emptying, pouch change, and use of night-drainage equipment

        Peristomal skin care

        Dietary and fluid modifications: importance of adequate fluid intake, foods that increase urine odor

        Prevention and management of urinary tract infection

        Prevention of stone formation

        Life-style issues (bathing; clothing; management of ostomy at work, during travel, during exercise and recreational activity, and during sexual activity; and disclosure issues)

        If applicable, potential alterations in sexual function

**20.** **c.** Pouch emptying and pouch change procedures

**21.** The patient may be taught to dust skin barrier powder onto the irritated areas; if necessary, skin sealants or water can be lightly blotted over the powder to ensure a nonpowdery pouching surface. The patient also must be instructed to contact the ET nurse for unusual or nonresponsive skin problems, as well as for pouching problems resulting in skin irritation.

**22.** **b.** 6 to 8 hours

**23.** Beans, cabbage, broccoli, brussels sprouts, and beer

**24.** Measures for odor control:
   **a.** Use odorproof pouch.
   **b.** Keep tail of drainable pouch clean.
   **c.** Use pouch deodorants if desired to reduce fecal odor when pouch is emptied; options include mouthwash, perineal cleansers, and commercial pouch deodorants.
   **d.** Use room deodorants when pouch is emptied or changed.
   **e.** Oral deodorizing agents (for some patients)
   **f.** Dietary manipulation
**25. a.** True
**26. d.** Patient with a jejunostomy
**27.** Sports drinks, broth or bouillon, fruit or vegetable juices, tea, and carbonated beverages
**28.** Measures to prevent food blockage:
   **a.** Omit high-fiber foods for the first 6 to 8 weeks after surgery.
   **b.** Add high-fiber foods one at a time in small amounts.
   **c.** Chew food well, and drink plenty of fluids.
   **d.** Monitor response to new foods.
**29.** Criteria for routine colostomy irrigation:
   **a.** The patient must have a descending or sigmoid colostomy.
   **b.** The patient should have normal bowel function, that is, soft to formed stool and fairly regular bowel elimination patterns.
   **c.** The patient must be able to learn to perform the procedure.
   **d.** The patient must choose irrigation as a management method.
**30. c.** Patient receiving pelvic radiation
**31. d.** Vasovagal reaction
**32. a.** Fluid volume deficit
**33.** Contraindications to management by diapering:
   **a.** High-volume or enzymatic output
   **b.** Persistent peristomal skin damage associated with diapering
   **c.** Fecal contamination of urinary stoma
**34. a.** True
**35. c.** Force fluids to prevent fluid-electrolyte imbalance
**36. a.** Repetitive lavage with 30 to 50 ml normal saline
**37.** Loss of bowel regulation:
   **a.** Reduced activity levels
   **b.** Reduced dietary bulk
   **c.** Aging process
**38. d.** Low-volume rectal enema
**39. d.** Catheterize the stoma using sterile technique
**40. c.** Patient with a history of uric acid stones

## REFERENCES

1. Becker KC, Stevens SA: Performing indepth abdominal assessment, *Nursing 88* 18(6):59, 1988.
2. Broadwell D: Gastrointestinal system. In Thompson M et al, editors, *Mosby's manual of clinical nursing*, ed 2, St Louis, 1989, Mosby–Year Book.
3. Brundage D: Renal system. In Thompson M et al, editors: *Mosby's manual of clinical nursing*, ed 2, St Louis, 1989, Mosby–Year Book.
4. Brunner L, Suddarth D, editors: *Textbook of medical-surgical nursing*, ed 5, Philadelphia, 1984, JB Lippincott.
5. Corman M: *Colon and rectal surgery*, ed 2, Philadelphia, 1989, JB Lippincott.
6. Erickson P: Ostomies: the art of pouching, *Nursing Clin North Am* 22:311, 1987.
7. Erwin-Toth P: Teaching ostomy care to the pediatric client: a developmental approach, *J Enterostom Ther* 15(3):126, 1988.
8. Ewing G: The nursing preparations of stoma patients for self-care, *J Adv Nurs* 14:411, 1989.
9. Fazio VW: Complications of intestinal stomas. In Fazio VW et al, editors: *Complications of colon and rectal surgery: prevention and management*, Philadelphia, 1985, WB Saunders.
10. Gray M, Dobkin K: Genitourinary system. In Thompson M et al, editors: *Mosby's manual of clinical nursing*, ed 2, St Louis, 1989, Mosby–Year Book.
11. Holmes J, Nichols R: Sepsis following colorectal surgery. In Fazio VW, editor: *Current therapy in colon and rectal surgery*, Philadelphia, 1990, BC Decker.
12. Ignatavicius D, Bayne M: *Medical-surgical nursing: a nursing process approach*, Philadelphia, 1991, WB Saunders.
13. Kodner I: Stoma complications. In Fazio V, editor: *Current therapy in colon and rectal surgery*, Philadelphia, 1990, BC Decker.
14. Lambert V, Lambert C: *Psychosocial care of the physically ill—what every nurse should know*, ed 2, Englewood Cliffs, NJ, 1985, Prentice-Hall.
15. Lewis C: *Aging: the health care challenge*, ed 2, Philadelphia, 1990, FA Davis.
16. Massoni M: Nurses' GI handbook, *Nursing 90* 20:65, 1990.
17. Moore E: Using self-efficacy in teaching self-care to the elderly, *Holistic Nurs Pract* 4(2):22, 1990.
18. Murray N, Vanderhoof JA: Short bowel syndrome in children and adults, *J Enterostom Ther* 14(4):168, 1987.
19. Petillo M: The patient with a urinary stoma: nursing management and patient education, *Nurs Clin North Am* 22:263, 1987.
20. Redman BK: *The process of patient education*, ed 6, St Louis, 1988, Mosby–Year Book.
21. Rideout B: The patient with an ileostomy: nursing management and patient education, *Nurs Clin North Am* 22:253, 1987.
22. Rorden J: *Nurses as health teachers: a practical guide*, Philadelphia, 1987, WB Saunders.
23. Ruzicki D: Realistically meeting the educational needs of hospitalized acute and short stay patients, *Nurs Clin North Am* 24:629, 1989.
24. Schultz N: Drug therapy and the ostomy patient, *J Enterostom Ther* 13(4):157, 1986.
25. Smith D, Johnson D: Stoma complications, *J Enterostom Ther* 11(1):35, 1984.
26. Standards of Care: *Patient with a colostomy*, Irvine, Calif, 1989, International Association for Enterostomal Therapy.
27. Thelan LA, Davie JK, Urden LD: *Textbook of critical care nursing: diagnosis and management*, St Louis, 1990, Mosby–Year Book.
28. Zarle N: Continuity of care: balancing care of elders between health care settings, *Nurs Clin North Am* 24:697, 1989.
29. Zink M: Double-lumen vs. single-lumen catheterization of ileal/colon conduits, *J Enterostom Ther* 11(5):190, 1984.

# 3

# Peristomal and Stomal Complications

BEVERLY G. HAMPTON

Stomal and peristomal complications occur less frequently than in the past because of improvements in surgical techniques and ostomy management. These complications still occur, however, and the nurse caring for the patient with an ostomy must be knowledgeable regarding preventive measures and must incorporate appropriate surveillance measures into outpatient follow-up. When such complications do occur, the nurse frequently must modify management of the patient's ostomy. Collaboration with the internist, surgeon, or dermatologist is often indicated.

The purposes of this chapter are (1) to describe peristomal and stomal complications that may occur, (2) to explain the causes of these complications and implications for prevention, and (3) to discuss appropriate management of the complications that develop, with an emphasis on nursing interventions.

## PERISTOMAL COMPLICATIONS

### Caput Medusae

Caput medusae refers to a bluish-purple discoloration of the skin caused by dilation of the cutaneous veins around a stoma (peristomal varices).[40] The discolored area blanches when pressed and displays irregular, small blood vessels (Plate 1). The name *caput medusae* comes from the resemblance of the dilated vessels to the head of the snake-haired Medusa.

Persons with a stoma and concomitant liver disease (such as sclerosing cholangitis, portal hypertension, or liver cirrhosis) are at risk for the development of these varices, as are patients with any disease that interferes with normal portal blood flow (see the box below). The high pressure in the venous network of the mesenteric veins enlarges channels communicating with veins in the abdominal wall. The dilated veins coursing away from the umbilicus or stoma create a vascular abnormality known as caput medusae.

Identification and management of the underlying disease is the first priority.[64] Minor peristomal bleeding or bleeding from the stomal surface usually resolves spontaneously. Occasionally direct pressure or topical hemostatic agents such as silver nitrate may be

---

### DISEASE PROCESSES AFFECTING PORTAL SYSTEM

**PREHEPATIC**
Congenital stenosis or atresia
Thrombosis of portal vein
Thrombosis of splenic vein
Extrinsic compression (i.e., tumors)

**HEPATIC**
Cirrhosis
Congenital hepatic fibrosis
Malaria
Syphilitic cirrhosis
Infectious viral hepatitis

Ingestion of poisons such as carbon
    tetrachloride
Sarcoidosis

**POSTHEPATIC**
Constrictive pericarditis
Budd-Chiari syndrome (obstruction of
    hepatic venous outflow, presumably
    resulting from spontaneous thrombosis
    of hepatic vein, possibly caused by birth
    control pills)

From Wright NE: Caput medusae in portal hypertension, *J Enterostom Ther* 8:17, 1981.

required.[46] More severe bleeding may require suture ligation or surgical intervention (injection sclerotherapy, mucocutaneous disconnection, and portosystemic shunts.)[16,30] In some patients it is necessary to relocate the stoma.[25] The nurse, patient, and family should be aware that patients with portal hypertension also are at risk for massive gastrointestinal bleeding.

**Nursing Interventions.** Gentle pouch removal technique and peristomal skin care are important. Adhesive products that are not essential should be avoided, since rubbing the skin to remove these products can increase the risk of trauma and bleeding. The use of hard faceplates and belts should be carefully evaluated, and these should be sized to prevent peristomal or stomal harm.

## Allergic Dermatitis

An allergic skin reaction is similar to the reaction in a person who is sensitive to poison ivy.[57] Should such a person come into contact with even a small amount of poison ivy, an allergic reaction (urticaria and swelling) occurs. An allergic response requires an initial exposure to a potential allergen; antibodies are then produced, and upon subsequent exposure(s) an allergic response is triggered. The agent encountered can be a part of the pouching equipment (such as faceplate, skin barrier, or belt) (Plate 2).

Damaged or inflamed peristomal skin is at increased risk for sensitization because the skin's immune system is overstimulated. The original skin problem may be denudation caused by an irritant dermatitis, specifically. The products used to treat the damaged skin may then create an allergic contact dermatitis. Once the sensitivity develops, it often lasts the rest of the patient's life.[57]

**Nursing Interventions.** Patients with preexisting and established allergies to food, medications, or other topical agents should be evaluated carefully for possible sensitivity to ostomy products. Skin testing may be accomplished by applying a small amount of the adhesive, barrier, pouch, or other suspect material on the patient's abdomen, occluding the substance,[37] labeling the occluded item, then examining the area 24 and 48 hours later for any skin reaction. Although the test also may be performed on a patient's back, the abdominal skin provides the most realistic "test" result because the skin thickness, temperature, and exposure to friction is the same as in the area where the ostomy has been or will be created.[48] Although preoperative skin testing in those persons who are particularly at risk is optimum, it is not always feasible. Skin testing can be performed after the surgery.

The nurse should suspect an allergic dermatitis whenever an area of inflammatory reaction corresponds precisely to the area covered by a particular product, for example, barrier, sealant, or adhesive. If doubt exists as to the particular allergen, repeat skin testing may be employed to identify the offending product.

The treatment of allergic dermatitis consists of (1) removal of the identified agent,[41] (2) use of corticosteroid agents (if prescribed after medical evaluation), (3) effluent containment, and (4) elimination of unnecessary products that contain potential allergens.[6,48,57,58]

## Irritant Dermatitis

When cells in the peristomal area sustain a direct toxic injury or become inflamed without developing specific allergic sensitization, the site is said to have developed irritant or contact dermatitis.[18] Fecal and urinary drainage, marked pH changes, enzymes, ostomy deodorants, or solvents may initiate the process. Tucker and Smith[57] described a two-step process in the development of this dermatitis. The defense mechanisms of the skin are first disturbed by an agent; this damage allows harmful substances to penetrate the skin, and the affected area then develops an inflammation. Once the skin is damaged, the inflammatory process may continue, although the agents that continue the process may not be the original irritants. Soaps, physical trauma, or even the mechanical action of cleansing the area can continue the inflammation that originally was activated by other agents.[8,15,18]

Long-standing dermatitis requires many months to heal, and as with the cells in scar formation, these damaged peristomal cells are altered. The cellular defenses are reduced, and agents that previously could be used freely on the stoma and the peristomal area may no longer be tolerated.

Areas of irritant dermatitis are usually erythematous, shallow, moist, and painful (Plate 3). Occasionally, severe weeping and discomfort can be managed with a compress of modified Burow's solution. Such therapy cannot be used concurrently with pouching, however, so it may not be appropriate when the stoma is functioning. The erythema and discomfort of severe irritant dermatitis may also be treated with corticosteroid creams. However, long-term or overzealous use of corticosteroid agents under the pouch may cause thinning of the skin, striae, and increased risk of infection. Corticosteroid creams usually provide rapid improvement, so only short term use is needed. The nurse should be aware that occlusion of these creams with adhesives intensifies their effects and increases the risk of damage to the skin.

**Nursing Interventions.** Irritant dermatitis is the most common type of peristomal skin complication and is often caused by stool leakage onto the skin. Treatment is directed at drying the skin with a skin barrier powder and evaluating the pouching system and technique. Because inappropriate product usage, effluent leakage, or abrasive materials in contact with the peristomal skin can initiate or maintain irritant or contact dermatitis, the nurse must review in detail all products and procedures used for ostomy management. (In an outpatient setting it is not unusual to see a patient who has been "opinion shopping" and incorporates all suggestions, deletes none, and may well be using eight to ten products in stoma care.) If possible, it may be helpful to discontinue everything but the essential products, such as the pouch and skin barrier.

## Folliculitis

Folliculitis is an inflammation within a hair follicle (Plate 4). Because folliculitis appears as an erythematous and sometimes pustular lesion, it may be confused with a yeast infection. Careful inspection shows the inflammation to be contained within hair follicles. The cause of folliculitis is traumatic hair removal that results from shaving the peristomal hair too frequently, indiscriminate shaving or dry shaving techniques, or careless pouch removal that damages the epidermis around the hair follicle. Infection of the hair follicles usually is caused by coagulase-positive staphylococci. Although the infection tends to be superficial, it may extend into the hair bulb.[50]

**Nursing Interventions.** The nurse should determine the patient's techniques for peristomal hair removal. If the patient uses a straight or blade-type razor, the nurse may suggest the use of an electric razor or scissors to clip the hair.[11] A depilatory also may be suggested, as is thorough washing and rinsing of the peristomal area after its use, but skin testing is recommended. In addition, the nurse should evaluate the patient's technique for pouch removal, since traumatic removal may initiate the problem.

In more severe cases *Staphylococcus aureus* can be cultured in specimens from the peristomal area; antibacterial powder may then be prescribed. Oral antibiotics rarely are needed.[1]

## Hernia

Peristomal hernia is a complication that may occur months or years after ostomy surgery. It is particularly common in patients with end colostomies and less frequently found in those with urinary conduit.[2,52] The hernia appears as a bulge around the stoma; the bulge represents loops of the intestine that protrude through the fascial defect around the stoma and into the subcutaneous tissue (Plate 5). The patient may be asymptomatic. If the bowel segment becomes incarcerated, however, the patient manifests symptoms of an acute abdomen (bowel obstruction, ischemic bowel, and abdominal pain). These symptoms mandate immediate consultation with a surgeon and emergency surgery.

Peristomal herniation has been attributed to the following causes: (1) placement of the stoma outside the rectus muscle, (2) an excessively large fascial defect, (3) placement of the stoma in the midline incision, (4) wound infection, (5) loss of muscle tone (as with weight gain or aging), or (6) an increase in intraabdominal pressure.

The use of the umbilicus for the stoma site has been suggested to provide stability and to reduce the chance of hernia formation.[16] This placement, however, may not be esthetically pleasing to the patient and should not be used in the patient with cancer who may require additional surgery for the management of a recurrence.[23]

**Nursing Interventions.** Nursing interventions for the patient with a peristomal hernia involves preventive measures, surveillance, and assistance with ostomy management.

Prevention includes an emphasis on measures to maintain abdominal muscle tone. The nurse should caution the patient against excessive weight gain and should explain that weight gain is a predisposing factor in stomal complications such as retraction and hernia formation. The patient also is instructed to avoid weight lifting and strenuous activity for the first 6 to 8 weeks after surgery, to allow the muscle layer to heal; once healing is complete, the patient is encouraged to begin abdominal exercises and slowly increase their intensity. The patient with poor abdominal muscle tone may benefit from the use of support belts designed to fit around the pouch and to provide support to the abdominal wall. These support devices also may benefit the patient with a chronic cough. (Coughing and sneezing increase intraabdominal pressure.)

Surveillance is another important nursing responsibility. Patients returning to the outpatient clinic should be evaluated for evidence of hernia formation. A hernia generally is apparent by visual inspection of the abdomen while the patient is sitting or standing. Palpation of the peristomal area with the patient in a recumbent position also reveals a fascial defect and hernia; these are also obvious when the patient raises his or her head. The patient also should be questioned regarding any noticeable swelling or bulge around the stoma.

Ostomy care for the patient with a hernia may require modification. Commonly required modifications include the use of support belts, a change in pouching equipment, and changes in irrigation techniques. Support belts, when used, need to be snug but not constricting and applied while the patient is lying down. Pouching equipment must conform to the protruberant abdominal surface; flexible systems (such as a two-piece pouch with floating flange) are more effective than rigid systems.

The patient who irrigates a colostomy and has a hernia often has delayed, prolonged, and incomplete evacuations. To reduce frustration, the patient should be encouraged to omit irrigations and to use bulk laxatives or stool softeners to maintain bowel function. Occasionally the patient prefers to continue "trying" to irrigate; if so, it is absolutely essential that a cone tip be used to instill the irrigant ( to prevent bowel perforation).

Surgical intervention is warranted when the bowel is incarcerated or when the patient prefers to have surgery. When the hernia is to be surgically repaired, a new stoma site should be selected.

## Pseudoverrucous Lesions (Hyperplasia)

Pseudoverrucous lesions are characterized by wartlike papules or nodules, or both, that have a white-gray or reddish brown discoloration (Plate 6). These lesions may be a single eruptive lesion or confluent and protrude from 2 mm to 10 mm above the skin level.[10] Pseudoverrucous lesions develop at the mucocutaneous border and conform to the shape of the discrepancy between the base of the stoma and the stomal opening in the pouch. In many cases these lesions are extremely painful to touch, so even minimal pressure produces discomfort.[32] Bleeding from the lesions is common. On microscopic examination these lesions show a thickened epidermis, hyperkeratosis, and acanthosis. No atypia or increased mitosis has been reported.[7]

Many terms have been used when discussing pseudoverrucous lesions: hyperplasia, hyperkeratosis, granulomas, chronic papillomatous dermatitis, pseudoepithelial hyperplasia, acanthosis, exuberant tissue growth, and proud flesh.[10,32,44,48] However, many of these terms reflect conditions that must be confirmed by tissue biopsy. Because biopsy is rarely necessary for selection of proper therapy, Jeter suggests identifying and using a term that is more descriptive of the macroscopic appearance of the affected area and scientifically accurate.[32] The term *pseudoverrucous lesions* has been proposed by Nordstrom, Borglund, and Nyman because it is more descriptive of the macroscopic appearance of the lesions and also supports histopathologic findings of the lesions. For example, although the term *hyperplasia* is commonly used to describe these lesions, hyperplasia describes an increase in the number of normal cells in normal arrangement; these observations have not been confirmed on histologic examination in pseudoverrucous lesions.[10,32,44]

Pseudoverrucous lesions are most commonly associated with urinary stomas, although they may also develop in the patient with an ileostomy or colostomy.[57] The height of the stoma also may influence the development of pseudoverrucous lesions. Nordstrom reported that pseudoverrucous lesions occurred only in patients with a stoma length of less than 10 mm. However, these lesions develop because the skin is chronically exposed to effluent (most commonly urine); therefore they may also develop in patients with nicely protruding stomas.

**Nursing Interventions.** The primary treatment of pseudoverrucous lesions is to correct the underlying problem, that is, chronic exposure of effluent to the skin. This exposure usually occurs because the pouching procedure or equipment is flawed and leaves effluent trapped against the skin. The most common situation precipitating pseudoverrucous lesions is an improperly sized pouch (i.e., the stomal opening in the pouch is too large). Effluent can also become trapped against the skin when the pouch leaks frequently and when the skin barrier dissolves quickly.

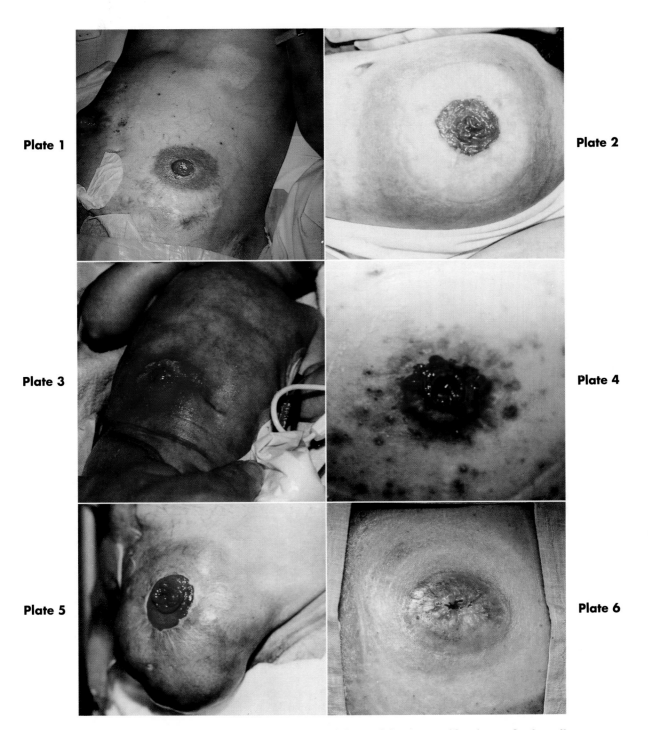

**Plate 1** Caput medusae in child with biliary atresia. Abdominal distention, dilated superficial capillaries, and purple hue encircling jejunostomy are evident. **Plate 2** Allergic contact dermatitis resulting from "picture-framing" pouch with tape. Immediate surrounding peristomal skin is clear because patient used skin barrier wafer. **Plate 3** Irritant (chemical) dermatitis in infant with ileostomy. Lumen opens at skin level, and skin is severely denuded and moist. **Plate 4** Folliculitis in peristomal skin. Pustular lesions arising from hair follicles are evident. **Plate 5** Parastomal hernia in man with colostomy. **Plate 6** Pseudoverrucous lesions in peristomal field completely overtaking ileal conduit mucosa.

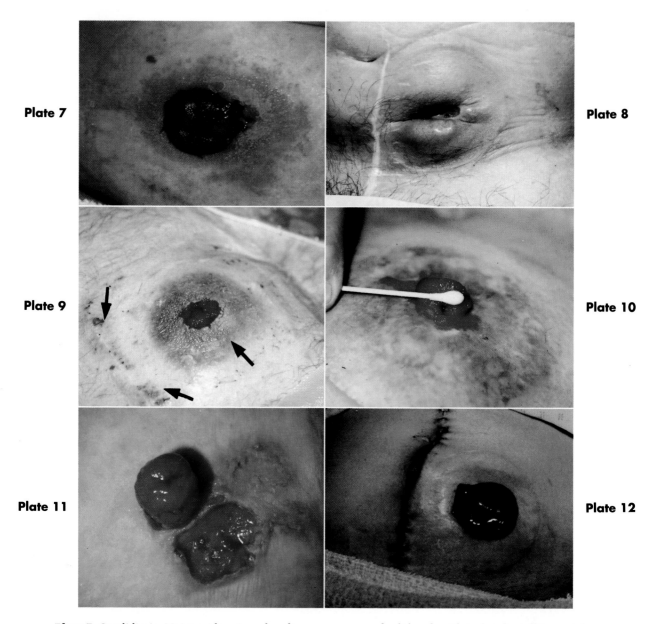

**Plate 7** Candidiasis. Moist epidermis and scaling appearance of solid rash with isolated satellite pustular lesions in periphery are evident. **Plate 8** Tumor recurrence at colostomy site, creating irregular skin surface. **Plate 9** Patient with flush ileal conduit stoma. Evidence of epidermal skin stripping caused by frequent removal of pouch adhesive outside immediate peristomal skin area can be seen at 7 o'clock to 10 o'clock position. Pseudoverrucous lesions surround stoma. **Plate 10** Ileostomy that had been surgically revised at same site. Suture fistula and "grafted" ileal mucosa onto peristomal skin are present. **Plate 11** Pyoderma gangrenosum near ileostomy. Characteristic halo of discoloration along border of ulcer and irregular, erythematous skin superior to pyoderma lesion suggest potential for progression of ulceration. **Plate 12** Stomal necrosis. Distinct band of necrosis is evident at mucocutaneous junction; lumen appears slightly better vascularized. Diffuse peristomal erythema and separation of surgical incision suggest that patient's ability to heal is impaired.

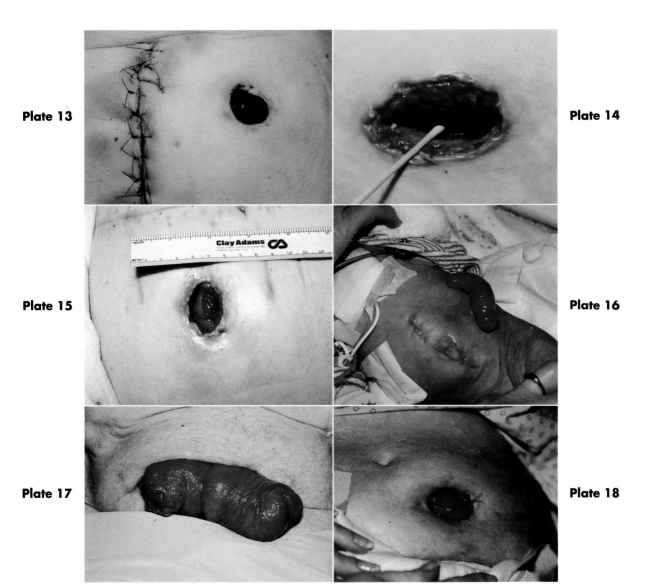

**Plate 13** Melanosis coli. **Plate 14** Complete circumferential mucocutaneous separation with complete retraction of stoma. **Plate 15** Complete separation of mucocutaneous junction in colostomy. Mild retraction of stoma is evident. **Plate 16** Prolapse of both limbs of loop colostomy in infant. **Plate 17** Prolapse of loop colostomy in adult. **Plate 18** Peristomal skin is retracted at mucocutaneous junction, yet stoma still protrudes above skin level. Erythema also present at mucocutaneous junction warrants monitoring for potential separation.

**Plate 1** from Emory University, Atlanta. **Plates 2, 4, 5, 6, 8, 11, 13, 14, 17, 19, and 24** from MD Anderson Cancer Center, Houston. **Plates 3, 7, 12, 16, 18, 20, and 24** from Abbott Northwestern Hospital, Minneapolis. **Plates 9, 10, 15, and 21** from Karen and Victor Alterescu, San Francisco.

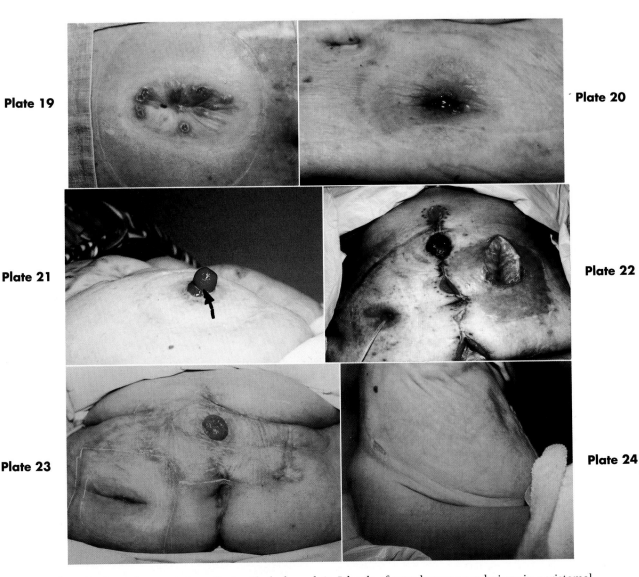

**Plate 19** Stomal stenosis in patient with ileal conduit. Islands of pseudoverrucous lesions in peristomal field were precipitated by cutting ostomy pouch too large, which allowed urine to macerate immediately surrounding skin. **Plate 20** Stenosis and retraction occurring in sigmoid colostomy after sloughing of necrotic stoma. Patient had partial bowel obstruction, and surgical revision was required. **Plate 21** Stomal laceration as evidenced by the white-yellow band on medial aspect of ileostomy. Laceration developed as result of improperly sized faceplate. **Plate 22** Woman who required total pelvic exenteration for recurrent cervical cancer. Internal radiation implantation and external beam radiation therapy had been employed previously. Ileal conduit is located in right lower quadrant. Colostomy required revision and relocation to midline incision after necrosis extending below fascial level developed. Pale color of subcutaneous tissue in old colostomy site (suggesting that tissue had received substantial prior radiation), healthy appearance of subcutaneous tissue where the midline incision was left open (suggesting that this tissue received much less radiation), and dark but viable stoma color can be seen. Skin surrounding initial colostomy site is also tanned. **Plate 23** Patient in Plate 22 is shown several months later. **Plate 24** Boy with prune-belly syndrome. Wrinkled abdomen and end ureterostomy are present.

The nurse should ensure that the pouch opening is correctly sized to minimize or eliminate skin exposure to effluent. The effectiveness of the pouching system should also be assessed and modified as needed to achieve a secure pouch seal. If the skin barrier in use is dissolved by the effluent in a short time, a more resistant skin barrier should be selected. Occasionally, with certain types of pouching systems for urinary stomas, it is possible to completely eliminate the skin barrier. Selection of proper equipment must also address financial concerns, since some patients leave pouching systems in place for an excessively long time because of cost considerations. Patients should be encouraged to increase their fluid intake in an attempt to acidify the urine, although pseudoverrucous lesions have been associated with both an acid and an alkaline urine pH.[7]

Specific measures of prevention and treatment of urine-induced pseudoverrucous lesions are discussed in Chapter 2.

## Bacterial Infections

Bacterial infection caused by *S. aureus* may appear as a large, patchy, erythematous crusty area with plaques.[11] Cultures of specimens from the affected area are suggested so that specific therapy such as topical or systemic antibiotics can be initiated. Extensive bacterial infections may be complicated by pustules, ulcers, abscesses, or cellulitis.[48]

**Nursing Interventions.** Patients may be unable to maintain a secure pouch seal if the infected areas are draining heavily. It may be necessary to increase the frequency of pouch changes to prevent leakage and to apply any prescribed topical medications. It may be beneficial to use a nonadhesive pouch or a pouch with a narrow skin barrier ring (after removing the attached adhesive tape), both of which can be secured with a belt. Infected areas can then be treated as needed with minimal disruption of the pouching system.

Occasionally areas that are draining heavily may be included in the pouch opening, provided that an excessive amount of peristomal skin is not exposed to effluent. Drying the area with a hair dryer on the cool setting may be necessary to obtain a secure seal. Once the bacterial infection is resolved, the usual self-care practices can be resumed.

## Candidal Infections

*Candida* is a genus of yeastlike, imperfect fungi that are a part of the normal floral of the mouth, intestine, and vagina. In the right situations *Candida* can be spread easily to the skin. *Candida albicans*, sometimes referred to as *Monilia*, is the most frequent agent of candidiasis and thrives in dark, damp sites. A leaking ostomy pouch, body perspiration, and denuded skin all provide optimum environments for candidiasis to develop on the skin. Other predisposing conditions include diabetes mellitus, immunosuppression, myelosuppression, use of oral contraceptives, topical corticosteroid therapy, and iatrogenic hypersteroidisms.[29] Antibiotic therapy also sets the stage for candidiasis because the body's normal flora are altered.

*Candida* infects only the stratum corneum, and the initial lesion is a pustule.[29] Friction disrupts the pustule, leaving papules and erythema. Often the infection forms a plaque with a sealing, advancing border and distinct, characteristic pustules outside the plaque (satellite lesions) (Plate 7). Dry skin usually stops the advancing border of the infection. Patients typically have pruritis at the site. The Latin name for candidiasis, *Monilia*, means *glowing white*; severe, extensive infections actually develop a white-coated appearance that indicates the presence of inflammatory cells. Once the nurse has seen this infection, he or she easily recognizes it in the future; however, positive identification can be made by a culture or by skin scrapings stained with potassium hydroxide.

**Nursing Interventions.** Treatment involves elimination of moisture and use of an antifungal medication (such as powder or lotion). The powder form is used more commonly because it is less likely to interfere with pouch adherence. Nystatin (Mycostatin), a prescribed antifungal powder, is applied sparingly to the affected area during pouch changes.[53] The excess powder should be brushed away; a sealant may be applied to enhance the pouch seal. The antifungal agent should be reapplied with each routine pouch change until the area is clear. Use of an antifungal agent on a prophylactic basis is not advised.[57] The pouch is evaluated and modified as indicated to prevent leakage. Pouch covers, gauze, or absorbent powders may be used to absorb perspiration trapped under pouch material.

### Malignancy in the Peristomal Area

A malignancy at the stoma site is uncommon and may indicate a potentially fatal complication.[5] This situation may be due to tumor implants at the time of the bowel resection, inadequate margins of the resection, or a second primary lesion.[9,16,22,36] Rothstein[48] discussed a primary basal cell epithelioma developing at a sigmoid colostomy, although this occurrence is rare. The initial symptoms of a peristomal malignancy may include bleeding, skin ulceration, and a palpable mass. The surgical treatment may consist of resection of the stoma or a wide excision of the skin on the abdominal wall, with the placement of the stoma in a new location.[16,36,42] Firm "lumps," which can suggest areas of abscess, also may appear around the stoma; however, a biopsy specimen of the area should be obtained if any question exists (Plate 8). Radiation therapy may also be warranted.

**Nursing Interventions.** The patient may describe an inability to maintain the pouch seal, particularly with the use of a hard faceplate or a skin barrier wafer with flange (with or without an insert). A flexible pouching system that molds and conforms to the irregular skin surface is suggested. The area of tumor may enlarge, drain, and slough, requiring a pouch with a cutting surface large enough to encompass the stoma and affected peristomal areas; in some cases it may be necessary to use a wound pouch that can be attached to bedside drainage. Deodorant products also may be needed.

### Mechanical Trauma

Damage to the peristomal skin may result from mechanical trauma. Common causes include abrasive cleansing techniques and traumatic tape removal that results in epidermal "stripping"; continued friction or pressure from ill-fitting equipment also may cause damage to the peristomal area. The affected skin is painful, and the moist, bleeding areas undermine the pouch seal, resulting in frequent pouch changes and further exacerbation of the problem (Plate 9). Lesions are typically shallow and irregularly shaped.

Mechanical trauma can be prevented by teaching the patient appropriate pouch removal and cleansing techniques. The patient is encouraged to limit the amount of adhesive used for securing the pouch and is taught to prevent traumatic removal by pushing down the skin while gently pulling up the pouch adhesive surface (the "push-pull" technique). Patients with sensitive skin may benefit from the use of skin sealants under adhesives and, in *carefully* selected situations, the use of solvents for adhesive removal. Inappropriate use of solvents and subsequent occlusion by the skin barrier or faceplate of a pouch can result in chemical or irritant dermatitis; thus, the patient needs to rinse the area with plain water thoroughly before reapplying the equipment.

Patients also must be instructed to avoid scrubbing or "picking" the peristomal area to remove residual amounts of skin barriers, pastes, and adhesives. Residual amounts of these items do not need to be removed if in doing so the skin is further damaged. In fact, the pouch seal generally is not affected by these residues.

Although not an injury of the immediate peristomal area, rubbing from belts worn too tightly or the hardware on a faceplate may cause mechanical trauma (such as a pressure ulcer).

**Nursing Interventions.** The nurse must evaluate the patient's techniques for pouch removal and peristomal skin care and must reeducate the patient if indicated. The nurse also must examine the fit of all faceplates, belts, and pouches; factors that contribute to poor fit and mechanical trauma include weight gain, weight loss, peristomal hernia, and prolapse.

Denuded areas usually require the use of a skin barrier powder; a skin sealant sometimes is used over the powder to create an effective adhesive surface. It is wise, however, to check the contents of any products used: most skin sealants contain alcohol or other substances that create a burning sensation when applied to denuded skin.

## Mucosal Transplantation

Occasionally, viable intestinal mucosa is transplanted to the abdominal surface in the immediate peristomal area (Plate 10). Mucosal transplantation is seldom an emergency situation requiring immediate attention or removal of the tissue; however, it may result in persistent mucus secretion and problems in maintaining a pouch seal. Muscosal transplantation (also known as seeding) is most often recognized to be precipitated by suturing the bowel to the epidermis, although other factors may also be present. Proper stoma construction (i.e., securing the bowel to the dermis) is important to reduce the risk of mucosal transplantation[16] (see Fig. 11-8).

**Nursing Interventions.** The goal must be to create a dry environment so that an effective seal can be obtained. This is most often accomplished by using absorptive powders over the lesion. It usually is helpful to use either a patch or a wafer of a solid skin barrier over the lesion as well.

Islets of mucosa transplanted to the skin also may bleed when touched. Careful pouch removal and cleansing is advised. The areas may also burn or itch if they come into contact with glues or other agents used in ostomy management.

## Pyoderma Gangrenosum

In 1930 Brunsting[13] first described pyoderma gangrenosum (PG) and thought that streptococci and staphylococci were the causative agents (Plate 11). Although all etiologic factors of PG are still unknown, it is established that the cause is not infection. Lesion cultures may reveal gram-positive or gram-negative organisms, but this result probably represents a secondary infection.[63]

Pyoderma gangrenosum is a rare inflammatory skin disease that can be destructive and extensive.[28] The lesions may appear as solitary or multiple tender, red lesions (macule, papule, pustule, nodule, or bullae) that become indurated and ulcerated.[29] The base of the

---

## PYODERMA GANGRENOSUM TREATMENT PROTOCOL

1. Flush area with normal saline.
2. Apply antinflammatory cream to base of lesion (if ordered).
3. Fill lesions with absorptive powder or granules.
4. Cover areas to create a dry surface for pouch adhesion (such as SteriStrips, paper tape, gauze, or skin barrier paste).
5. Apply appropriately sized pouch.

---

lesion enlarges, discharging purulent and hemorrhogic exudate.[17,60] The lesions appear raised with dusty red to purplish margins, ragged, erythematous borders, and irregular shapes. The base of the lesion is deep red and is often painful, and peristomal lesions may communicate with nearby structures such as bowel. Sites commonly affected are the lower extremities, buttocks, abdomen, and face. Although the mucous membranes usually are not at risk, they may be involved. Once the disease is active, even minor trauma (e.g., skin abrasions) may initiate new lesions.[21]

Diseases associated with PG include ulcerative colitis, Crohn's disease, arthritis, leukemia (acute and chronic myelogenous and acute lymphocytic), polycythemia vera, and multiple myeloma. Because the disease is seen in association with these systemic disorders, various researchers have considered an altered immune process to be the cause; this is not, however, established, nor is there any definitive laboratory test for the diagnosis of PG.

**Nursing Interventions.** The initial symptom of patients with peristomal PG often is pouch leakage resulting from undermining caused by the draining lesions, as well as pain at the site. Occasionally leakage of effluent may cause a superinfection of the ulcers in addition to the denudation of the surrounding skin.[38] The nurse should refer the patient for the management of the underlying systemic disease (such as Crohn's disease); once the systemic disease improves, the PG usually improves as well. Systemic corticosteroids are most consistent in resolving lesions.[29] Sulfonamides, 6-mercaptopurine, azathioprine, and clofazimine have also been used with varying results.[4,63] Topical management involves the use of absorptive powders and modification of the pouching system as needed to maintain an effective seal. Topical corticosteroids may also be used. The box above presents a suggested PG treatment protocol.

Complications of PG, such as fistula formation, may result in the need for more aggressive surgical management or even relocation of the stoma to another site.[43]

## Unusual Peristomal Complications

Various unusual dermatologic complications have been reported in the peristomal area,[45,57,62] although the nurse infrequently encounters these situations. Certainly in caring for the patient with a stoma, the nurse can encounter any condition in which a cutaneous or mucosal manifestation can occur.[61] In presenting these unusual situations here, it is hoped that the nurse will become aware of the need to adequately review the patient's history for documentation of diseases that may be accompanied by skin lesions. Any unusual skin lesion and any lesion not responding to traditional therapy should be referred to the dermatologist for evaluation and recommendations.

**Dermatomyositis.** Dermatomyositis is an unusual collagen disease affecting the skin with edematous and erythematous lesions that appear primarily in the face and eyelids.[47,57] Papules may cover the knuckles of the fingers and are known as Gottron's papules. Progressive symptoms include muscle weakness, atrophy, and telangiectatic contractures; skin telangiectasias and atrophy; and generalized organ involvement, leading to death in 50% of the afflicted persons. A relationship may exist between dermatomyositis and adenocarcinoma.

In the one case of dermatomyositis in an ostomy patient reported in the literature a malleable, soft, two-piece pouching system was described as effective in adhering to the patient's firm abdomen and in containing effluent.[57]

**Herpesvirus Infection.** Herpes simplex virus (HSV) and varicella zoster virus (VZV) precipitate similar skin lesions. HSV infections are common on the lips, in the mouth, and in the genital regions; however, other cutaneous sites such as the buttocks are becoming more prevalent. After the initial infection HSV becomes dormant in the ganglion at that site. Stress, fever, fatigue, and local trauma may reactivate the dormant HSV. Within 12 to 24 hours lesions progress from erythema to papules to uniformly shaped vesicles. The center of the vesicles subsequently umbilicate (that is, depress) and rupture, revealing crust-covered erosions. When the crust sheds (in approximately 7 to 12 days), the surface of the lesions is reepithelialized without scarring.

Herpes zoster, also known as shingles, is an infection caused by a reactivation of VZV (the virus that causes chicken pox). During chicken pox the varicella virus enters the cutaneous nerves, where it becomes dormant in the dorsal root ganglion. Older age, immuno-compromise, lymphoma, radiation therapy, fatigue, and emotional distress may reactivate the virus.

Although both herpesvirus infections are manifested by vesicles and crust formation, herpes zoster is quite distinct from HSV on clinical examination. First, zoster infections begin with pain and burning sensations (hyperesthesia) in intact skin. Second, a zoster infection involves only the skin that follows the affected dermatome. Third, the clusters of vesicles that develop amidst the red, swollen plaques are of various sizes and shapes. Fourth, some zoster eruptions can be quite extensive and can result in skin necrosis, bacterial infection, or excessive scarring.[29] Finally, zoster is quite painful, and the incidence and duration increase with age. Although the mechanism of this pain is poorly understood, it is not related to severity of the infection.[29]

If a patient with an ostomy develops either type of herpesvirus infection in the peristomal field, the pouching system must be evaluated with the intent of maintaining an effective pouching system while also facilitating local treatment of the infection. Nonadhesive pouching systems and pouches secured with a belt should be considered. If an adhesive pouch is being used, skin barrier powders and skin barrier wafers may be needed to provide a suitable adhesive surface. Oral corticosteroids and topical aluminum acetate (Burow's solution) may be effective in controlling pain. Acyclovir, an antiviral medication, may be administered intravenously, orally, or topically to reduce pain, inflammation, and viral shedding.[29]

**Mycosis Fungoides.** Mycosis fungoides is a cutaneous T (thymus-derived)–cell lymphocyte dysplasia. (It is not, as the name may imply, fungal in origin.) Cutaneous T-cell lymphoma (CTCL) includes not only mycosis fungoides but also Sézary syndrome, lymphoma cutis, and reticulum carcinoma of the skin.[24] The three stages of mycosis fungoides are patch, plaque, and tumor; although they occur in this order, all three may be present simultaneously.[20,50] The first stage resemble atopic eczema and psoriasis; red, flat, scaly patches with sharply demarcated margins. The plaque phase is characterized by severe itching. Patches become elevated, may become indurated, and may develop an area of central clearing resulting in ring-shaped lesions within the plaque. Characteristics of the tumor stage are the following: tumor growths on the skin (often mushroom-shaped), ulceration of these growths, secondary bacterial infection, and lymph node and internal organ involvement.[4,24,29]

Medical treatment of mycosis fungoides depends on the disease stage, but it may include topical or systemic chemotherapy, ultraviolet therapy, total body irradiation, and administration of monoclonal antibodies.[50] This disorder is not common; approximately 800 to 1000 new cases occur per year.[24]

In the patient with an ostomy, general peristomal skin management includes protecting the skin from leakage of the effluent, fitting equipment properly, and assessing the patient's self-care ability in response to his or her current treatment plan for the disease.

**Pemphigus.** Pemphigus, one of a group of bullous disease, is a rare immunologic disorder in which circulating antibodies attach to the intercellular substance of the epidermis.[29] In some forms it is potentially fatal. The most common form in North America is pemphigus vulgaris. This disease is distinct from bullous pemphigoid and epidermolysis bullosa. For further information on these diseases, the reader is encouraged to refer to a dermatology textbook.[29]

Patients with pemphigus usually are 50 to 60 years of age and also may have lupus erythematosus, rheumatoid arthritis, pernicious anemia, malignant disorders, or thyroiditis.[4,50] The literature contains one report of a patient with an ostomy performed because of colon cancer who manifested this skin disorder in the peristomal area.[47]

Weeks before blisters develop on the skin, oral erosions are often present. The early skin lesions of pemphigus are small bullae or vesicles and appear on normal skin.[29] These bullae, when untreated, enlarge and spread. Because the roof of the vesicle is thin, the blisters rupture easily. Healing of unroofed pemphigus vulgaris lesions requires several weeks and results in brown hyperpigmentation. Historically lesions became infected and death occured in all cases.[29] Today treatment may consist of corticosteroid therapy, antibiotics, and topical compresses.

The patient with an ostomy requires evaluation for a nonadhesive pouch. As with any lesion that does not heal, appropriate consultation should be sought. A biopsy should provide the diagnosis.

**Psoriasis.** Psoriasis, a chronic, recurring skin disorder, may be present in 4% to 6% of the general population. Psoriasis is characterized by whitish scaly patches of various sizes on the elbows, knees, scalp, and nails. The scale is thick and bleeds at minute points when removed (Auspitz's sign). The cause is unknown; however, one third of the patients with psoriasis report a family history of the disease. The average age at which psoriasis occurs is 27 years, but it may develop at any time from infancy to advanced age; it is more prevalent in white than in black persons, and it is not seen in native Americans or native Filipinos. Warm weather and sunlight improve the disorder, whereas drugs such as beta blockers, lithium, antimalarial agents, and nonsteroidal antiinflammatory agents, as well as stress, pregnancy, and arthritis, exacerbate it.[39,47,55] Active psoriasis may develop in areas of minor trauma (Koebner's phenomenon) such as surgical incisions, sunburn, abrasions, and chemical or mechanical injuries.

Because psoriasis is prevalent in the general population, it is reasonable to expect that it would occur in the peristomal area, and the nursing literature contains several such reports.[47,55,57]

Psoriasis has been successfully treated topically with corticosteroid creams and occlusive dressings.[27] This approach works well in the peristomal area because a skin barrier wafer is occlusive and a common component of most pouching systems. Corticosteroids become less effective with continued use and also result in atrophy of the skin and telangiectasia. Gentle skin cleansing and adhesive removal should be encouraged, to reduce trauma. Pouch security should be evaluated and appropriate consultation provided. Becoming attuned to the entire disease process aids the nurse in correct identification and appropriate consultation.

## STOMAL COMPLICATIONS

### Bleeding

Hemorrhage from the stoma site during the immediate postoperative period is caused by inadequate hemostasis during stoma construction. The bleeding originates from small vessels of the mucosa, the mesentery, or the exit site of the stoma on the abdominal wall (Plate 14).

Portal hypertension is another cause of stomal hemorrhage.[27] Portal hypertension occurs when damage to the liver obliterates or narrows many of its vascular channels, resulting in obstruction of venous blood draining from the bowel into the liver through the portal vein.[1,16,25] Portal hypertension may be caused by cirrhosis or by sclerosing cholangitis; sometimes it is associated with inflammatory bowel disease or malignancies involving the liver. Portal hypertension results in dilation of the veins (varices) in the gastrointestinal tract, and erosion into these dilated vessels can cause massive bleeding. Possible treatments of severe stomal bleeding caused by portal hypertension include injection sclerotherapy with agents such as polidocanol, phenol in almond oil, or tetradecyl sulfate; local therapy often is ineffective, however, and portosystemic shunting is required.[16]

Trauma is another cause of stomal bleeding. Pouches that are improperly sized or improperly applied may injure the mucosa, leading to bleeding.[3] Patients may inadvertently damage the stoma if they use incorrect technique while shaving the peristomal skin with a safety razor. Forceful use of irrigation tips or tubes, as well as some sports-related injuries, can also cause stomal bleeding.

Diseases such as recurrent inflammatory bowel disease, pyoderma gangrenosum, polyps, diverticulae, or recurrent malignancy can cause bleeding of the stoma. Certain medications or therapies also may cause bleeding.

**Nursing Interventions.** Stomal bleeding is a symptom that should initiate the nurse's detective skills. Minor superficial bleeding during the pouch change procedure seldom requires therapy and stops spontaneously. Superficial bleeding that does not stop spontaneously may require cauterization (suture placement or topical hemostatic agents) or direct pressure. Massive or repetitive bleeding requires correction of the causal factor. For example, the patient with inadequate intraoperative hemostasis may require reoperation, and the patient with portal hypertension may require sclerotherapy or portosystemic shunting.[16]

Trauma to the stoma necessitates elimination of the traumatic events; large hematomas on the stoma may require needle drainage.

Nursing responsibilities include assessment of the severity and source of the bleeding (stomal or within the lumen of the bowel), physician notification, and measures to control the bleeding and maintain hemodynamic stability. It sometimes is difficult to determine the source of the bleeding, especially when the bleeding is intermittent. For example, the patient may report that he or she found a significant amount of blood in the pouch, but that bleeding did not recur when he or she removed the pouch to check the stoma. Such an occurrence warrants further medical evaluation.

Bleeding resulting from stomal trauma requires careful assessment of the patient's self-care techniques. These procedures should be modified and the patient reeducated as indicated.

The nurse should question the patient regarding any prescription or over-the-counter medications taken or used in the pouch that might cause bleeding. For example, in the past, patients sometimes were taught to place aspirin in the pouch to control odor; this is now known to cause mucosal ulceration and bleeding.

### Necrosis

The normal stoma is beefy red or pink, with a shiny appearance, similar to the mucosa within the person's mouth. Evaluating the stoma color, size, and condition is an ongoing process for the patient and the nurse and is particularly important during the early postoperative period, when necrosis is most likely to occur. Ischemia and necrosis may result from the following: (1) excessive tension on the mesentery, which compromises arterial inflow or venous outflow, or both; (2) interruption of blood supply to the stoma, such as an embolus; (3) excessive devascularization; or (4) narrowly spaced sutures, sutures tied too snugly around the stoma, or continuous, constricting sutures.[16,35]

Damage to the stoma is variable. Necrosis may be circumferential or scattered on the mucosa; the depth may be quite superficial and limited to the visible mucosa or deep, extending down to the fascial level or below. When necrosis extends below the fascia, the danger of perforation and ensuing peritonitis exists. This situation requires a second laparotomy and reconstruction of the stoma, potentially in another abdominal site. The stoma that is necrotic sloughs, creates odor, and results in stomal stenosis or retraction, or both (Plate 12). Often a mucocutaneous separation also develops.

**Nursing Interventions.** The primary nursing responsibilities are ongoing assessment of stomal viability and prompt physician notification should significant ischemia develop. Assessment is facilitated by the use of transparent pouches during the initial postoperative period. Pouch openings should be sized to clear the stoma and to prevent constriction, which could further impair circulation to the stoma. Odor control, frequent pouch changes, superficial debridement of the slough, and reassurance of the patient are also important interventions. The management of stomal necrosis is further discussed in Chapter 2.

### Melanosis Coli

The viable stoma that appears buff to dark brown or black may be the result either of fecal stasis or of the overuse of anthracene-containing cathartics, or of both (Plate 13). Melanosis coli was first described in 1830, but the name *melanosis coli* was not applied to it until 1858.[56] Brockos, Willard, and Bank[12] in 1933 reported this benign condition of dark-colored bowel in 41 patients; the researchers related it to the extended use of cathartics such as cascara. Additional anthracene agents that, when used excessively, may cause bowel pigmentation are sagrada, senna, aloe, rhubarb, and frangula. Other authors have described the bowel mucosa appearance as resembling that of the back of toads or the skin of tigers.[12,56]

The initial documentation of these pigmented areas may occur when the bowel mucosa is examined during a proctosigmoidoscopy. However, other areas (the terminal ileum, appendix, or mesenteric lymph nodes) may also be pigmented and may be identified during surgery.[24]

**Nursing Interventions.** Melanosis coli is not an emergency; it need only be recognized. The results of a recent proctosigmoidoscopic examination should be reviewed to ascertain whether any excessively dark or pigmented areas were detected. A discussion with patients regarding their prior bowel habits, including the types of laxatives used and the frequency with which they were used, may provide data useful in determining the origin of an unusually dark or necrotic-appearing stoma.

Certainly, postoperative identification of a dark stoma should prompt careful examination, documentation, and discussion with the surgeon. Patient and nursing staff education regarding the color of the stoma and the cause of the color is important. Placement of a label on the pouch indicating that the stoma is viable and noting the cause of its unusual appearance, as well as chart documentation in the chart and care plan, may eliminate frantic telephone calls to the nurse who is directing the patient's care. It also is wise to document the information on home-care referrals, to alleviate the further alarm and surprise of any other health care providers.

## Mucocutaneous Separation

The stoma may separate from the skin, leaving a defect that must heal by scar formation. This complication can occur in any patient with compromised healing, for example, the malnourished patient, the patient receiving corticosteroids, the patient who has excessive tension at the stoma-skin suture line, or the patient with poorly perfused tissue.[23] Mucocutaneous separation also can result when the defect in the skin, through which the bowel is fashioned into a stoma, is oversized.[1,16] Mucocutaneous separation can be circumferential or limited to a portion of the junction; it may be superficial or deep (Plates 14 and 15).

**Nursing Interventions.** Mucocutaneous separation is best prevented by maximizing the patient's nutritional state before surgery and by constructing a stoma without tension. The patient who is on a regimen of corticosteroids before surgery may benefit from the administration of intravenous vitamin A to counteract the negative effects these medications have on wound repair.[19]

After surgery it also is important to monitor the mucocutaneous suture line and to notify the surgeon of any breakdown. Erythema or induration at the mucocutaneous junction often precedes separation. A suggested procedure for managing this complication is discussed in Chapter 2.

## Prolapse

Prolapse may complicate any abdominal stoma but occurs more frequently in loop stomas than in end stomas. In a loop stoma the prolapse may develop in either the distal or proximal segments, but it occurs more frequently in the distal portion of the bowel.[23,35] The prolapse is a telescoping of the bowel out through the stoma (Plates 16 and 17).

A number of etiologic factors have been cited for prolapses, including the following[16,23,31]: (1) an excessively large opening in the abdominal wall, which may be a result of surgical technique or an edematous bowel at the time of stoma construction; (2) inadequate fixation of the bowel to the abdominal wall; (3) poorly developed fascial support (such as with infants); and (4) increased abdominal pressure associated with tumors or resulting from coughing or crying (particulary in infants).

**Nursing Interventions.** Prolapse may require surgical intervention or may be managed conservatively. Surgical correction is required for prolapse complicated by ischemia or bowel obstruction or for prolapse that is recurrent or severe. Surgical correction may consist of excising the bowel from surrounding tissue to the fascial level or to the level of the peritoneum, removing the excess length, and then recreating the stoma.[23] A progressive prolapse requires a laparotomy, then resuturing of the mesentery to the bowel wall, the peritoneum, and the fascia. A prolapsed loop colostomy may be converted to an end stoma and a mucous fistula.

Mild prolapse not associated with ischemia or obstruction usually is managed conservatively. Conservative management sometimes is preferred for the patient who has a viable, nonobstructed stoma and who may be a poor surgical candidate, as well as for the patient with a temporary stoma that is prolapsed. In many instances the prolapse can be reduced by having the patient lie down (this reduces the intraabdominal pressure), then applying gentle, continuous pressure against the most distal portion of the stoma, thus returning the bowel to its intraperitoneal place. If the bowel is edematous, cold compresses may be used to alleviate the edema, thus facilitating reduction of the prolapse. Once the prolapse has been reduced, support over the stoma must be applied to prevent recurrence (such as with an abdominal binder or prolapse belt).

When a prolapse is managed conservatively, the patient requires emotional support, education, and frequent reevaluation of his or her management routine. Patients may be repulsed by the appearance of the prolapsed stoma and the associated management difficulties.

Because the prolapsed stoma extends into the pouch and increases in diameter, the patient's pouching technique and equipment must be reevaluated. Ill-fitting equipment may rub the mucosal surface, resulting in bleeding, mechanical trauma, interference with the pouch seal, and the development of irritant contact dermatitis. Two-piece equipment must be used cautiously to prevent a segment of the bowel from becoming pinched between the securing devices. Faceplates and convex inserts also should be used cautiously because the stoma may rub against the protruding lip of the equipment.

Complications such as ischemia or abdominal pain suggest an incarcerated bowel (stoma) and must be reported to the surgeon (Plate 14). Immediate surgical intervention usually is required.

## Retraction

A retracted stoma frequently causes management problems because of the difficulty in obtaining and maintaining a pouch seal (Plates 14 and 18). Retraction may be caused by any of the following: (1) excessive scar formation (such as with a mucocutaneous separation, a necrotic stoma, or chronic peristomal skin infections), (2) surgical technique (insufficient mobilization of the mesentery or excessive tension on the suture line at the fascial layer), (3) premature removal of the support device for loop stoma, and (4) weight gain.[31] Obesity, radiation damage to the bowel and mesentery, and recurrent malignancies all make it technically difficult (if not impossible) to mobilize the bowel and mesentery to create a healthy and tension-free stoma.

**Nursing Interventions.** Because stomal necrosis and mucocutaneous separation often precede stomal retraction, stomas developing these complications in the immediate postoperative period should be monitored for retraction. Circumferential mucocutaneous separation concurrent with stomal retraction below the fascia constitutes a surgical emergency.

Stomal retraction is primarily a nursing management problem. Retraction can consist of retraction of the entire stoma, resulting in a concave defect in the abdomen, where the stoma is located (Plate 14). Retraction also may be limited to the mucocutaneous junction; appropriate stomal protrusion is usually present (Plate 18). The patient should be assessed for retraction in the sitting position before hospital discharge and at every outpatient appointment. Pouching options for retracted stomas are discussed in Chapter 2 and include use of convexity, support belts and binders, and customized reusable faceplates, depending on the severity of the retraction.

Convexity (with belts, inserts, or faceplates) is essential to maintain an adequate seal and prevent undermining. Barrier pastes also can be used to fill small indentations.

There has been a tendency to avoid the use of custom-made, reusable faceplates in recent years, but these are an excellent choice for the patient because they are a one-step item rather than one with multiple inserts in flanges, which often involve overuse of pastes, adhesives, and "build-up" procedures and are not "user friendly" for many patients.

If pouching modifications do not provide a secure pouch seal, the patient should be referred for surgical evaluation and possible surgical revision of the stoma. Surgical revision can sometimes be accomplished by making an incision around the stoma, dissecting down to the fascial layer, and advancing the bowel sufficiently to create a stoma without tension. More frequently a laparotomy is required to provide sufficient mobilization of the bowel and mesentery. It must be realized that surgical revision does not produce a more manageable stoma unless the conditions causing the retraction have been corrected.

## Stenosis

Stenosis is a narrowing of the lumen of an ostomy and typically occurs at either the fascial or cutaneous level (Plates 19 and 20). Stenosis that occurs early in the postoperative period can be a result of inadequate suturing of the fascial layer, inadequate excision of the skin during the construction of the stoma, or a mucocutaneous separation.[2,16] It may also result from serositis or edema that results when the stoma is not matured primarily. Newer surgical techniques, however, specifically the Brooke eversion technique, have reduced the incidence of this complication.

Stenosis that develops later may be caused by disease (Crohn's disease or tumor), excessive scar tissue formation at the skin or fascial level that commonly occurs with repeated instrumentation (dilation) of the stoma, trauma resulting from improperly fitting equipment, pseudoverrucous lesions (hyperplasia), or chronic irritant dermatitis of the peristomal skin.[2] Urinary conduit stenosis may develop as a result of chronic inflammation caused by alkaline urine and prior irradiation of the bowel segment.[33,34]

---

## SIGNS AND SYMPTOMS OF PARTIAL STOMAL OBSTRUCTION

**DESCENDING OR SIGMOID COLOSTOMY**
Abdominal cramps
Explosive passage of stool
Excessive flatus
Narrowed caliber of stool
Episodes of diarrhea

**ILEOSTOMY**
Abdominal cramps
Episodes of nausea

Diarrhea
Stool passed from stoma in projectile
   fashion

**URINARY CONDUIT**
Recurring urinary tract infections
Urine passed from stoma in projectile
   fashion
High residuals of urine in conduit
Decreased urinary output
Flank pain

---

**Nursing Interventions.** The main focus of nursing care is to minimize risk factors that contribute to stenosis development. Preventive measures include maintenance of a secure pouch seal to prevent peristomal skin breakdown, urine acidification measures, and prompt treatment of epithelial "hyperplasia," as well as avoidance of daily stoma dilation.

Surveillance for the development of stenosis is another important nursing responsibility, particularly with patients who have had stomal necrosis, weight gain, or a mucocutaneous junction separation. Pouching equipment should be removed when patients return to the outpatient area so that a careful assessment of the stoma can be made. A digital examination should always be performed. The patient should be questioned regarding symptoms of partial obstruction (see the box above).

The patient with severe stomal stenosis should be referred for surgical evaluation. Surgical revision usually is required for any patient with stenosis that produces partial obstruction. Stenosis at the skin level frequently can be corrected by administering local anesthesia and then excising the peristomal skin and resuturing the stoma to the peristomal skin. Stenosis at the fascial level may require a laparotomy. The person with a urinary conduit may require reconstruction of the conduit if extensive narrowing is present; when a small area is involved, the stenotic area only may be resected.

## Laceration

Stomal lacerations develop most often as a result of pouching technique; they may also develop in conjunction with trauma such as a car accident. Although lacerations may be severe enough to penetrate through the bowel wall, they are most often quite shallow. Because the stoma does not contain nerve endings, the patient generally does not have pain with the laceration. A laceration is usually a yellow to white linear discoloration in the stomal mucosa (Plate 21). Bleeding may be present; the patient often reports the presence of fresh blood in the pouch and no clear reason for the bleeding.

**Nursing Interventions.** A stomal laceration is diagnosed during close visual inspection of the stoma. However, because a stomal laceration is typically a secondary problem (i.e., the patient is primarily seeking assistance because of such things as stomal bleeding, pouch leakage, or peristomal skin denudation), it is a complication that may be overlooked. Stomal laceration frequently is associated with other complications such as hernia and prolapse.

Treatment of a stomal laceration is simply to identify and eliminate the factor causing the laceration. Typically the pouch is sized too small, or a generously protruding stoma (Fig. 2-1) rubs against a rim such as a flange or a convex insert. Occasionally, altering clothing (such as tight-fitting jeans) may be necessary because of the excessive pressure being exerted against the stoma and, ultimately, the pouching equipment. Hemostatic measures (such as silver nitrate) are seldom necessary to control bleeding. Once the causative agent is eliminated, the laceration heals spontaneously and symptoms cease.

## SUMMARY

Stomal and peristomal complications can be the result of surgical techniques, disease processes, medical management, or patient self-care practices.[49] Effective nursing care must be directed toward recognizing and understanding these complications, as well as initiating early interventions and teaching patients and other nurses. Patients must be examined periodically to identify and correct techniques that may place them at risk for the developement of complications. Once complications develop, close surveillance (daily, weekly, or biweekly) is essential to monitor the status of the complication and the effectiveness of interventions.

## SELF-EVALUATION

### QUESTIONS

1. Which of the following may develop in the patient with impaired portal blood flow?
   a. Dermatomyositis
   b. Caput medusae
   c. Mycosis fungoides
   d. Malignancy
2. Folliculitis may develop in the peristomal area as a result of:
   a. Yeast
   b. *Candida*
   c. Shaving
   d. Psoriasis
3. In the ostomy patient an oversized aperture in a urinary pouch may cause predisposition to:
   a. Prolapse
   b. Hernia
   c. Pseudoverrucous lesions
   d. Mucocutaneous separation
4. The patient with multiple areas of tumor growth in the peristomal area may require what type of ostomy equipment?
5. Denuded skin resulting from incorrect removal of an ostomy pouch is an example of:
   a. Irritant dermatitis
   b. Allergic dermatitis
   c. Mechanical trauma
   d. Dermatomyositis
6. Describe mucosal transplantation and the reason it may develop.
7. When skin testing an ostomy product, it should be placed on the:
   a. Forearm
   b. Inner thigh
   c. Abdominal surface
   d. All of above
8. A peristomal irritant dermatitis results from:
   a. Allergic sensitization
   b. Failure to allow a skin sealant to dry properly
   c. Shaving peristomal skin
   d. Using a belt to secure the pouch
9. Melanosis coli develops as a result of long-term use of:
   a. Antacids
   b. Antihistamines
   c. Anthracene-containing laxatives
   d. Bulk-forming laxatives

10. The patient with a colostomy and a peristomal hernia may be instructed to do all of the following except:
    a. Wear a girdle or a support belt
    b. Restrict lifting activities
    c. Increase the volume and velocity of irrigant
    d. Delete the irrigation procedure

11. A prolapse may develop as a result of:
    a. Bowel edema with an oversized abdominal exit site
    b. Rigid appliances that are held in place with tight belts
    c. Chronic peristomal dermatitis
    d. Forceful colostomy irrigations

12. The portion of a loop stoma most likely to prolapse is:
    a. Proximal loop of bowel
    b. Distal loop of bowel
    c. Both bowel segments are equally vulnerable
    d. Common on end stomas only

13. The patient with an ischemic colostomy should be monitored closely for which of the following?
    a. Mucocutaneous separation
    b. Hernia
    c. Prolapse
    d. Laceration

14. Mycosis fungoides is:
    a. An unusual colon cancer
    b. An irritant dermatitis
    c. Herpesvirus
    d. Cutaneous T-cell lymphoma

# SELF-EVALUATION

**ANSWERS**

1. **b.** Caput medusae
2. **c.** Shaving
3. **c.** Pseudoverrucous lesions
4. Flexible equipment that conforms to the area on an uneven abdominal surface
5. **c.** Mechanical trauma
6. Mucosal transplantation is thought to be the seeding of mucosa onto the epidermis as a result of suturing the bowel to the epidermis instead of the dermis.
7. **c.** Abdominal surface
8. **b.** Failure to allow a skin sealant to dry properly
9. **c.** Arthracene-containing laxatives
10. **c.** Increase the volume and velocity of irrigant
11. **a.** Bowel edema with an oversized abdominal exit site
12. **b.** Distal loop of bowel
13. **a.** Mucocutaneous separation
14. **d.** Cutaneous T-cell lymphoma

## REFERENCES

1. Abrams JS: *Abdominal stomas: indications for operative techniques and patient care*, Boston, 1984, PSG Publishing.
2. Allen-Mersh TG, Thomson JPS: Surgical treatment of colostomy complications, *Br J Surg* 75:416, 1988.
3. Alterescu V: Stoma lacerations, *J Enterostom Ther* 12:217, 1985.
4. Arnold HL, Odom RB, James WD, editors: *Andrews' diseases of the skin*, ed 8, Philadelphia, 1990, WB Saunders.
5. Baciewicz F et al: Adenocarcinoma of an ileostomy site with skin invasion, *Gastroenterology* 84:168, 1983.
6. Beck MH et al: Allergic contact dermatitis to epoxy resin ostomy bags, *Br J Surg* 72:202, 1985.
7. Bergman B et al: Chronic papillomatous dermatitis as a pertistomal complication in conduit urinary diversion, *Scand J Urol Nephrol* 13:201, 1979.
8. Bergman B, Löwhagen GB, Mobacken H: Irritant skin reactions to urostomal adhesives, *Urol Res* 10:153, 1982.
9. Blake DP, Scheithauer BW, van Haerden JA: Metastasis to a Brooke ileostomy: an unusual cause of stomal dysfunction, *Dis Colon Rectum* 24:644, 1981.
10. Borglund E, Nordström GM, Nyman CR: Classification of peristomal skin changes in patients with urostomy, *J Am Acad Dermatol* 19:623, 1988.
11. Broadwell DC: Peristomal skin integrity, *Nurs Clin North Am* 2:321, 1987.
12. Brockos HL, Willard JH, Bank J: Melanosis coli: the etiologic significance of the anthracene laxatives: a report of 41 cases, *JAMA* 101:1, 1933.
13. Brunsting LA et al: Pyoderma (ecthyma) gangrenosum: clinical and experimental observations in five cases occurring in adults, *Arch Dermatol* 22:655, 1930.
14. Celestin LR: *A color atlas of the surgery and management of intestinal stomas*, St Louis, 1987, Mosby–Year Book.
15. Colwell JC: Karaya sensitivity, *J Enterostom Ther* 11:159, 1984.
16. Corman ML: *Colon and rectal surgery*, ed 2, Philadelphia, 1989, JB Lippincott.
17. Cuttino C: Pyoderma gangrenosum: an innovative wound care protocol, *J Enterostom Ther* 14:216, 1987.
18. Davis MG: Contact dermatitis from an ostomy deodorant, *Contact Dermatitis* 4:11, 1978.
19. Doughty DB: Principles of wound healing and wound management. In Bryant R, editor: A*cute and chronic wounds: nursing management*, St Louis, 1992, Mosby–Year Book.
20. Edelsow RL: Cutaneous T-cell lymphoma. In Fitzpatrick TB et al, editors: *Update: dermatology in general medicine*, New York, 1983, McGraw-Hill.
21. Finkel SI, Janowitz, HD: Trauma and the pyoderma gangrenosum of inflammatory bowel disease, *Gut* 22:410, 1981.
22. Gergold BS, Januzzi JL: Paracolostomy carcinoma, *Am J Proctol Gastroenterol Colon Rectum Surg* 35:9, 1984.
23. Gershenson DM, Smith DB: Enteric diversions. In Smith DB, Johnson DG, editors: *Ostomy care and the cancer patient*, Orlando, Fla, 1986, Grune & Stratton.
24. Gilyon K, Kuzel TM: Cutaneous T-cell lymphoma, *Oncol Nurs Forum* 18:901, 1981.
25. Goldstein WZ, Edoga J, Crystal R: Management of colostomal hemorrage resulting from portal hypertension, *Dis Colon Rectum* 26:86, 1980.
26. Goode PS: Nursing management of disorders of the gastrointestinal system. In Broadwell DC, Jackson BS: *Principles of ostomy care*, St Louis, 1982, Mosby–Year Book.
27. Graeber GM, Ratner MH, Ackerman NB: Massive hemorrhage from ileostomy and colostomy stomas due to mucocutaneous varices in patients with coexisting cirrhosis, *Surgery* 79:107, 1976.
28. Greenstein AJ, Janowitz HD, Sachar DB: The extra-intestinal complications of Crohn's disease and ulcerative colitis: a study of 700 patients, *Medicine*, 55:401, 1976.
29. Habif TP: *Clinical dermatology: a color guide to diagnosis and therapy*, ed 2, St Louis, 1990, Mosby–Year Book.
30. Hesterberg R, Stahlknecht CD, Roher H: Sclerotherapy for massive enterostomy bleeding resulting from portal hypertension, *Dis Colon Rectum* 29:275, 1986.

31. Hill HL: *Ileostomy: surgery, physiology and management,* New York, 1976, Grune & Stratton.
32. Jeter KF: Hyperplasia or what? *J Enterostom Ther* 10:181, 1983.
33. Johnson DG, Smith DB: Urinary diversions. In Smith DB, Johnson DG, editors: *Ostomy care and the cancer patient,* Orlando, Fla, 1986, Grune & Stratton.
34. Johnson J et al: Special problems posed by cancer treatments. In Smith DB, Johnson DG, editors: *Ostomy care and the cancer patient,* Orlando, Fla, 1986, Grune & Stratton.
35. Kodner IJ: Colostomy and ileostomy, *Clin Symp* 30:2, 1978.
36. Kretschmer K: *The intestinal stoma,* Philadelphia, 1975, WB Saunders.
37. Landman LA, Ramos-Wilson O: Patch testing, *J Enterostom Ther* 16:131, 1989.
38. Last M et al: Conservative management of paraileostomy ulcers in patients with Crohn's disease, *Dis Colon Rectum* 27:779, 1984.
39. Lipman S: Koebner reaction: colostomy bag, *Int Psor Bull* 8:5, 1985.
40. Lo RK, Johnson DT, Smith DB: Massive bleeding from an ileal conduit caput medusae, *J Urol* 131:114, 1984.
41. Mann RJ, Stewart E, Peachey RDG: Sensitivity to urostomy pouch plastic, *Contact Dermatitis* 9:80, 1983.
42. Martin PJ, Spratt JS: Stomas and their care. In Spratt JS, editor: *Neoplasms of the colon and rectum,* Philadelphia, 1984, WB Saunders.
43. McGarity, WC, Robertson DB, McKeown PP: Pyoderma gangrenosum at the parastomal site in patients with Crohn's disease, *Arch Surg* 119:1186, 1984.
44. Nordström GM, Borglund E, Nyman CR: Local status of the urinary stoma: the relation to peristomal skin complications, *Scand J Urol Nephrol* 24:117, 1990.
45. Polano MK: A case of cutaneous ameebiosis, *Dermatologica* 151:253, 1975.
46. Roberts L et al: Bleeding stomal varices, *Dis Colon Rectum* 33:547, 1990.
47. Rodriguez, DB: Treatment for three ostomy patients with systemic skin disorders: psoriasis, pemphigus, and dermatomyositis, *J Enterostom Ther* 8:31, 1981.
48. Rothstein MS: Dermatologic considerations of stoma care, *J Am Acad Dermatol* 15:411, 1986.
49. Rowbotham JL: Managing colostomies, *CA* 31:6, 1981.
50. Sauer GC: *Manual of skin diseases,* ed 5, Philadelphia, 1985, JB Lippincott.
51. Schoetz DJ, Coller JA, Veidenheimer MC: Pyoderma gangrenosum and Crohn's disease: eight cases and a review of the literature, *Dis Colon Rectum* 26:155, 1983.
52. Sjodahl K, Anderberg B, Bolin T: Parastomal hernia in relation to site of the abdominal stoma, *Br J Surg* 75:334, 1988.
53. Smith DB: Multiple stomas, fistulas, and draining wounds. In Smith DB, Johnson DG, editors: *Ostomy care and the cancer patient,* Orlando, Fla, 1986, Grune & Stratton.
54. Reference deleted in proofs.
55. Storey V: Persistent peristomal skin reaction: a case of psoriasis, *J Enterostom Ther* 9:63, 1982.
56. Thayer WR, Denusa T: Miscellaneous diseases of the large bowel and anal canal. In Kirsner JB, Shorter RG, editors: *Diseases of the colon, rectum, and anal canal,* Baltimore, 1988, Williams & Wilkins.
57. Tucker SB, Smith DB: Dermatologic conditions and complication ostomy care. In Smith DB, Johnson DG, editors: *Ostomy care and the cancer patient,* Orlando, Fla, 1986, Grune & Stratton.
58. van Ketel WG, van de Burg CKH, de Haan P: Sensitization to expoxy resin from an ileostomy bag, *Contact Dermatitis* 9:516, 1983.
59. Reference deleted in proofs.
60. Williams S: Recognizing peristomal pyoderma gangrenosum, *J Enterostom Ther* 11:77, 1984.
61. Williams SG, Halpin-Landry JE: Caring for the person with a stoma and systemic lupus erythematous, *J Enterostom Ther* 17:128, 1990.
62. Wilson CB: Phycomycotic gangrenous cellulitis, *Arch Surg* 111:532, 1976.
63. Wolf K, Stingl G: Pyoderma gangrenosum. In Fitzpatrick TB et al, editors: *Update: dermatology in general medicine,* New York, 1983, McGraw-Hill.
64. Wright NE: Caput medusae in portal hypertension, *J Enterostom Ther* 8:17, 1981.

# 4 Continent Diversions and Reservoirs

BONNIE SUE ROLSTAD
KATHRYN HOYMAN

## OBJECTIVES

1. Describe the historical development of continent reservoirs.

2. Describe the anatomic structures and bowel segments used to create continent diversions and reservoirs.

3. Identify the criteria for patient selection with the following procedures:
   a. Ileoanal reservoir
   b. Kock continent ileostomy
   c. Kock urinary reservoir
   d. Ileocecal urinary reservoir

4. Compare and contrast the perioperative and discharge planning needs of the patient with a continent reservoir.

5. Identify complications associated with each type of continent reservoir.

6. Discuss patient teaching information that should be included for the person who will have or has had a continent diversion or reservoir.

Some life-saving surgeries result in the necessity to establish permanent stomas; this outcome has an undeniable physical and emotional effect on the patient's life. For these patients the presence of the stoma and external pouching system may be lifelong reminders of the societal stigmas regarding elimination. The need to provide long-term physical and emotional support for many of these patients also has resulted in significant costs for the health care system. Although most patients with permanent stomas adjust well, complications that include peristomal skin irritation, pouching system dysfunction, stoma problems, renal deterioration (in patients with a urinary diversion), social inhibition, depression, and sexual dysfunction also have been reported.*

The underlying issue is continence: the ability to control and evacuate feces, flatus, or urine at socially acceptable times and places. In fecal continence the definition extends to being able also to distinguish between gas and stool. Surgeries resulting in traditional abdominal stomas render the patient incontinent. The use of a pouching system provides a measure of continence or control over elimination. Even infrequent leakage and odor, however, are frank reminders of underlying incontinence.

The quest for fecal and urinary continence has resulted in numerous and varied continent diversion techniques. A better understanding of physiology, improved technical skills, and advances in technology have resulted in improved procedures for continent diversions, some of which are performed routinely today. These procedures continue to evolve because of research and surgical refinements.

This chapter focuses on the most frequently performed continent diversions: construction, perioperative issues, complications, and anticipated outcomes. Discussion is limited to continent diversions that employ the use of reservoirs, with or without cutaneous stomas.

In the strictest sense, continent diversions could include any diversion of the urinary or fecal stream that provides a mechanism for containing effluent within the body. This definition includes cutaneous stomas without reservoirs, which provide continence because of passive or active implanted devices used to occlude the stoma. Examples of these procedures include the sigmoid colostomy, with an implantable sphincter prosthesis, and the continent ostomy valve, which occludes the opening of a conventional or continent ileostomy. Conservative occlusion may be obtained through use of a plugging device (e.g., Conseal plug or Conseal colostomy system, (Colorplast, Inc., Tampa, Florida). Most of the aforementioned surgical approaches are considered experimental in the United States and are used only infrequently.

Interest in continent diversions originates from patients and the health care professionals caring for them. In a 1985 study[65] from the Mayo Clinic, 40% of 675 patients with Brooke ileostomies who were aware of alternatives to permanent stomas stated that they desired or would consider a change. The authors concluded that regardless of the success these patients had with the ileostomies, there remains a need to be continent. Research in this area also has been motivated by the prolonged survival of these patients. With operative survival routine and cure of cancer common, patients are living longer and therefore are willing to have a type of surgery that promises a more "natural" result. That is, patients no longer are universally grateful to be alive; they also seek an improved quality of life.

As with all newer procedures, a collaborative approach among knowledgeable caregivers is essential. The health care team needs to share an appreciation of the technical, educative, and emotional components of rehabilitation. The nurse who specializes in the care of ostomy patients collaborates to develop and provide education for all the caregivers involved. Large medical centers generally are the preferred providers of continent diversion surgeries because of their expertise in performing the procedures, in managing complications, and in providing long-term follow-up. The counseling role of the nurse is particularly important during the care of patients with continent diversions. Because many of these patients have endured long-term illness, the anticipated fears, concerns, and anxieties related to surgery may be intensified. The new surgical techniques recommended to these patients may make them feel isolated and unique. Further, these feelings may be height-

---

*References 8, 17, 24, 28, 45, 66, 71, and 87.

ened when the patient realizes that most health care providers are not acquainted with the surgery. Nursing interventions that may help these patients are discussed in Chapter 1; in addition, an excellent resource and source of support are persons who have recuperated from a similar surgery. Even patient visitors who have had complications with their surgery may be reassuring because they are reminders that successful rehabilitation after complications is possible. For example, in response to patients' needs, support and education groups for persons with ileoanal reservoirs are being developed in various parts of the United States.

Ethical issues relative to informed consent are major considerations with any new surgical procedure. Thorough education and opportunities for follow-up during the decision-making phase are essential to patient understanding. All appropriate surgical options should be discussed with the patient, including perioperative care, potential complications, and anticipated outcomes. Anticipated outcomes of traditional surgical approaches should be compared with those of continent diversions in order to provide a reference point for the patient. For example, in a discussion of the Kock urinary reservoir the potential outcomes of the traditional ileal conduit should be compared and explained. The final decision to have a continent diversion rests with the patient.

Successful outcomes begin with preoperative assessment and planning. Patient assessments are similar to those reviewed in Chapter 1. With continent diversions the emphasis is placed on assessment of patient motivation and ability to master self-care skills. Highly motivated patients usually are more compliant and tend to participate in postoperative problem solving. However, it is the responsibility of the physician and nurse in the preoperative period to be certain that the patient has an accurate understanding of anticipated outcomes. Self-care procedures are not necessarily more difficult than those involved with caring for an external pouching system, but they may require more time and attention. For this reason the continent diversion that requires intubation may be contraindicated if the patient, because of poor vision or disabling arthritis, must rely on a caregiver to perform intubations. When intubation is required, patients themselves should be responsible for intubating their continent diversion; significant others, who commonly may have the same anxieties as the patient, are included in teaching sessions with the physician and nurse.[47,80]

## INTESTINAL CONTINENT DIVERSIONS

Major advances in small-bowel, colon, and rectal surgery in the past 50 years have greatly affected surgical options for patients with chronic ulcerative colitis and familial adenomatous polyposis (FAP). Two surgical alternatives to a permanent stoma that result in continent diversions are the ileoanal reservoir (IAR) (also referred to as restorative proctocolectomy, ileal pouch–anal anastomosis, or pelvic pouch) and the Kock continent ileostomy.

### Indications

Many factors must be considered for a patient to be eligible for an IAR or a Kock continent ileostomy. Diagnosis and clinical course of the disease are considered first. These procedures are universally accepted as appropriate for chronic ulcerative colitis and FAP. The patient with chronic ulcerative colitis may require an emergency surgical procedure (because of free perforation, massive hemorrhage, or toxic megacolon) or, more commonly, an elective or urgent procedure (because of intractable disease). Because persons with FAP and long-standing pancolitis (10 years or more) are at an increased risk for the development of cancer,[57] they are also candidates for this type of surgery. Therefore the IAR and Kock continent ileostomy are also indicated to manage the risk of carcinoma of the colon and rectum in these patients. Occasionally, patients have total colectomy to control some of the extracolonic complications associated with ulcerative colitis, such as pyoderma gangrenosum, uveitis, and periarteritis nodosa.[91,92] Extracolonic manifestations of FAP are unaffected by colon resection.

Whether continent diversions are appropriate in the patient with Crohn's disease continues to be debated. Because Crohn's disease is a transmural disease that can involve any or all of the gastrointestinal tract and is associated with a high rate of recurrence after surgery, the risk of recurrence in the remaining small bowel may result in the need for further resection, leading to possible short-bowel syndrome.[79] Crohn's disease can be difficult to identify; undifferentiated colitis occurs in approximately 10% to 15% of patients with inflammatory bowel disease.[34] In the patient with Crohn's disease who is misdiagnosed and has an IAR, for example, complications such as fisulta-in-ano, rectovaginal fistula, or sepsis may develop and often necessitate ileoanal pouch excision.[7,27,76] Although some patients with Crohn's disease who have had lengthy remissions have had a Kock continent ileostomy constructed,[25] results of long-term research on these patients are not available.

After consideration of diagnosis and clinical course of the disease, other patient selection criteria include absence of concomitant carcinoma of the colon, patient motivation and compliance, emotional stability, and the patient's ability to make an informed decision. Anorectal continence is imperative when patients are considering an IAR, and preoperative anal manometry may be necessary. Relative contraindications either to the Kock continent ileostomy or to the IAR are obesity and age. Most commonly these procedures are performed in young patients (between 20 and 45 years of age). Although the decision regarding surgical alternatives is individualized, patients over 50 years of age require careful evaluation.

The decision concerning which type of surgical procedure to perform in a patient with chronic ulcerative colitis or FAP ultimately rests with the patient and physician (see Table 11-1 for a comparison of gastrointestinal surgical procedures). Preservation of the anus and rectum, when possible, is a priority.

The restorative IAR is an option for patients that accomplishes preservation of essential continence-related structures and removal of disease. If the IAR fails, a continent ileostomy or Brooke ileostomy may then be performed. An IAR, however, cannot be constructed once the anus and rectum have been removed (such as with a total proctocolectomy). In this situation a Brooke ileostomy may be converted to a continent ileostomy.[4,58]

## Ileoanal Reservoir

**Historical Evolution.** The evolution of the IAR is linked to the Kock continent ileostomy because one component of the IAR is an ileal reservoir similar to that devised by Kock. Two concepts guided the development of the IAR. (1) Anal continence could be preserved after rectal mucosal stripping and ileoanal anastomosis, and (2) anal continence could be enhanced through addition of an ileal reservoir.[93]

Restorative procedures originated with ileoanal pull-through procedures, first reported in 1933 by Nissen.[61] However, the prototype of the ileoanal anastomosis was pioneered in the late 1940s by Ravitch and Sabiston,[68] who performed rectal mucosal stripping in dogs in conjunction with a total colectomy and anastomosis of the distal ileum to the anus. In the years after this report, other researchers performed similar procedures in patients with chronic ulcerative colitis and FAP, with successful maintenance of continence.[20,89] The reported failure rate was 40%, resulting from stool frequency, perianal skin denudation, and perianal sepsis.

In 1964, Soave[82] and Boley[10] simultaneously reported use of a coloanal pull-through procedure for the treatment of Hirschsprung's disease (see Fig. 10-3). In 1977, Martin, LeCoultre, and Schubert[54] reported satisfactory results with 15 of 17 young patients with ulcerative colitis using the pull-through technique. After these findings numerous researchers reported on the straight ileoanal anastomosis.[5,34,85] Whereas it appeared that children did quite well with the straight ileoanal procedure, adults had ongoing problems associated with frequent stools and incontinence.[84]

In 1955, Valiente and Bacon[89] proposed a triple-limb ileal pouch to increase capacity and decrease stool frequency. Karlan, McPherson, and Watman,[43] in 1959, demonstrated the efficacy of a double ileal isoperistaltic pouch to enhance continence, but it was not until the pioneering work of Kock[48] in 1969 and use of the continent ileostomy in the following decade that the efficacy of a continent ileal reservoir was actually established. In addition to these developments, increasing knowledge of anorectal physiology ultimately led Parks and Nicholls[63] in 1978 to combine the two concepts of ileoanal anastomosis and continent ileal reservoir construction. The result was a total proctocolectomy with rectal mucosal stripping and a triple-limb, S-shaped pouch with ileoanal anastomosis as shown in Fig. 4-1. In 1980, Utsunomiya[88] reported a J-shaped pouch design (Fig. 4-2), and Fonkalsrud[29] later reported a lateral reservoir (Fig. 4-3). The W-shaped reservoir and other refinements continue to be reported.[46,60] Today the most frequent type of reservoir configuration is J or S shaped.

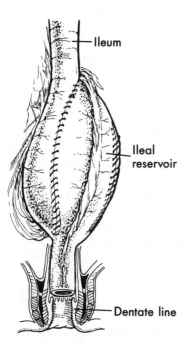

**Fig. 4-1** S-shaped configuration for IAR. Three 10-cm limbs of ileum are used, antimesenteric surface of each limb opened, and adjacent bowel walls anastomosed.

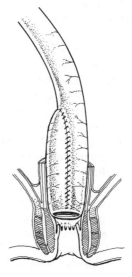

**Fig. 4-2** J-shaped configuration for IAR. Distal ileum is aligned in J shape; antimesenteric surface of J shape is opened, and adjacent bowel walls anastomosed. Side-to-end anastomosis of bowel to dentate line is evident.

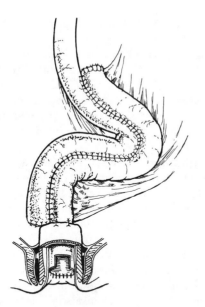

**Fig. 4-3** Lateral or side-by-side ileoanal pouch configuration.

**Preoperative Considerations.** A lengthy recovery period is associated with construction of an ileoanal reservoir. These patients frequently require two surgical procedures performed approximately 8 to 12 weeks apart. The initial procedure (stage 1) is a major operation and typically includes colectomy, rectal mucosectomy, ileal reservoir construction, ileoanal anastomosis, and temporary ileostomy (end or loop). The second surgery (stage 2) is less extensive and involves closure of the ileostomy (takedown), which then functionalizes the reservoir. Reservoir adaptation occurs during the subsequent 3 to 6 months, enhancing the patient's ability to control stool.[22] Additional surgery may be required if certain complications develop. Therefore the relationship between the nurse and the patient having an IAR will be long-term. It is important that a therapeutic relationship be established early in the preoperative period so that supportive counsel can be provided on a long-term basis. Teaching materials that illustrate the complex procedure and address the numerous self-care considerations are useful.[70,73] Topics of particular importance for these patients are fecal continence, perianal skin care, reservoir function, fluid and electrolyte maintenance, and ostomy care.

Although the IAR is most often performed in two stages as described previously, it may also be completed in three stages and in one single stage, largely depending on the condition of the patient and surgical expertise. Patients with acute disease who require emergency surgery and patients with chronic disease who do not have access to larger medical centers may be best served with a three-stage approach. In such cases the initial procedure usually involves only the abdominal colectomy with Hartmann's pouch or mucous fistula and a temporary ileostomy; thus the diseased colon is removed, and the fecal stream is diverted. Because anorectal continence structures are left intact, the patient is able to recover from the operation and illness and consider surgical options to be conducted at a later date. Patients then have the opportunity to confer with their physicians, an ET (enterostomal therapy) nurse, a person with an IAR, and a person with an ileostomy.

In carefully selected patients, the surgeon may elect to perform the IAR without an ileostomy, hence a one-stage surgical procedure. Most commonly this option is considered only when the patient (such as the FAP patient) is healthy before surgery or in patients with chronic ulcerative colitis who are healthy and are not receiving corticosteroid therapy.

Regardless of the staging decision, the stoma site must be selected before surgery. The stoma site is marked in the traditional manner, usually in the right lower quadrant of the abdomen, as described in Chapter 1.

### Stage 1 Procedure

*Preoperative preparations.* The technique of IAR is complex and requires an experienced, well-coordinated surgical team. The surgical procedure takes approximately 3 to 4 hours. Preoperative bowel preparation includes a full mechanical preparation of polyethylene glycol (e.g., Golytely or Colyte), which may be modified or omitted depending on the patient's condition. Administration of oral antibiotics is based on physician protocol. If oral antibiotics are used (there is a trend toward omitting preoperative oral antibiotics), neomycin and erythromycin base or neomycin and metronidazole may be drug combinations of choice. Intravenous antibiotic preparations include a second preoperative dose of a second-generation cephalosporin, occasionally with a second dose after surgery. A peripheral or central intravenous catheter and urinary catheter are routinely inserted in the preoperative holding room; a nasogastric tube may be used.

*Operative procedure.* The ileoanal reservoir procedure comprises five basic steps. First, an abdominal colectomy is performed through a midline abdominal incision with the patient in modified lithotomy position. Attention is directed to preserve the hypogastric and parasympathetic nerves so that impotence and bladder dysfunction are avoided. Second, a rectal mucosectomy is performed, which may be accomplished through various techniques. A transanal excision of approximately 4 to 6 cm of the rectal mucosa and submucosa beginning at the dentate line may be undertaken. The extent of the mucosectomy however, is controversial. Some surgeons think that leaving the transitional epithelium intact may improve the patient's sensation.[75] Third, the ileal pouch is designed in an S- or a J-shaped configuration. The S-shaped pouch requires the use of approximately 30 cm of distal ileum (three 10-cm limbs for the pouch with 1 to 2 cm for the spout). Slightly less bowel is used for construction of a J pouch. The length of the mesentery must be sufficient so that the spout can reach the dentate line without tension. The pouch is constructed by opening the antimesenteric surface of the ileum, allowing anastomosis of adjacent walls. Fourth, a pouch-anal anastomosis is performed by lowering the reservoir into the pelvis through the muscle sleeve; anastomosis of the spout and dentate line is then possible. A pelvic drain such as the Jackson Pratt may exit the perineal region or, more commonly, the lower left quadrant of the abdomen. Finally, a temporary end or loop ileostomy is constructed at the premarked site in the lower right quadrant of the abdomen.[76]

*Postoperative care.* Postoperative care includes routine observations for patients who have had major abdominal surgery. In addition, stoma viability, the mucocutaneous juncture, and peristomal skin integrity must be monitored. Output from a traditional ileostomy (i.e., without reservoir construction) in the early postoperative period is 1000 to 1500 ml/24 hr.[65] However, because a more proximal portion of the bowel is used to create the ileostomy in IAR procedures, output initially may be as high as 1500 to 2000 ml/24 hr. Patients are observed for signs of hemorrhage, abdominal abscess, small-bowel obstruction, dehydration, and other related complications. As bowel function returns, the nasogastric tube, if used, is removed and oral intake is instituted. Drainage from the abdominal drain site may vary in amount and character; initially, daily drainage output averages 100 to 150 ml of serosanguineous fluid. Most medical centers do not recommend routine irrigation of this drain, which generally is removed within 2 to 4 days of the operation. The urinary catheter is removed on the second to fifth day after surgery. Systemic antibiotics are discontinued within 24 hours of the operation, and corticosteroids, if used, are tapered.

Occasionally the patient may have the urge to defecate, which is accompanied by mucus discharge. Both these occurrences are normal. The basis for the urge to defecate stems from mucus secretion from the bowel wall (including the reservoir), which eventually causes distention and stimulates the intact anorectal continence mechanisms. The volume and consistency of mucus discharge varies.

Postoperatively the patient also may have transient incontinence. This phenomenon is the result of intraoperative manipulation of the anal canal. With new intraoperative techniques, however, transient incontinence is less common. Before surgery, patients are informed about this possibility and its transient nature; reassurance and a review of the components of continence are helpful to allay anxiety. When transient incontinence occurs, it usually resolves in 4 to 8 weeks or before ileostomy takedown. Kegel exercises are suggested later to strengthen the pelvic floor and sphincter muscles; they are not recommended in the immediate postoperative period.

---

## ILEOANAL RESERVOIR IRRIGATION PROCEDURE

Intubation, irrigation, or both are not routinely performed; they are performed only upon recommendation from the physician or ET nurse. Pouch intubation may be indicated to remove thick mucus, to test continence during sphincter training, to dilute thick stool, and to facilitate stool evacuation through a stricture in the anal canal.

1. Gather supplies:
   Catheter (usually No. 28F Silastic, cut 7 to 8 inches in length)
   Water-soluble lubricant
   60-ml catheter-tipped syringe
   Mild soap
2. If an irrigation is being performed, fill the syringe with 60 ml tepid tap water. Set aside.
3. Lubricate the catheter.
4. Sit on the toilet, and tip to one side to insert the catheter into the anal canal. (Men may prefer to stand with one foot on the toilet seat for easier access to the anal opening.)
5. Gently insert the catheter into the anus, and advance it approximately 3 to 4 inches. If resistance is met, remove the catheter and begin again. A gentle twisting motion may

be helpful. Direct the catheter slightly backward after insertion. Effluent will enter the catheter, signaling entry into the pouch. (If this is the first intubation, remove the catheter and mark with indelible ink or a piece of tape to indicate how far the catheter should be inserted. Some patients will mark the correct spot for holding the catheter and then advance the catheter until the fingers are almost touching the anal skin.)

6. If intubation alone is being performed, allow the contents to drain and remove the catheter. When irrigation is being performed, attach the syringe and instill approximately 60 ml tap water. Remove the catheter and syringe. The Valsalva maneuver may facilitate emptying.
7. Clean the catheter by rinsing it in warm water and washing it with a mild soap. Strong detergents and bleach cause the catheter to become brittle. Allow the catheter to dry. It generally is not necessary to carry the catheter at all times. If needed, however, supplies may be carried in a plastic bag, makeup case, or small shaving kit.

Irrigation of the reservoir may be indicated to remove malodorous mucus and is performed with a No. 28F catheter (such as the Continent Ileo Pouch Catheter, Mentor Corporation, Santa Barbara, California) (see the box on p. 136). The Medena (Möindal, Sweden) and the Ileal Reservoir Catheter (Weber and Judd Drugs, Rochester, Minnesota) also may be used. This procedure should be undertaken only after a radiographic study indicates healed pouch suture lines. Because of new reservoir configurations with shorter outlets, pouch irrigation to remove mucus rarely is indicated.

Perianal skin care should be implemented to protect the epidermis from mucus discharge and maceration. Patients are instructed to gently rinse the skin with water and dry thoroughly with soft tissues immediately after mucus discharge. If preferred, a gentle cleansing solution may be used. When further perianal skin protection is desired, a skin sealant or ointment may be used. Some patients may require a perineal pad or a cotton wad placed at the anal opening to absorb drainage.

The type of ileostomy constructed during this procedure may be loop or end; currently the most frequently performed is the loop. A loop ileostomy presents a pouching challenge because it frequently bows inferiorly or retracts, resulting in effluent contact with the skin and denudation. Pouching systems with minimal to moderate convexity are indicated in these cases. Because the distal segment of the loop (the mucous fistula) secretes mucus, the pouch aperture must clear the mucous fistula opening. Maintaining intact peristomal skin also is difficult when the mucous fistula is at skin level. If a supporting device is used under the loop ileostomy, it may be removed on the fifth to seventh postoperative day. A fascial bridge often is preferred to secure the stoma because no external devices are required. The preceding discussion illustrates that it may be preferable to construct temporary stomas with the distal limb closed and anchored within the subcutaneous tissue[72,92] (see Fig. 11-2).

Before the patient is discharged from the hospital, self-care instructions are reviewed and written information is provided. Critical content specific to the patient with an IAR includes the following material:

1. Measures to maintain fluid-electrolyte balance and hydration. Fluid intake of 10 to 12 (240 ml) 8-ounce glasses daily is recommended to replace fluid lost in ileal output. A normally functioning, established ileostomy excretes about 500 ml of water and 60 mEq of sodium per day, which represents two to three times the amount found in the feces of individuals with intact colons. Primary potassium depletion is uncommon; when it occurs, it is secondary to sodium depletion.[38] As previously stated, a newly constructed, "high" ileostomy (such as with the IAR) may discharge 1500 to 2000 ml/24 hr. Therefore increased intake of fluids and salt is required. Patients are encouraged to salt foods liberally and to respond to thirst. Patients also may be encouraged to drink fluids that contain electrolytes, such as Gatorade.

2. Measures to prevent food blockage. Conservative dietary guidelines include continuing a soft diet for 2 weeks after hospitalization, with a gradual increase in fiber content. As with traditional ileostomies, high-fiber foods are identified as potential causes of small-bowel obstruction. Patients are instructed to limit high-fiber foods, to add new foods to the diet one at a time, and to ingest food in small quantities (six small meals per day). Chewing well and drinking fluids also are recommended when eating fibrous foods.

3. Measure to prevent peristomal or incisional hernia. Restricting lifting to no more than 5 pounds during the initial 4 weeks after surgery is recommended to avoid abdominal tension that could result in a hernia.

4. Measures to increase stamina and resume normal activities of living. Patients are encouraged to walk daily for exercise and to avoid activities that strain abdominal muscles. Sexual activity may be resumed when strength returns. Anal sex, however, is contraindicated, as are enema tips, suppositories, and catheters that have not been recommended by the physician or ET nurse. Self-care instructions pertinent to routine ileostomy care are discussed in Chapter 2.

Outpatient follow-up with the ET nurse is scheduled within 1 to 2 weeks of discharge and within 1 month after the first visit. Follow-up visits focus on evaluation of the pouching system, reinforcement in self-care, and emotional support. Patients who are scheduled for radiographic studies of the reservoir or who may need to perform irrigations are instructed to order a reservoir catheter. Routine irrigations, however, rarely are necessary.

### Stage 2 Procedure

*Preoperative considerations.* Before ileostomy takedown, a radiographic study is performed to ensure that suture lines are healed and to determine the position of the reservoir in the pelvis. This study, which usually takes place 8 to 10 weeks after the original operation, is performed with water-soluble media; often the patient's reservoir catheter is used. If the radiology staff is unfamiliar with the IAR, information about the patient's altered anatomy should be provided. Patient teaching (such as perianal skin care and diet) can be reinforced at this time.

After the radiographic study, Kegel exercises may be instituted. The patient should perform the exercises five to ten times a day, with 20 to 30 repetitions each. Some medical centers suggest that patients instill fluid into the reservoir and then perform Kegel exercises to improve continence. Reservoir irrigation, when used, usually is suggested only once a day during exercises. Irrigation may not be necessary, however, if the patient is able to control mucus output.

Bowel preparation for ileostomy takedown usually includes clear liquids for 24 hours before the operation, an oral cathartic, and an antibiotic administered intravenously. The surgical procedure usually requires approximately 1 hour.

*Postoperative care.* Ileostomy takedown usually requires a 4- to 6-day hospitalization. A nasogastric tube and urinary catheter generally are not required. If, however, evidence of bowel obstruction, dilation, or multiple adhesions occurs, a nasogastric tube may be necessary. Fecal output begins when intestinal peristalsis returns (usually 2 to 3 days); then oral intake is initiated slowly. Stool frequency and urgency typically follow. Therefore prompt, aggressive perianal skin care is necessary.

The key to effective perianal skin protection is to begin early in the postoperative period with a consistent program and effective products and to involve the patient and caregivers. When the reservoir starts functioning, use of skin sealants or moisture barrier preparations must be initiated. Soft tissues are used to avoid mechanical trauma during cleaning. Patients are instructed to moisten tissues with tap water and to dab rather than rub the skin. Hospital toilet paper should *not* be used. Chemicals (e.g., soaps, solvents, and medications) are to be avoided. If perianal skin denudation occurs, a "no-touch" perineal spraying device may be suggested. If a pad becomes necessary, it is instituted early and changed with each staining to avoid continued contact with the skin and the potential for development of maceration and candidiasis.

Patients empty the reservoir spontaneously and may be advised to chart frequency of stool evacuations. After an elective ileostomy takedown, patients usually are clinically healthy and highly motivated to participate in care.

As the diet is advanced, the patient should be cautioned to avoid large meals and high fiber in the diet. These measures help avoid obstructive symptoms brought on by a prolonged ileus or mechanical bowel obstruction. Dietary indiscretions may result in nausea and vomiting and a prolonged hospital stay. Fluid intake of at least 10 to 12 glasses per day is recommended. The patient is informed of the types of food that thicken stool and loosen stool consistently (see the box in Chapter 2, p. 69).

On discharge from the hospital, the patient is given written instructions similar to those given after the stage I procedure, with the exception of ileostomy care. A follow-up appointment with the ET nurse should be arranged for 1 to 2 weeks after hospital discharge.

*Complications.* More than 1000 ileoanal reservoir procedures have been reported from various centers, with rare operative mortality.[60] Overall morbidity rates, however, average from 40% to 50%.[92] A significant factor in this high morbidity rate may be the learning curve inherent in new procedures; in other words, as the procedure becomes more commonplace, morbidity decreases. Current data[93] reflect a decreasing postoperative complication rate. The incidence of major pelvic sepsis is about 5% to 8% in patients with ileoanal reservoir. This complication is potentially devastating, considering that 50% of patients who require laparotomy for treatment of sepsis ultimately require reservoir removal. Septic complications of lesser magnitude include cuff abscess and pouch-anal fistula. Other complications related to ileoanal reservoir include intestinal obstruction, ileoanal stricture, pouchitis, perianal skin denudation, sexual and bladder dysfunction, metabolic complications, stoma complications, and functional failures.[22,92,93]

*Functional results.* Function of the ileoanal reservoir improves with time. Initially patients have frequent (10 to 12 per day) small-volume bowel movements. Bowel movements decrease as solid foods are taken and the reservoir expands. Expansion of the reservoir and increasing capacity are known as adaptation. Information on functional results is similar from one institution to another, even when different configurations of reservoirs have been performed.[6,27,40,93]

In a recent long-term follow-up (16 to 88 months) study the University of Minnesota Hospital and Clinics reported on the functional results in 114 patients.[90] Most patients evacuate spontaneously. A small percentage (8%), however, of S pouches constructed with long pouch outlets (a configuration popular before 1984) require catheterization to evacuate pouch contents. Stool frequency generally stabilizes at approximately six per day, including one at night. Continence usually is complete or nearly complete in 81% of patients; 91% of patients have perfect or near-perfect continence during waking hours, but this decreases to 76% during sleep. Most patients without total stool continence (39% during the day and 57% at night) report pad staining rather than frank incontinence. More than half the patients wear a pad during the day, as well as at night, for "security." Nearly 70% of patients require no dietary modification; those who do modify their diet have few limitations. To modify bowel function, 50% of patients take medications, including loperamide hydrochloride or diphenoxylate hydrochloride and atropine. Patients also use bulking agents such as psyllium hydrophilic mucilloid (21% of patients). As long as 2 years after surgery, patients report improvements in function, such as decreased or absent nocturnal leakage and decreased bowel movements during the day and night.

Before surgery 86% of patients were sexually active. Most report no change or increased levels of sexual activity; 2% report severe limitations or no sexual encounters because of seepage or no partner. No cases of impotence and one case of suspected retrograde ejaculation were reported. Three patients have subsequently become pregnant and delivered successfully by cesarean section. (Vaginal delivery also is an option for reservoir patients.) Most patients have returned to previous employment and educational pursuits.

Ninety-eight percent of patients report no limitations in daily activities. Eighty-one percent state that their social activities are not limited. Those who do have activity limitations report restrictions in activities such as hiking, hunting, and fishing only because of the lack of proximity to a bathroom for several hours.

Thirteen percent of the patients had subsequent permanent ileostomy surgery as a result of pouchitis, Crohn's disease, mesenteric desmoid tumor, postoperative hemorrhage, or pelvic sepsis. No reservoir failures have occurred in this series of patients since 1986. Ninety-five percent of patients, including half of those whose reservoirs ultimately were excised, stated in retrospect that they would again select an ileoanal reservoir over permanent ileostomy.[90]

***Long-term management considerations.*** Fluid and electrolyte imbalance, dehydration, and perianal skin denudation may develop in patients who have frequent bowel movements (i.e., more than six to seven per day). Stool frequency is a result of diet, reservoir function, and reservoir capacity after an ileostomy takedown. As the reservoir expands and adapts, stools decrease in number and bowel activity becomes more predictable. Stool frequency subsequently may increase because of gastroenteritis, diet, pouchitis, mechanical problems, and unidentified factors.[72]

Management of postoperative problems begins with a patient history. Of particular importance is identification of time since surgery, bowel patterns, onset of the problem, and actions taken to eliminate the problem and their results. Differentiating between gastroenteritis and pouchitis may be difficult. Pouchitis is an inflammation of the reservoir caused by bacterial overgrowth of unknown cause. Pouchitis usually is characterized by sudden onset of increased stool frequency, hematochezia, fever, malaise, pelvic discomfort, and inflammation of the mucosal surface of the reservoir. Treatment of pouchitis includes the administration of antibiotics (particularly metronidazole) and possibly tap water reservoir irrigations three times daily in an attempt to decrease bacteria.

Measures used to decrease stool frequency include antidiarrheal medications, bulk-forming agents, and diet. Dietary assessment also is important. Bran and fiber from fresh fruits and vegetables usually are not recommended because these foods may cause bloating and increased frequency. Some patients, because of personal preferences, eat foods that may cause frequency (e.g., caffeinated beverages, chocolate, spicy foods, raw fruits and vegetables, and alcoholic beverages) or flatus (e.g., beans, cabbage, beer, carbonated beverages, milk and milk products, and onions). For these persons, 8 to 10 stools daily may be normal. Those patients who wish to decrease frequency should be informed about constipating foods. Applesauce, bananas, boiled rice, cheese, creamy peanut butter, and tapioca are foods that may thicken the stool. The patient may be able to identify other constipating foods from personal experience.

Incontinence is considered on the basis of severity and is referred to as either incontinence or seepage. The incidence of incontinence is lower (4% to 6%) than that of seepage (29% to 53%).[44] Incontinence is thought to be due to lowered internal sphincter resting pressures caused by manipulation of the anorectal tissue during the operation. As with other patients with incontinence, assessment of the incontinent episodes is performed and should guide treatment. Stool character is an important assessment and can easily be modified. Assessment of incontinence in an anorectal physiology laboratory may be indicated. Studies may include manometry, electromyelography, and dynamic radiographic assessment of function.

Interventions to reduce or eliminate incontinence must be individualized. Bulk-forming agents bind stool and minimize liquid output, so they are useful inasmuch as seepage is more likely to occur when stool is liquid. Incontinence also may be treated by antidiarrheal medications and food limitations before bedtime. Frequency and incontinence may result from ileoanal anastomosis strictures and from structural characteristics of the reservoir. Patients with strictures may require dilation and may benefit from reservoir irrigation. Of particular importance for the patient with incontinence are prevention and treatment of perianal skin denudation that may result from frequency and seepage.[69]

Patient satisfaction with IAR surgery has been high because the IAR approximates normal anatomy and eliminates the need for a permanent stoma. However, the need for perioperative education and emotional support from the nurse cannot be overstated. As with other patients who have long-term illness and surgical intervention, a short-term mental health consultation may be indicated.

## KOCK CONTINENT ILEOSTOMY

**Preoperative Considerations.** Preoperative teaching includes providing information regarding perioperative care and issues unique to Kock pouch management.[18,35,52,81] The operation usually takes 3 to 4 hours. An abdominal colectomy, proctectomy, ileal pouch construction with continent nipple valve, and permanent ileostomy are performed. A catheter is placed into the stoma during the operation to evacuate effluent without suture-line distention once peristalsis returns. Depending on the physician's protocol, the catheter

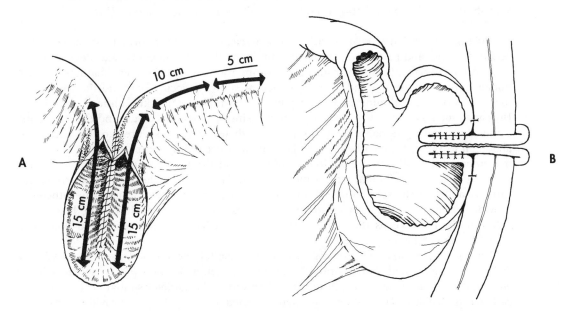

**Fig. 4-4** Construction of Kock continent ileostomy. **A,** Two 15-cm limbs are used to create pouch, and one 15-cm limb is used to fashion a nipple valve and stoma. **B,** Distal limb is intussuscepted into reservoir to create one-way valve and accomplish continence. Sutures or staples, or both, are placed to stabilize and maintain intussuscepted nipple. Anterior surface of reservoir is anchored to anterior peritoneal wall.

may remain in the pouch for 3 to 4 weeks after surgery or even longer. Postoperative irrigations are performed every 2 to 4 hours to rinse mucus from the pouch. Once the catheter is removed, the pouch is intubated at gradually lengthened intervals, which allows the pouch gradually to increase capacity (e.g., week 1, every 2 hours; week 2, every 3 hours). Eventually the pouch expands to a capacity of 400 to 800 ml and is emptied by means of intubation two to four times a day.[3] A small dressing or bandage is recommended to cover the stoma.

Abdominal assessment and stoma site marking are performed by the ET nurse. Depending on the surgeon's preference and the patient's abdominal contours, the stoma may be located above the pubic hair line in the lower right quadrant or at the position for a conventional ileostomy. The stoma may be flush, although slight protrusion is preferable.

Preoperative bowel preparation is similar to that described for patients receiving an ileoanal reservoir.

**Operative Procedure.** A colectomy and proctectomy are performed. The distal 45 cm of ileum is used to construct an ileal pouch, nipple valve, outflow tract (i.e., efferent limb), and stoma. Two 15-cm limbs are fashioned into a U-shaped 30-cm ileal loop, and the antimesenteric borders of adjacent limbs are opened and sutured together (Fig. 4-4, *A*). A nipple valve is created by intussuscepting the distal 10 cm of ileal segment. Sutures or staples, or both, with or without a polyglycolic acid mesh are used to stabilize the intussuscepted portion of ileum, thus securing the nipple valve (Fig. 4-4, *B*). The anterior portion of the pouch is then sutured to the anterior abdominal wall directly under the stoma. Thus the outflow tract is kept short to facilitate intubation directly into the reservoir via the stoma (Fig. 4-4, *B*).[21]

**Postoperative Care.** Postoperative uses of nasogastric tube, urinary catheter, intravenous feeding, and pain medications are similar to those for patients with ileoanal reservoirs. After the patient returns from the operating room, a No. 28F pouch catheter is positioned through the stoma and into the pouch. A suture is secured around the catheter to indicate correct positioning of the catheter in the pouch. (No skin sutures are placed.) Dressings such as a split 4- × 4-inch gauze dressing are then placed around the stoma and catheter to absorb drainage. Next, the pouch catheter must be secured to the side of the abdomen to prevent the catheter from bending and occluding and to prevent "in-and-out" movement of the catheter. A combination of foam and Montgomery straps is one method of securing the catheter.[86] First, a thick piece of foam (4 × 4 × 1 inches) is placed around the catheter and over the split gauze. Montgomery straps are then tied around the catheter to provide stabilization; the straps also hold the gauze and foam in position. The height provided by the foam keeps the catheter from kinking when the catheter is laid down and secured to the abdomen.

During preparation for discharge from the hospital the method used to secure the catheter is reevaluated. If the stoma is located in such a position that a pouch will not adhere, the patient must be taught to carefully position the catheter so that occlusion of the catheter is avoided. The catheter is then attached to a leg bag to provide continuous drainage. (On discharge the foam pad is no longer used, for esthetic reasons and because its bulk prevents patients from wearing their usual clothes.) However, if the patient has adequate peristomal adhesive surface, a two-piece pouching system is more convenient. The flange is cut to the size of the stoma and applied. A long suture is then placed around the catheter, and the strings are positioned to lay across the flange. When the flange and pouch are snapped together, the suture (hence the catheter) is secured in place. The catheter then drains into the two-piece pouch, and the patient is taught the correct procedure for emptying the two-piece pouch. The patient is observed for early postoperative complications, which may include bowel obstruction (2% to 17%), hemorrhage (0.5% to 5%), sepsis (2% to 11%), and fistula (1% to 7%).[26]

The pouch catheter is connected to low intermittent suction or to gravity drainage. Fecal drainage onto peristomal skin may be caused by a catheter that is dislodged, occluded, or adhering to the wall of the pouch. In this case the catheter should be inspected. Some surgeons order irrigations of the catheter every 2 hours for the first 24 hours. Most commonly, the catheter is routinely irrigated with 30 ml of normal saline every 3 to 4 hours, beginning the day after the operation. A plugged catheter should be suspected if the patient complains of fullness, cramping pains, or nausea; catheter irrigations should be undertaken, given these symptoms.

As the patient recovers and gastrointestinal function resumes, the diet may be advanced and intravenous fluids gradually discontinued. Patients are encouraged to drink 2.5 to 3 L of fluid daily to keep the consistency of the stool loose and to maintain good hydration. The catheter typically remains in the pouch for approximately 4 to 6 weeks to keep the pouch decompressed and to prevent distention of the sutures or the nipple valve. Once the catheter is removed, instruction of the intubation technique begins (see the box below). In some medical centers, however, this instruction begins approximately 10 to 12 days after surgery.[86] Under the supervision of the ET nurse the patient may learn to gently irrigate, drain, remove, and insert the catheter. While the catheter is out, the patient may bathe; the catheter is then reinserted until the next practice session. It is advised that the catheter

---

### KOCK CONTINENT ILEOSTOMY INTUBATION PROCEDURE

1. Gather supplies:
   Catheter (usually No. 28F Silastic)
   Water-soluble lubricant
   60-ml catheter-tipped syringe
   Gauze dressing and tape
   Mild soap
   Bag for supplies
2. Sit or stand at the toilet. (Sit on a chair near the toilet if the perineal area is uncomfortable.)
3. Lubricate the catheter. Slowly insert the catheter into the stoma so that it passes directly into the pouch. If difficulty is encountered, take deep breaths and apply gentle pressure to the catheter, advancing it into the pouch while exhaling. Insert to the premarked site indicated on the catheter.
4. Draining the pouch usually takes approximately 5 minutes. When the stool is thick, time needed to drain the pouch increases. It is helpful to dilute pouch contents by instilling a small amount (20 to 25 ml) of tepid tap water.
5. Clean the catheter by rinsing it in warm water and washing it with mild soap. Avoid strong detergents. Allow catheter to dry. Supplies may be carried in a plastic bag, makeup case, or small shaving kit.

Other hints: If the catheter will not go into the pouch, relax. Be sure the catheter is well lubricated. Change position: lie down or stand up. Using the syringe, instill air or water into the catheter to relax the pouch valve. If the pouch is full and attempts to empty are unsuccessful a few hours afterward, call the physician.

not be removed from the pouch for more than 30 minutes.[18,71,81,86]

In conjunction with intubation the catheter also may be clamped to begin gentle distention of the pouch (when suture lines are healed).[40] The patient is instructed to intubate the pouch on a predetermined schedule based on the physician's protocol. A catheter and water-soluble lubricant are used cautiously to avoid forcing the catheter or introducing it too far. Most instructions advise irrigating with tap water at least once per day, before retiring at night, to reduce baterial counts. Frequently used protocols instruct patients to intubate every 2 hours during the day, beginning with the fifth week after the operation, and to connect the catheter to straight drainage during the night. This schedule is advanced to every 3 hours the following week and is gradually increased to intubations every 6 hours by

---

### KOCK CONTINENT ILEOSTOMY INTUBATION SCHEDULE

1. Leave the catheter in the pouch for 4 weeks from the day of surgery, except during your daily bath or shower. Catheter out (Date) _____
2. Fifth week (Date) _____ Intubate every 2 hours. Attach catheter to drainage at night.
3. Sixth week (Date) _____ Intubate every 3 hours. Attach catheter to drainage at night or waken at 3 AM or 4 AM to intubate.
4. Seventh week (Date) _____ Intubate every 4 hours. You should be able to sleep 6 to 8 hours at night.
5. Eighth week (Date) _____ Intubate every 5 hours during the day.
6. Ninth week (Date) _____ Intubate every 6 hours during the day. Maintain this schedule.

From Mayo Foundation for Medical Education and Research, Rochester, Minn., 1991.

---

### KOCK CONTINENT ILEOSTOMY SCHEDULE FOR CLAMPING THE CATHETER

1. Leaving the catheter in the pouch with continuous drainage for 2 to 3 weeks. Catheter out (Date) _____
2. Third week (Date) _____ During the day, clamp the catheter for 2 hours, open, and drain. Connect the catheter to continuous drainage at night.
3. Fourth week (Date) _____ During the day, clamp the tube for 3 hours, open, and drain. Connect the catheter to continuous drainage at night.
4. Fifth week (Date) _____ During the day, clamp the catheter for 4 hours, open, and drian. Open and drain the catheter once during the night.
5. Sixth week (Date) _____ During the day, clamp the catheter for 5 hours, open, and drain. Drain the cathter during the night if necessary.
6. Seventh week (Date) _____ During the day, clamp the catheter for 6 hours, open, and drain. Drain the catheter during the night if necessary.
7. Eighth week (Date) _____ Remove the catheter and intubate 3 or 4 times in a 24-hour period. Maintain this schedule.

From Mayo Foundation for Medical Education and Research, Rochester, Minn., 1991.

the ninth week. An intubation schedule and a clamping schedule are given in the boxes on p. 144.

Discharge instructions are similar to those used with the IAR relative to fluid intake, dietary precautions, and lifting restrictions. Patients are instructed to carry the catheter with them at all times. Some may wish to use a small pouch for supplies. A medical-alert identification bracelet also is recommended. Follow-up visits with the ET nurse are scheduled within 1 to 2 weeks after hospital discharge.

**Functional Results.** As in other continent diversions, function improves with time as pouch size increases and adaptation occurs. The principal late complications are pouchitis, fistula, and nipple valve extrusion. In a Mayo Clinic study[65] the most common of these complications are pouchitis, which occurred in 7% of patients, and nipple valve extrusion, which required surgical revision in 22% of patients. These complications affected function by increasing intubation frequency and compromising pouch continence. Three percent of patients required the use of an external pouching system, 75% of patients were completely continent for stool and gas, with 23% having occasional leakage. Six months after the operation, patients were performing intubation three to six times in 24 hours. Excision of the pouch occurred in approximately 5% of patients as a result of nipple valve failure, recurrent fistula, pouchitis, and suspected Crohn's disease.[21] Both the Mayo Clinic and the Cleveland Clinic report high patient satisfaction with the procedure (89% and 93%, respectively).[3,26]

**Management Considerations.** Management issues that necessitate additional teaching and emotional support are related to intubation, diet, and pouch function. Intubation technique requires manual dexterity, practice, and a commitment to the intubation schedule. Evaluation with the physician and ET nurse is undertaken at regular follow-up visits. Diet modifications sometimes are indicated, particularly if excess flatus is the complaint. Food choices should be evaluated for patients who have related problems. Of particular importance for the patient with the Kock continent ileostomy is the avoidance of high-fiber food that may plug the catheter or cause obstruction. Examples of fibrous foods to limit or avoid are mushrooms, sauerkraut, nuts, raw celery, corn, apple peelings, and peas. Good hydration and thorough chewing of food are essential. Occasionally stool may become too thick to pass through the catheter. Drinking large amounts of prune or grape juice will help loosen stool consistency. The patient is encouraged to respond to the sensation of fullness by emptying the pouch; prolonged overdistention of the pouch is thought to harm the nipple valve.[86]

## CONTINENT URINARY DIVERSIONS

### Historical Evolution

In 1950 two separate surgical teams reported methods of creating urinary diversions. Bricker[12] described the traditional ileal conduit; Gilchrist and colleagues[32] described an internal pouch. For reasons lost to history the Bricker ileal conduit became the more common surgery. In the 1960s Nils G. Kock, a surgeon from the University of Göteborg in Sweden, adapted his highly successful Kock pouch ileostomy procedure for use as a urinary diversion. Use of this surgery did not spread rapidly, however, because of the procedure's surgical difficulty, lengthy operative time, and high revision rate.

In 1985, Rowland, Mitchell, and Rihrle[78] reported a modification of the original

Gilchrist procedure to create the continent Indiana pouch. The Gilchrist procedure and its multiple variations are gaining acceptance rapidly because of their relative surgical simplicity and low morbidity and mortality rates.[83]

Today there is renewed interest in continent diversion and bladder reconstruction, which can be attributed to three factors. First, long-term negative consequences associated with the ileal conduit have been demonstrated. Pernet and Jonas,[66] for example, report a high rate of renal deterioration in these patients. As long-term patient survival increases, these negative outcomes become more of a concern. Second, long-term survival has made the continent diversion more desirable to patients who want urinary elimination to be as normal as possible. Third, and perhaps underrated as an influencing factor, is the acceptance of clean intermittent catheterization as a viable management option. Gilchrist's procedure called for clean catheterization in the 1950s, when sterile technique was the accepted standard.

## Indications

Patient selection for a continent urinary diversion should be made carefully. These continent procedures commonly necessitate an operative time approximately $1\frac{1}{2}$ to $2\frac{1}{2}$ hours longer than the time required for the traditional ileal conduit and therefore require a patient who can endure a more lengthy operation. Because more bowel is used, the patient also must have a sufficient amount of healthy bowel, which may be a prohibitive factor in patients with a history of multiple bowel resections, bowel disease, or radiation damage. These criteria reflect common practice, but they are not universally accepted. Ahlering, Weinberg, and Razor[1] wrote that physical status, prognosis, and history of pelvic irradiation should not exclude patients from candidacy. As experience and comfort with the new surgeries increase, barriers to candidacy probably will be removed gradually.

An evaluation also must be made of the patient's motivation and ability to master the self-care skills involved in the continent ostomy.[13] If a patient already has a colostomy or is having fecal and urinary diversion at the same time, pouching skills will transfer. When both a fecal ostomy and a continent urinary reservoir are created, however, the patient is required to learn two nearly exclusive sets of skills.

## Preoperative Considerations

Preparation for the operation is similar to preparation for any major abdominal exploration. The patient needs to be informed about the preoperative bowel preparation and the usual preoperative and postoperative routines, including an explanation of postoperative tubes. Specifically, the patient needs to be informed of the expected surgical outcomes. Despite preoperative teaching, patients may hear only that they will not need an external pouch and will have a "new bladder." Patients need to be aware that this "new bladder" will not function identically to the natural bladder. Their responsibilities in maintaining the new reservoir need to be clear so that unrealistic expectations do not lead to frustration.

Selection of the stoma site should also take place if an abdominal outlet is planned. Some authors suggest a low stoma site, near the pubic hair line.[50] Although aesthetically pleasing, there are two limitations to this low stoma position. First, the stoma needs to be easily visible to the patient; intubation is more difficult if performed by touch rather than by sight. Second, temporary pouching may be required while pouch capacity is expanding or later, if the continence mechanism fails. Therefore the stoma should be marked in a location that will support a pouch.

There are many surgical variations in the construction of a continent urinary diversion, but the aim of all continent diversions is the same. They should create a "continent, low-pressure reservoir to collect and store urine, allow expulsion of urine under voluntary control and at convenient intervals, protect the upper urinary tracts from obstruction and reflux of urine and avoid significant shifts of water and electrolytes."[33]

Comparative factors among the surgeries are the portion of bowel used to create the reservoir, the location of the reservoir, the mechanisms of continence, and the antireflux mechanism. Although preoperative and postoperative care for the two most commonly performed continent urinary reservoir procedures (the Kock pouch and the ileocecal pouch) and all other variations is similar, each is discussed separately in the following section. Variations in nursing care after the two surgeries depend more on institutional preference than on the procedures themselves.

## Classifications of Surgeries

**Kock Pouch.** The Kock urinary reservoir was developed as a variation of the Kock continent ileostomy. To construct a reservoir, which is located in the abdominal cavity, 60 to 80 cm of ileum is used. As with the Kock continent ileostomy, the continence mechanism at the stoma site is achieved by an intussuscepted nipple valve. A second nipple valve is constructed at the other end of ileum and the ureters implanted; this second valve is intended to prevent reflux into the ureters (Fig. 4-5).

Although Kock performed this procedure as early as 1975[19,50] and several others researchers[11,30] also have reported experiences with this type of surgery, the surgery is not widely preformed, perhaps because of the surgical difficulty and high reported complication rate of the procedure. Loss of continence appears to be the most serious and most common complication of this surgery. Reoperative rates vary from 10% to 30%.[19] Most sur-

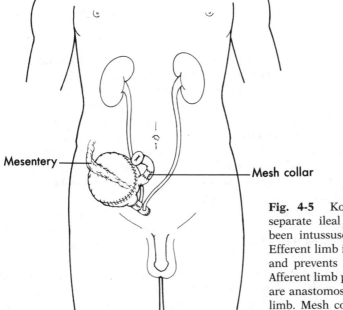

Mesentery

Mesh collar

**Fig. 4-5** Kock continent urostomy. Two separate ileal limbs are present: each has been intussuscepted to create nipple valve. Efferent limb is brought out to skin as stoma and prevents leakage of urine from pouch. Afferent limb prevents reflux of urine; ureters are anastomosed to distal portion of afferent limb. Mesh collar is placed to secure intussuscepted nipple valves.

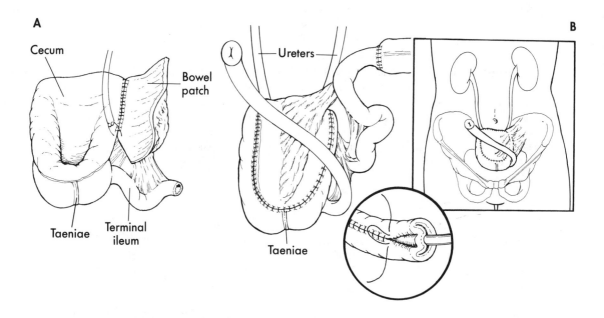

**Fig. 4-6**   Construction of Indiana urinary pouch. **A,** Cecum and terminal ileum segment of ileum are isolated from gastrointestinal tract; another segment of bowel is resected to use as patch. Antimesenteric borders of cecum and bowel segment are opened; bowel patch is sewn to open edges of cecum. **B,** Ureters have been tunneled into taeniae coli along posterior aspect of pouch. Terminal ileum has been plicated to fit catheter and stoma created at predetermined stoma site.

geons agree that the operative time is 1 to 2 hours longer than with the traditional ileal conduit.

**Ileocecal Pouches.**   The ileocecal pouches are modifications of the original Gilchrist procedure of the 1950s. The most common of these ileocecal pouches is the Indiana pouch. The Indiana reservoir is constructed from approximately 20 cm of cecum and 15 cm of terminal ileum.[77] Another segment of bowel (either ileum or colon) is resected to use as a patch (Fig. 4-6, *A*). The distal portion of the ileum is anastomosed to the colon to reestablish bowel continuity. The patch and the cecal segment are opened along the antimesenteric borders, and the patch is sutured to the cecal segment. This creates a moderate-volume pouch and interrupts the organized contractions that can occur in intact bowel segments (Fig. 4-6, *B*).[16] If the patient already has an ileal conduit, it may be possible to use the ileum of the conduit as the ileal patch, thus preventing further bowel loss.[62,77]

Continence is maintained both by the ileocecal valve and by the remaining length of ileum, which is plicated (pleated or made smaller) to create a long outflow tract and stoma. A No. 12F catheter is placed through the ileal segment, and the ileum is folded or pleated to fit the diameter of the catheter (Fig. 4-6, *B*).

The ureters are tunneled into the taeniae of the colonic segment to prevent reflux. The reservoir itself can be positioned in the pelvis or in the abdomen. For an abdominal reservoir the plicated ileum is brought through the abdominal wall and a stoma is created (Fig.

4-6, *B*). For a pelvic urinary reservoir the plicated ileum can be managed in a number of ways, as discussed in the section, Neobladder.

Most surgeons report that the Indiana pouch requires an additional 30 minutes to 1½ hours of surgical time over that required for the traditional ileal conduit. However, Ahlering, Weinberg, and Razor[1] report that, with experience, operative time gradually decreases until it is similar to that for the traditional conduit procedure. Complication rates and reoperative rates generally are reported to be as low as and similar to rates for the ileal conduit.[1] The other variations of ileocecal pouches, such as the Miami pouch, involve variations of surgical technique but are identical from a care and teaching standpoint.

**Other Surgical Variations.** The Kock and ileocecal pouches are the two procedures most commonly reported. With increasing numbers of medical centers performing continent diversions, however, many variations of surgical technique have developed.[51,53] Although some of the fine points of surgical technique do not directly affect nursing care, awareness of the surgical variations is important. For example, the aforementioned variations in stoma-site placement may affect nursing care. In addition, some surgeons prefer to use the umbilicus as the ostomy site. Although a small, flush stoma at the umbilicus has aesthetic advantages, this positioning may pose pouching hurdles. Should the continence mechanism fail, an umbilical stoma can be difficult to pouch effectively.

Because the continence mechanism at the outlet has been most problematic in the development of the surgery, it is not surprising that a number of variations in outlet construction exist.[39] Mitrofanoff, in 1980, reported using the appendix or the ureter as a catheterizable entry into a natural bladder, augmented bladder, or substitute reservoir.[36] Duckett and Snyder[23] also have reported the use of the appendix as the catheterizable segment. This stoma is much smaller than stomas created in other surgical variations. Guzman and colleagues[36] have used invaginated ileum, which results in a serosal stoma. In addition, other parts of the intestinal system, such as the transverse colon and gastric segments, are being tried as reservoir components.

It is probable that surgical variations will continue to appear. Eventually, surgical experience will identify which techniques lead to optimum long-term outcomes, and the number of variations in use will begin to decrease. Under these circumstances, it is impossible to predict the surgical procedure that will be common in 5 to 10 years. The general principles of care, adjustment, and teaching, however, remain constant.

## Postoperative Considerations

Postoperative care includes all the general principles of care for patients who have had major abdominal surgery and is similar to the care of the patient receiving an ileal conduit. As in traditional conduit surgery, the stoma should be assessed for viability. Any sign of loss of vascular supply, such as a dark or dry stoma, should be reported to the physician immediately.

The patient has either a gastrostomy or nasogastric tube until peristalsis returns and flatus is passed. In addition, a surgical drain (either a Penrose or a Jackson Pratt) is used to remove drainage from the surgical cavity. Care of these tubes is identical to that after other abdominal surgeries.

Some of the tubes present during the immediate postoperative period are unique to continent urinary reservoir procedures and deserve special mention. Ureteral stents, which originate in the pelvis of the kidneys and extend through the ureter and into the reservoir, are placed intraoperatively. The stents exit the reservoir either through the stoma or through separate stab wounds. Depending on length, type of tubing used, and exit site, the stents may be placed to dependent drainage or may be contained within a pouching system.

Unobstructed drainage from the reservoir is essential. This drainage may be accomplished by two types of drainage tubes. A Kock pouch has a primary drainage tube exiting through the stoma. The Kock pouch drainage tube usually is a No. 22F to 28F catheter. The ileocecal pouches usually have a cecostomy tube (i.e., reservoir tube) exiting through a separate stab wound. This primary drainage tube most commonly is a No. 22F to 24F Malecot. In addition, the ileocecal pouches may have a secondary drainage tube exiting the stoma; this tube is smaller (usually No. 12F) because the diameter of the ileum has been narrowed.

The primary drainage tube empties any urine that passes around the stents, as well as any mucus that accumulates in the pouch. The primary tube is placed to dependent drainage and irrigated at intervals varying from every 2 to every 8 hours, depending on the surgeon's preference. The purpose of irrigation is to remove accumulated mucus and to ensure a free flow of urine. Distention must be avoided during the postoperative phase to allow suture lines to heal. Therefore irrigation is performed gently, as needed, with use of approximately 60 ml of normal saline. Irrigation is repeated until mucus evacuation stops and clear returns are obtained.

Tubes and drains are removed as soon as their purpose is completed. Ureteral stents are removed about 7 to 10 days after surgery, with radiologic confirmation of open ureters. The primary drain tube remains in place postoperatively for about 3 weeks[37]; the tube usually remains in place in the period immediately after discharge from the hospital. If a secondary tube is present, it may be removed with the stents or it may be left until the end of the 3-week interval.

After surgery, patients have several educational needs. First, they must understand the purpose of all the tubes and drains. Second, they must learn self-care skills. Patients should be taught to care for the pouch tube (if it is still in place after discharge), and they must be able to irrigate mucus from the pouch. In some settings the stents or secondary stoma tube also remains at discharge; patients must be able to care for these tubes, or arrangements must be made for a caregiver to provide this service.

Because the patient does not require an external collecting system, it is easy to assume that emotional needs are fewer in this group than in patients having a traditional ileal conduit. The patient with a continent urinary reservoir, however, has lost a body part and may have a grief reaction to that loss. The surgical incision and stoma also represent a change in body image with which the patient must deal.

A patient who sought a "pouchless" alternative may regard the presence of a temporary pouching system—containing the stents or pouch tubes, or both—as a negative outcome. Clear preoperative discussion of outcomes and expectations minimizes this reaction.

## Recovery Period

The recovery period is defined as the period from discharge until the patient masters self-care techniques and integrates changes in body image. This period usually entails the patient resuming a normal diet, gaining strength, returning to presurgical activity, and practicing care skills until he or she is confident in handling common situations.

The patient usually returns to the clinic or hospital about 3 weeks after the operation for testing of reservoir continuity and continence and for self-intubation teaching. By this time

---

## CONTINENT URINARY RESERVOIR INTUBATION PROCEDURE

**EQUIPMENT NEEDED**
Catheter size _____
Water-soluble lubricant: *Do not use a petroleum-based lubricant.*
Gauze and tape (or other stoma covering)
Washcloth or towelette

**PROCEDURE**
Wash hands.
Remove the stoma covering.
Wipe away any mucus that has accumulated with washcloth or towelette.
Moisten catheter tip with water or lubricant.
Place large end of catheter into drainage container, or position it over the toilet.

Place the lubricated end of the catheter through the stoma until urine is flowing easily. If resistance is met, pause and then continue with gentle pressure, moving the catheter slightly until it passes into the pouch.
Hold the catheter in place until urine stops flowing. Take a few deep breaths, and move the catheter around to check whether the pouch is empty.
Start to withdraw the catheter, slowly allowing additional urine, if present, to drain.
Pinch the catheter before removing it from the stoma to prevent drips of urine on clothing.

---

the patient usually is tube-free, except for the presence of the primary drainage tube, and also should have gained some skill and comfort in maintaining and irrigating the drainage tube.

Before the pouch is allowed to function as a reservoir, a "pouchogram," which is roughly equivalent to a cystogram, is performed. This study tests the ability of the reservoir to hold fluid without leaking from anastomoses or stoma and verifies the antireflux mechanism of the pouch.

Once pouch integrity is confirmed, the patient can be taught to intubate the reservoir through the stoma (see the box above). A No. 16F to 18F red rubber catheter is commonly used to intubate the stoma. A coudé catheter may prove helpful for intubation if the reservoir does not allow easy access.[37] Opportunities for the patient to practice intubation must be provided. In some settings it is standard to readmit patients to the hospital for intubation teaching; usually, however, teaching takes place on an outpatient basis.[14]

There are some inherent difficulties in teaching intubation in the clinic setting. For example, it is difficult to ascertain if the intubation is performed correctly unless urine is obtained. To remedy this situation, practice sessions in a clinic situation can be facilitated by instilling about 100 ml of normal saline through the catheter. Then, when the pouch is intubated, the patient can be rewarded by draining fluid. This procedure can be repeated several times until the patient has overcome any initial nervousness. If the primary drainage tube does not exit through the stoma, the tube should be clamped and left in place during the learning period to serve as a back-up option for emptying the reservoir. However, if the primary drainage tube originally exits from the stoma, the tube must be removed before teaching begins.

With the Kock pouch, catheterization may become more difficult as the pouch fills. An overdistended pouch exerts pressure against the nipple valve, which makes passing the catheter more difficult. If all the techniques to facilitate catheter passage (as described in

## CATHETERIZATION: PATIENT GUIDELINES

Carry catheterization and irrigation supplies with you at all times. For women a small cosmetic bag is convenient. For men a small camera case that clips on a belt may be workable.

If you cannot wash a catheter immediately after catheterization, return it to a plastic bag. Wash the catheter when possible. Do not use a bag that has stored a soiled catheter for storing a clean one.

Be sure to empty pouch whenever you feel full. If your fluid intake has been high, do not wait for the scheduled time.

Drink at least 8 glasses of fluid a day (8-oz glasses). This helps prevent infections.

If your skin becomes moist from mucus, use a skin-sealant wipe on the skin around your stoma for protection.

Replace catheters on a regular basis, at least once a month and more often if they show cracks, softness, or discolorations.

Always wear a medical-alert identification bracelet or necklace. (You will receive an application with correct wording.) Also carry a card giving instructions for inserting the catheter.

If you are having difficulty passing the catheter, try these hints:

Relax, take a few deep breaths, and try again.

Change position: sit down, stand up, or lie down.

Stop, and try again in 5 minutes.

If you feel full and cannot pass a catheter, contact your physician or go to an emergency room.

---

the box, Catheterization: Patient Guidelines, above) the patient needs to seek medical attention as soon as possible.

The patient also needs to practice irrigating the catheter after it has been passed into the reservoir (see the box on p 153, *top*). If the patient was discharged with instructions to irrigate a postoperative pouch tube, this skill will transfer to intermittent catheter irrigation.

In addition to the actual intubation and irrigation skills, the patient needs to learn to clean and store the catheters and to purchase additional catheters (see the box on p. 153, *bottom*). After use, the catheter must be washed with detergent, rinsed well, and allowed to dry. Some centers recommend disinfecting the catheter between use by boiling or soaking it in alcohol or povidone-iodine (Betadine). Once dry, it can be stored in a clean Ziploc-type plastic bag until it is needed again. The patient who may not be able to clean the catheter immediately in a public rest room can return the catheter to a plastic bag and wash it in the usual manner when possible. Patients need to be cautioned to keep soiled plastic storage bags separate from those that will hold clean catheters.

Catheters become spongy or less pliable with time and usually need to be replaced every 2 months. Infection-prone patients (such as immunosuppressed patients) should replace the catheter every 1 to 2 weeks.

As a safety measure the patient should be encouraged to wear identification that includes medical information and to always carry information about the continent urinary reservoir. In the event of trauma the patient with a urinary reservoir may pose confusing problems for emergency personnel in their assessments of urine output, especially if the patient has retained the original bladder. Another safety consideration recommended by many centers is to avoid any use of self-retaining catheters (with inflated balloon) for

## CONTINENT URINARY RESERVOIR IRRIGATION PROCEDURE

**EQUIPMENT NEEDED**
Bulb syringe or piston-type syringe
Water or normal saline
Container for holding water or saline
Equipment for draining catheter

**PROCEDURE**
Wash hands.
Lubricate the catheter, and drain the pouch following the routine procedure.
Leave the catheter in place when finished.
Fill the syringe with water or saline.
Insert syringe into free end of catheter.

Push saline into pouch.
Withdraw fluid gently with syringe, or remove syringe from catheter and allow fluid and mucus to drain.
Repeat until fluid returns clear (no more mucus).
Do not instill more fluid if instilled fluid does not return.
Use only enough pressure when instilling and withdrawing fluid to break up mucus; using excessive force is unnecessary and may cause injury.

## GUIDELINES FOR CLEANING AND STORING CATHETERS

Wash catheters with soap and water, using hand to clean catheter.
Rinse soap and water through inside of catheter.
Rinse catheter well.

Hang catheters to drip dry over a clean surface, such as a towel.
When catheters are dry, place them into a *clean* Ziplock-type plastic bag to store.

straight drainage through the stoma. Many surgeons believe that the pressure of the inflated balloon against the continence valves may cause necrosis and subsequent incontinence. Straight catheters, secured by taping to the skin, may be passed through the stoma and left in place to continuously drain the reservoir.

Passing a catheter through a stoma appears to be a fairly straightforward procedure; however, to many patients it is a frightening and unnerving experience. With the ileocecal pouch the entire length of the catheter may need to be passed before urine is reached. The sensation of passing a catheter, although not painful, is different from anything the patient has previously experienced. To allay anxiety and to maintain control, the patient who cannot pass the catheter should be aware of back-up suggestions as discussed in the box, Catheterization: Patient Guidelines, on p. 152.

### Rehabilitation

All continent reservoirs continue to expand over time, reaching a capacity of 600 to 1000 ml. During pouch expansion the time between catheterizations is lengthened (see the box on p. 154). Among the difficulties that may occur during this time are pouch spasms

## URINARY RESERVOIR EMPTYING SCHEDULE

NOTE: The internal pouch should be emptied at regular intervals to prevent overdistention. As the capacity of the pouch increases, the intervals can be lengthened. Individual surgeons may prefer modifications of the catheterization and irrigation schedule. Regardless of printed schedules, the patient also must respond to feelings of fullness by emptying. The person with more than average mucus production must irrigate more frequently than average.

**FIRST WEEK**
Catheterize every 2 to 3 hours while awake and once at night.
Irrigate with each catheterization.

**SECOND WEEK**
Catheterize every 3 to 4 hours while awake and once at night.
Irrigate with each catheterization.

**THIRD WEEK**
Catheterize every 4 hours while awake and once at night.
Irrigate morning and evening and as needed in between.

**FOURTH WEEK AND BEYOND**
Catheterize every 4 hours while awake.
Irrigate morning and evening and as needed in between.

Modified from Heneghan GM et al: The Indiana pouch: a continent urinary diversion, *J Enterostom Ther* 17:231, 1990.

that may overcome the outflow pressures and a failure of the continence mechanism, both of which result in incontinence. Therefore the patient needs to know how to apply a simple pouch or how to contact an ET nurse until incontinence is corrected.

During the rehabilitation period the patient begins to become more independent. A regular catheterization schedule can provide patients with the structure they desire. Patients also need to be aware, however, that a printed schedule does not take into account their life-styles. The person who drinks four cups of coffee with breakfast needs to empty the pouch earlier than scheduled, as does the patient who occasionally or regularly enjoys a few cans of beer. With time patients learn to recognize what a full reservoir feels like and thus to modify the catheterization routine to fit their intake habits. Most persons with continent urinary reservoirs eventually are able to sleep through the night, emptying immediately before retiring and again upon waking. Intake patterns or capacity of the individual reservoir, however, may require some persons to set an alarm clock and empty during the night to prevent overdistention or leakage. Mastering self-care skills in the general community requires practice, hints from knowledgeable caregivers, and guidance from persons successful with continent reservoirs.

### Neobladder

The term *neobladder* describes an internal urinary reservoir that empties through the urethra. Because the urine stream has not been diverted, the surgery falls outside the scope of ET nursing practice. However, inasmuch as the surgery is an alternative to diversion and is closely related both to undiversion surgery and to augmentation cystoplasty, it is of interest to the ET nurse.[56]

The principles for neobladder construction are the same as those for an internal reservoir that empties through an abdominal stoma. Variations most commonly used are the Indiana pouch with pelvic outlet to the urethra and the Camey procedure, which uses a U-shaped segment of ileum with the ureters entering the upper ends of the U and the urethra anastomosed at the dependent segment of the U.[9]

The primary difference between continent urinary diversions and neobladders lies in the mechanism of continence. Unless the lower portion of the bladder can be spared, continence depends soley on the urethra and external sphincter.[2] This means that total bladder substitution usually is limited to men.[55] Even with male patients, most surgeons report a significant problem with nocturnal enuresis, which can affect up to 50% of patients.[9,15]

Opinion varies as to the safety of leaving the urethra intact when cancer is the cause of the cystectomy.[31,41] Tumor recurrence in the urethra is a concern when the urethra remains. For patients in whom the urethra must be resected, an artificial sphincter together with a reconstructed neourethra may be used. Again, this surgery is more suitable for men than for women.

Postoperative care and monitoring for neobladder patients are similar to those for patients receiving a continent urinary reservoir with abdominal stoma. The primary difference is that a catheter passed through the urethra into the reservoir takes the place of the stoma tube. This catheter provides a stent for the anastomosis between urethra and neobladder, as well as a secondary urinary outlet (a suprapubic or "pouch" tube is the primary outlet).

When all tubes are removed, emptying the neobladder and avoiding urine stasis are important. Neobladder drainage in most procedures relies on passive emptying when the external sphincter is relaxed and on abdominal straining.[2] If these techniques are not sufficient, the patient must learn intermittent self-catheterization. In general, however, patient satisfaction with the neobladder procedure is high, despite the aforementioned problems. The value of maintaining "normal" anatomy is difficult to underestimate.

## SUMMARY

Continent diversions are not suitable for every patient. It is evident, however, that patient interest and satisfaction with these procedures continue to be compelling forces in the ongoing evolution of these alternatives to permanent incontinent stomas. Patients with continent diversion incur significant physical, emotional, and financial costs; however, those who have elected these procedures have realized considerable benefits related to personal dignity and self-esteem. Further research, which will assist in developing new and better operations and aspects of postoperative ET nursing management, is required. At this time the ET nurse's role continues to be one of maintaining specialized knowledge in surgical alternatives and their perioperative technical, educational, and emotional management.

# SELF-EVALUATION

## QUESTIONS

1. The ileoanal reservoir and Kock continent ileostomy are surgical options for patients with:
   a. Diverticulitis
   b. Crohn's disease
   c. Chronic ulcerative colitis and familial adenomatous polyposis
   d. Recurrent cancer

2. What surgical procedures typically are performed during the first stage of an ileoanal reservoir?

3. The length of bowel used to construct the S-shaped ileoanal reservoir is approximately:
   a. 10 cm
   b. 20 cm
   c. 30 cm
   d. 40 cm

4. Identify information that should be provided to a patient after the final surgical procedure for the ileoanal reservoir.

5. A complication of the ileoanal reservoir may be:
   a. Limitation of activities
   b. Chronic constipation
   c. Nausea
   d. Pouchitis

6. The length of bowel used to construct a Kock continent ileostomy is approximately:
   a. 45 cm
   b. 35 cm
   c. 25 cm
   d. 15 cm

7. How long does a catheter typically remain in place after a Kock continent ileostomy?

8. The anticipated capacity of a Kock ileostomy is:
   a. 100 to 400 ml
   b. 400 to 800 ml
   c. 800 to 1000 ml
   d. 1000 to 1200 ml

9. The ideal stoma site for a continent urinary reservoir is near the pubic hair line.
   a. True
   b. False

10. After a stage 1 IAR procedure, what range of stool output is typical of the newly constructed loop ileostomy?
    a. 500 to 1000 cc/24 hr
    b. 1000 to 1500 cc/24 hr
    c. 1500 to 2000 cc/24 hr
    d. 2000 to 2500 cc/24 hr

11. The patient with a loop ileostomy after a stage 1 IAR should be instructed to do all of the following *except*:
    a. Consume large quantities of fiber in small, frequent meals to thicken ileostomy output
    b. Wait to practice Kegel exercises until the surgeon or ET nurse gives approval
    c. Return to the ET nurse–outpatient clinic in 10 to 14 days for evaluation of the pouching system
    d. Replace fluid losses with electrolyte solutions to prevent dehydration
12. The length of bowel used to construct a Kock urinary reservoir is:
    a. 20 to 40 cm
    b. 40 to 60 cm
    c. 60 to 80 cm
    d. 80 to 100 cm
13. List two differences between the Kock urinary reservoir and the ileocecal pouch.
14. Explain the purpose of postoperative irrigation of a Kock urinary reservoir or an ileocecal urinary pouch.
15. What size catheter is used to intubate:
    a. Continent ileostomy
    b. Continent urinary diversion
16. The Indiana pouch can be constructed as an abdominal reservoir with urine exiting through the stoma or as a pelvic reservoir with urine exiting through the urethra.
    a. True
    b. False
17. A self-retaining (balloon) catheter may be inserted into a continent urinary diversion to facilitate continuous urine drainage.
    a. True
    b. False
18. Neobladder drainage relies on what mechanism?

# SELF-EVALUATION

## ANSWERS

1. **c.** Chronic ulcerative colitis and familial adenomatous polyposis
2. **a.** Abdominal colectomy
   **b.** Rectal mucosectomy
   **c.** Ileal reservoir construction
   **d.** Pouch-anal anastomosis
   **e.** Temporary ileostomy
3. **c.** 30 cm
4. **a.** Perianal skin protection and cleansing
   **b.** Dietary and fluid intake
   **c.** Symptoms of dehydration
   **d.** Symptoms of pouchitis
   **e.** Sexual activity
5. **d.** Pouchitis
6. **a.** 45 cm
7. A catheter often remains in place for 3 to 4 weeks.
8. **b.** 400 to 800 ml
9. **b.** False
10. **c.** 1500 to 2000 cc/24 hr
11. **a.** Consume large quantities of fiber in small, frequent meals to thicken ileostomy output
12. **c.** 60 to 80 cm
13. **a.** The ileocecal pouch is constructed of 20 cm of cecum and 15 cm of terminal ileum, whereas the Kock urinary reservoir requires 60 to 80 cm of ileum.
    **b.** Continence with the Kock urinary reservoir depends on an intussuscepted nipple valve; with the ileocecal reservoir, continence depends on the ileocecal valve and plicated ileum.
    **c.** Reflux in the Kock urinary reservoir is prevented by creating a second intussuscepted nipple valve, whereas the ileocecal reservoir tunnels the ureters into the taeniae of the colonic segment to prevent reflux.
14. Mucus is created by the bowel segments used to create these urinary reservoirs. Unless removed routinely, it can obstruct urinary outflow and cause the reservoir to overdistend, thereby placing stress on the suture lines and on the continence mechanisms and increasing the risk of internal leakage.
15. Catheter size:
    **a.** No. 28F
    **b.** No. 16F to 18F
16. **a.** True
17. **b.** False. The balloon may cause necrosis if left against the pouch for long periods or may damage the continence valve mechanism. A straight catheter should be inserted and secured with tape if continuous drainage is necessary.
18. Relaxation of the external sphincter and abdominal straining facilitate passive emptying of the neobladder. If relaxation is insufficient, self-catheterization may be necessary.

# REFERENCES

1. Ahlering TE, Weinberg AC, Razor B: A comparative study of the ileal conduit, Koch pouch, and modified Indiana pouch, *J Urol* 142:1193, 1989.
2. Alcini E et al: Ileocaeco-urethroplasty after total cystectomy for bladder cancer, *Br J Urol* 57:160, 1985.
3. Ambroze WL, Pemberton JH, Dozois RR: Surgical alternatives to ileostomy or colostomy, *Adv Intern Med* 35:375, 1990.
4. Barnett WO: Current experiences with the continent intestinal reservoir, *Surg Gynecol Obstet* 168:1, 1989.
5. Beart RW, Dozois RR, Kelly KA: Ileoanal anastomosis in the adult, *Surg Gynecol Obstet* 154:826, 1982.
6. Beart RW et al: The J ileal pouch-anal anastomosis: the Mayo Clinic experience. In Dozois RR, editor: *Alternatives to conventional ileostomy*, Chicago, 1985, Mosby–Year Book.
7. Becker JM, Raymond JL: Ileal pouch-anal anastomosis, *Ann Surg* 204:375, 1986.
8. Bloom DA, Grossman HB, Konnak JW: Stomal construction and reconstruction, *Urol Clin North Am* 13:275, 1986.
9. Boccon-Gibod L et al: Continent substitution enterocystoplasty using a low-pressure detubularized ileal reservoir, *World J Urol* 6:179, 1988.
10. Boley SJ: New modification for the surgical treatment of Hirschsprung's disease, *Surgery* 56:1015, 1964.
11. Boyd SD, Skinner DG, Kieskovsky G: Ongoing experience with the Kock continent ileal reservoir for urinary diversion, *World J Urol* 3:155, 1985.
12. Bricker EM: Bladder substitution after pelvic evisceration, *Surg Clin North Am* 30:1511, 1950.
13. Brogna L, Lakaszawski M: The continent urostomy, *Am J Nurs* 86:160, 1986.
14. Brogna L, Lakaszawski M: Nursing management: the continent urostomy, *J Enterostom Ther* 13:139, 1986.
15. Camey M: Bladder replacement by ileocystoplasty following radical cystectomy, *World J Urol* 3:161, 1985.
16. Carroll PR et al: Functional characteristics of the continent ileocecal urinary reservoir: mechanisms of urinary continence, *J Urol* 142:1032, 1989.
17. Coe M, Kluka S: Concerns of clients and spouses regarding ostomy surgery for cancer, *J Enterostom Ther* 15:232, 1988.
18. Cox BG, Wentworth AA: *The ileal pouch procedure*, Rochester, Minn, 1977, Mayo Comprehensive Cancer Center.
19. deKernion JB et al: The Kock pouch as a urinary reservoir: pitfalls and perspectives, *Am J Surg* 150:83, 1985.
20. Devine J, Webb R: Resection of the rectal mucosa, colectomy and anal ileostomy with normal continence, *Surg Gynecol Obstet* 92:437, 1951.
21. Dozois RR et al: Continent ileostomy: the Mayo clinic experience. In Dozois RR, editor: *Alternatives to conventional ileostomy*, Chicago, 1985, Mosby–Year Book.
22. Dozois RR et al: Restorative proctocolectomy with ileal reservoir (symposium), *Int J Colorect Dis* 1:2, 1986.
23. Duckett JW, Snyder HM: Use of the Mitrofanoff principle in urinary reconstruction, *World J Urol* 3:191, 1985.
24. Dyk RB, Sutherland AM: Adaptation of the spouse and other family members to the colostomy patient, *Cancer* 9:123, 1956.
25. Fazio VW: Comments on Kock NG et al: Continent ileostomy: the Swedish experience. In Dozois RR, editor: *Alternatives to conventional ileostomy*, Chicago, 1985, Mosby–Year Book.
26. Fazio VW, Church JM: Complication and function of the continent ileostomy at the Cleveland Clinic, *World J Surg* 12:148, 1988.
27. Fleshman JW et al: The ileal reservoir and ileoanal anastomosis procedure: factors affecting technical and functional outcome, *Dis Colon Rectum* 31:10, 1988.
28. Follick M, Smith T, Turk D: Psychosocial adjustment following ostomy, *Health Psychol* 3:505, 1984.

29. Fonkalsrud EW: Total colectomy and endorectal ileal pull-through with internal ileal reservoir for ulcerative colitis, *Surg Gynecol Obstet* 150:1, 1980.

30. Gerber A: The Kock continent ileal reservoir: an alternative to the conventional urostomy, *J Enterostom Ther* 12:15, 1985.

31. Gerber WL: Is urethral sparing at cystectomy a safe procedure? *Urology* 36:303, 1990.

32. Gilchrist RK et al: Construction of a substitute bladder and urethra, *Surg Gynecol Obstet* 90:752, 1950.

33. Goldwasser B, Webster GD: Continent urinary diversion, *J Urol* 134:227, 1985.

34. Goligher JC: The quest of continence in the surgical treatment of ulcerative colitis, *Adv Surg* 14:53, 1980.

35. Griffith SA: *The continent ileostomy,* Irvine, Calif, 1983, United Ostomy Association.

36. Guzman JM et al: Modified Benchekroun technique for continent ileal stoma, *J Urol* 142:1431, 1989.

37. Heneghan GM et al: The Indiana pouch: a continent urinary diversion, *J Enterostom Ther* 17:231, 1990.

38. Hill GL: Physiology of conventional ileostomy. In Dozois RR, editor: *Alternatives to conventional ileostomy,* Chicago, 1985, Mosby–Year Book.

39. Hinman F: Functional classification of conduits for continent diversion, *J Urol* 144:27, 1990.

40. Hulten L: The continent ileostomy (Kock's pouch) versus the restorative proctocolectomy (pelvic pouch), *World J Surg* 9:952, 1985.

41. Johnson DE, Smith DB: Future considerations. In Smith DB, Johnson DE, editors: *Ostomy care and the cancer patient,* Orlando, Fla, 1986, Grune & Stratton.

42. Kälble T et al: Ureterosigmoidostomy: long-term results, risk of carcinoma and etiological factors for carcinogenesis, *J Urol* 144:1110, 1990.

43. Karlan M, McPherson RC, Watman RN: An experimental evaluation of fecal continence—sphincter and reservoir—in the dog, *Surg Gynecol Obstet* 108:469, 1959.

44. Keighley MRB: Abdominal mucosectomy reduces the incidence of soiling and sphincter damage after restorative proctocolectomy and J-pouch, *Dis Colon Rectum* 30:386, 1987.

45. Kennedy HJ: Quality of life in patients with an ileostomy, *Int Disabil Stud* 10:175, 1988.

46. King DW, Lubowski DZ, Cook TA: Anal canal mucosa in restorative proctocolectomy for ulcerative colitis, *Br J Surg* 76:970, 1989.

47. Kobza L: Impact of ostomy upon the spouse, *J Enterostom Ther* 10:54, 1983.

48. Kock NG: Intra-abdominal "reservoir" in patients with permanent ileostomy: preliminary observations on a procedure resulting in fecal "continence" in five ileostomy patients, *Arch Surg* 99:223, 1969.

49. Kock NG et al: The continent ileal reservoir (Kock pouch) for urinary diversion, *World J Urol* 3:146, 1985.

50. LaFollette SS: A continent urostomy, *AORN J* 40:207, 1984.

51. Leonard MP, Gearhart JP, Jeffs RD: Continent urinary reservoirs in pediatric urological practice, *J Urol* 144:330, 1990.

52. MacClelland DC: Kock pouch: a new type of ileostomy, *AORN J* 32:191, 1980.

53. Mansson A, Colleen S, Sundin T: Continent caecal reservoir in urinary diversion, *Br J Urol* 56:359, 1984.

54. Martin LW, LeCoultre C, Schubert WK: Total colectomy and mucosal proctocolectomy with preservation of continence in ulcerative colitis, *Ann Surg* 186:477, 1977.

55. Montie JE: Changing concepts in urinary diversions, *Ostomy/Wound Management* 12:10, 1986.

56. Morin JM: Urinary undiversion, *J Enterostom Ther* 12:125, 1985.

57. Morson BC, Dawson IMP: Adenomas and the adenomacarcinoma sequence. In *Gastrointestinal pathology,* ed 2, Oxford, UK, 1979, Blackwell Scientific Publications.

58. Nemer FD, Rolstad, BS: Ileoanal reservoir in patients with ulcerative colitis and familial polyposis, *J Enterostom Ther* 12:74, 1985.

59. Nicholls RJ, Moskowitz RL, Shephard NA: Restorative proctocolectomy with ileal reservoir, *Br J Surg* 72:76 (suppl), 1985.

60. Nicholls RJ, Pezim ME: Restorative proctocolectomy with ileal reservoir for ulcerative colitis and familial adenomatous polyposis: a comparison of three reservoir designs, *Br J Surg* 72:470, 1985.

61. Nissen R: Meeting of the Berlin Surgical Society, Zentralbl Chir 15:888, 1933. Cited in Ravitch MM: Anal ileostomy with sphincter preservation in patients requiring total colectomy for benign conditions, *Surgery* 24:170, 1948.

62. Oesterling JE, Gearhart JP: Utilization of ileal conduit in construction of continent urinary reservoir, *Urology* 36:15, 1990.

63. Parks AG, Nicholls RJ: Proctocolectomy without ileostomy for ulcerative colitis, *Br Med J* 2:85, 1978.

64. Pemberton JH: Management of conventional ileostomies, *World J Surg* 12:203, 1988.

65. Pemberton JH et al: Current clinical results. In Dozois RR, editor: *Alternatives to conventional ileostomy*, Chicago, 1985, Mosby–Year Book.

66. Pernet FPPM, Jonas U: Ileal conduit urinary diversion: early and late results of 132 cases in a 25 year period, *World J Urol* 3:140, 1985.

67. Pressel P: The continent urostomy: an interview with Drs. Joeseph Kaufman and Alex Gerber, *J Enterostom Ther* 11:152, 1984.

68. Ravitch MM, Sabiston DC: Anal ileostomy with sphincter preservation in patients requiring total colectomy for benign conditions, *Surgery* 24:170, 1948.

69. Rolstad BS: Ileoanal reservoir: functional results and management, *South Med J* 77:1535, 1984.

70. Rolstad BS: Ileoanal reservoir: an overview for patients, *Ostomy Q* 23:81, 1986.

71. Rolstad BS: Innovative surgical procedures and stoma care in the future, *Nurs Clin North Am* 22:341, 1987.

72. Rolstad BS, Nemer FD: Management problems associated with ileoanal reservoir, *J Enterostom Ther* 12:41, 1985.

73. Rolstad BS, Rothenberger DA: *Ileoanal reservoir: a patient resource*, Kalamazoo, Mich, 1986, Upjohn.

74. Rolstad BS, Wilson G, Rothenberger DA: Sexual concerns in the patient with ileostomy, *Dis Colon Rectum* 26:170, 1983.

75. Rothenberger DA: *Controversies in ileoanal pouch construction*. Lecture presented at the fifty-third Principles of Colon and Rectal Surgery course, University of Minnesota Medical School, Minneapolis, Oct 1990.

76. Rothenberger DA et al: The S ileal pouch-anal anastomosis. In Dozois RR, editor: *Alternatives to conventional ileostomy*, Chicago, 1985, Mosby–Year Book.

77. Rowland RG: Continent urinary reservoirs. In Rous SN, editor: *Urology annual*, vol I, Norwalk, Conn, 1987, Appleton & Lange.

78. Rowland RG, Mitchell ME, and Rihrle R: The cecoileal continent urinary reservoir, *World J Urol* 3:185, 1985.

79. Schoetz DJ Jr, Coller JA, Veidenheimer MC: Proctocolectomy with ileoanal reservoir: an alternative to permanent ileostomy, *Postgrad Med* 75:123, 1984.

80. Schover L: Sexual rehabilitation of the ostomy patient. In Smith DB & DE Johnson, editors: *Ostomy care and the cancer patient*, Orlando, Fla, 1986, Grune & Stratton.

81. Sivly PM et al: Enterostomal care after ileostomy: continent ileostomy or ileoanal anastomosis. In Dozois RR, editor: *Alternatives to conventional ilesotomy*, Chicago, 1985, Mosby–Year Book.

82. Soave F: A new surgical technique for treatment of Hirschsprung's disease, *Surgery* 56:1007, 1964.

83. Sullivan H, Gilchrist RK, Merricks JW: Ileocecal substitute bladder: long-term follow-up, *J Urol* 109:43, 1973.

84. Telander RL, Perrault J: Total colectomy with rectal mucosectomy and ileoanal anastomosis for chronic ulcerative colitis in children and young adults, *Mayo Clin Proc* 55:420, 1980.

85. Telander RL, Perrault J: Colectomy with rectal mucosectomy and ileoanal anastomosis in your patients, *Arch Surg* 116:623, 1981.

86. Todd D: Personal communication, Jan 1992.

87. Tucker SB, Smith DB: Dermatologic conditions complicating ostomy care. In Smith DB and DE Johnson, editors: *Ostomy care and the cancer patient*, Orlando, Fla, 1986, Grune & Stratton.

88. Utsunomiya J et al: Total colectomy, proctocolectomy and ileoanal anastomosis, *Dis Colon Rectum* 23:459, 1980.
89. Valiente MA, Bacon HE: Construction of pouch using "pantaloon" technique for pullthrough of ileum following total colectomy, *Am J Surg* 90:742, 1955.
90. Wexner SD et al: Long-term functional analysis of the ileoanal reservoir, *Dis Colon Rectum* 32:275, 1989.
91. Wolff BG, Culp CE, Dozois RR: Diagnosis and indications for ileostomy. In Dozois RR, editor: *Alternatives to conventional ileostomy*, Chicago, 1985, Mosby–Year Book.
92. Wong WD: *Ileoanal pouch—complications and functional failures*. Lecture presented at the Principles of Colon and Rectal Surgery course, Minneapolis, University of Minnesota, Oct. 1990.
93. Wong WD, Rothenberger DA, Goldberg SM: Ileoanal pouch procedures, *Curr Probl Surg* 22:1, 1985.

# 5 Principles of Cancer Therapy

CATHERINE R. RATLIFF

## OBJECTIVES

1. Describe the role of surgery in the treatment of cancer.
2. Discuss palliative surgical management.
3. Identify the types of chemotherapeutic agents and their effects on the cell cycle.
4. List primary side effects of chemotherapeutic agents.
5. Describe the uses of chemotherapy.
6. Identify the various types of radiation therapy used in cancer treatment, including external, internal, and intraoperative types.
7. Describe hyperthermia.
8. Discuss the use of biologic response modifiers.
9. Identify the use of bone marrow transplantation.

In the search for a term to describe malignant diseases, the ancient Romans turned to their word for crab, *cancer,* because such diseases "stretched out" in many directions like the legs of a crab. The term is used interchangeably with *malignant tumor* and *neoplasm.* The term *neoplasm* comes from the Greek word meaning *new growth.* Cell division is an orderly process; its purpose is development of the organism or replacement of dead cells. When cells divide without a purpose, they form neoplasms or tumors. *Oncology,* from the Greek word *onkos,* meaning mass, is a term used in the treatment and study of cancer.[36]

More than 200 diseases whose cells divide without a purpose are called cancer, which has existed since the beginning of time and affects human beings wherever they live and whatever their race, nationality, or socioeconomic status. In the past 40 years a 50% overall cure rate for cancer has been effected, along with a higher cancer incidence rate.[4] The estimate for new cancer cases in 1991 is 1,100,000; 514,000 of affected persons are expected to die of their disease. In 1987 cancer represented 23% of the total number of deaths in the United States, second only to heart disease.[3] The major cause of cancer deaths has been lung cancer, with other major sites being the colon and rectum, uterus, breast, skin, and buccal cavity and pharnyx.

Although not every ostomy is created as a result of cancer, a significant number of patients with a diagnosis of cancer have an ostomy. For example, a patient may have an ileostomy to treat ulcerative colitis and later a breast cancer may develop. More commonly, however, the ostomy is a result of the malignancy. Methods of cancer treatment include surgery, chemotherapy, radiation therapy, biotherapy, hyperthermia, and bone marrow transplantation. These methods of cancer treatment and implications for the ostomy patient are discussed in this chapter.

## SURGERY

Surgery is the oldest form of curative treatment for cancer. In approximately 1600 BC the Egyptians described the first recorded surgical excision of a tumor. In 1809 Ephraim McDowell excised a 22-pound ovarian tumor from a patient who then survived 30 years.[31] In 1826 Lisfranc excised a rectal carcinoma and constructed a perineal colostomy.[37] From 1860 to 1890 Billroth performed the first laryngectomy, gastrectomy, and esophagectomy.[31] In 1884 Maydl suggested the use of a goose-quill bridge to support a loop colostomy on the abdominal wall.[37] Radical exenterative surgery requiring either a fecal or a urinary ostomy was pioneered by Brunschwig, Bricker, and Appleby in the late 1940s. They demonstrated improved survival rates for patients receiving exenterative surgery for treatment of rectal and gynecologic cancers. Since then the number of these surgical procedures has increased; thus the number of ostomies has increased.[12]

Surgery, which is the primary treatment for most solid tumors, plays a role in prevention, tissue diagnosis, cure, and palliation.

### Prevention

The importance of surgery in the prevention of cancer often is underestimated. One approach is the excision of premalignant lesions. Another is prophylactic surgery for persons with congenital or genetic conditions that place them at risk for cancer. Familial polyposis results in colon cancer in 80% of affected patients. In extensive ulcerative colitis, colon cancer will develop within 25 years in one third of the patients.[12,35] Prophylactic removal of the colon and rectum provides protection for both types of patients.

### Diagnosis

The major purpose of surgery in the diagnosis of cancer is to obtain tissue for histologic diagnosis by incisional biopsy, excisional biopsy, needle biopsy, or endoscopy.[31] The type of technique used depends on the location, size, and growth characteristics of the tumor (see the box on p. 165).

### Staging

The treatment and prognosis of certain cancers, for example, lymphomas and ovarian cancer, depend on accurate staging of the disease, that is, careful determination of the exact extent of the cancer. Often, adequate staging can be achieved by physical examination, radi-

---

## DIAGNOSTIC SURGICAL TECHNIQUES

**INCISIONAL BIOPSY**
Removal of a portion of the tumor

**EXCISIONAL BIOPSY**
Removal of the entire tumor mass with a
  margin of surrounding normal tissue

**NEEDLE BIOPSY**
Aspiration of tissue samples through a
  special needle inserted into the tumor

**ENDOSCOPY**
Removal of small portions of the tumor
  with forceps after visual examination
  through a flexible endoscope

---

ologic studies and other noninvasive techniques. Surgical staging, however, is necessary for cancers that are inaccessible and difficult to stage by other means.

**Cure**

The primary goal of curative surgical oncology is to reduce the tumor burden. Surgical excision that encompasses a sufficient margin of normal tissue is adequate treatment for many solid tumors. Many tumors, however, may have vascular invasion or poorly differentiated histopathologic findings. In these cases surgery is used only for cytoreduction and, to effect a cure, must be accompanied by other therapies such as chemotherapy or radiation therapy. If the number of tumor cells can be reduced to a small amount by surgery, any remaining cancer cells subsequently may be destroyed by these other therapies.

The malignancies that most commonly require construction of a stoma include colorectal, bladder, and cervical cancer. A permanent stoma is required when the distal bowel and anal sphincter are removed or when the bladder is removed. A temporary stoma also may be constructed on a temporary basis to protect a bowel anastomosis lower in the colon or to provide decompression of a bowel partially or completely obstructed by tumor. If tumor is later irradiated or surgically excised, it may be possible to "take down" the stoma; if the tumor is not removed, the stoma provides palliation and relief from obstruction for the duration of the patient's life.

Because of the predictable, metastatic spread and centralized, slow growth pattern of cervical cancer, it is a tumor suitable for en bloc resection. A total pelvic exenteration is an attempt at a surgical cure. The surgery combines several major procedures: radical hysterectomy with pelvic lymph node dissection and bilateral salpingo-oophorectomy, vaginectomy, cystectomy, and abdominoperineal resection of the rectum. A colostomy and urinary diversion are created, and vaginal reconstruction may be performed.[15] Most medical centers with a large number of cases are reporting a 40% to 50% 5-year survival rate.[25] The indications for exenteration are those tumors that are centrally located in the pelvis and those that have failed to respond to previous irradiation. The patient requires physical and mental reserves adequate for recovery. Surgery risks, financial costs, ability to learn ostomy care, and emotional adjustment associated with pelvic exenteration are all important factors to be considered in the decision regarding the surgery.[18] The nursing care plan should be

**Table 5-1**   Ostomy patient needs

| Time | Information | Technical skills | Emotional support |
|------|-------------|------------------|-------------------|
| Preoperative | Nature of surgical procedure; expected postoperative course | Introduction to ostomy and related equipment | Worries concerning threats to survival; fears of pain; discussions of patient-introduced concerns |
| Postoperative | Surgical outcome; ostomy construction; anticipated recovery rate; ostomy self-help and visitor | Ostomy self-care skills | Exploration of ostomy experience |
| Discharge | Community resources When to seek help and from whom | Transfer of skills to home situation | Preparation for first month at home; closure on period of hospitalization |

From Watson PG: Meeting the needs of patients undergoing ostomy surgery, *J Enterostom Ther* 12:123, 1985.

developed on the basis of the needs and time frames of patients with ostomies, as described by Watson [43] (Table 5-1).

## Palliation

Palliative surgery is undertaken to improve the quality of life by relieving pain, perforation, or obstruction; to stop bleeding; or to drain sites of infection. The primary goal is not to prolong life but to ensure a more comfortable life.[43] Examples of palliation include decompression or bypass of obstructed bowel, insertion of enterostomy tubes for nutritional needs, diversion of the fecal stream above a colonic fistula (rectovaginal, rectovesical, or enterocutaneous), and excision of primary or metastatic lesions. Complications resulting from chemotherapy and radiation therapy, such as skin breakdown, fistulas, radiation proctitis, radiation cystitis, and obstruction and perforation, also may necessitate surgical intervention.

## Reconstruction

Reconstructive surgery involves the reconstruction of anatomic defects caused by the cancer surgery. The need to remove a margin of normal tissue around a tumor's border sometimes involves extensive surgical resection, with resulting disfigurement and dysfunction. Loss of perineal tissue as a result of extensive resection of recurrent rectal cancer may necessitate the use of myocutaneous flaps for tissue coverage. Use of gracilis muscle flaps is recommended over the use of rectus muscle flaps to preserve abdominal wall space for stoma placement.[43] The myocutaneous gracilis muscle graft also has been used in patients receiving total pelvic exenteration to create a functioning neovagina, necessitated by the vaginectomy performed during the surgical procedure.

Patients with cancer may have ostomies created for various reasons: some as part of curative therapy, others to manage complications, to palliate symptoms, or to treat an unrelated disease. The nurse may need to mark several possible stoma sites before surgery to allow the surgeon flexibility, depending on the surgical procedure, its purpose, and previous cancer therapy. Coordination of all members of the health care team is essential. Postoperative complications such as infection may be more common in the patient with cancer and may require prompt, aggressive treatment.

## CHEMOTHERAPY

Chemotherapy is the use of cytotoxic drugs for both the cure and the palliation of cancer. Presently, chemotherapy is the curative therapy for 14 types of cancer that account for 11% of the cancers in the United States.[6] In the 1950s chemotherapy was administered primarily as a single agent. Today chemotherapeutic agents are administered singly or in combination and can be given in a variety of settings: cancer centers, community hospitals, outpatient clinics, or physician offices.

During the last 15 years the introduction of new drugs to treat cancer has been minimal; the last major advances occurred in 1971 with the introduction of cisplatin and in the mid-1980s with etoposide.[14] Approximately 100 cytotoxic drugs are approved by the Federal Drug Administration. Recently several analogues of existing chemotherapeutic agents have been investigated for differences in mechanism of action, activity, and toxicity. The hope is that these analogues will be able to overcome the tumor cells resistant to currently available drugs.

### History

Early Egyptian papyruses contain descriptions of the use of various drugs to treat ulcerating skin tumors. Paul Ehrlich coined the term *chemotherapy* when using infected mice in the development of antibiotics. In the early 1900s George Clowes from Roswell Park developed a strain of inbred mice that could carry transplanted tumors. The work of both these researchers served as the starting point for testing potential cancer chemotherapy agents.[9]

The modern age of cancer chemotherapy began with the use of hormonal therapy for breast and prostate cancer in the early 1940s.[21] Research on poisonous gas during World War II linked nitrogen mustard as a tumorigenic initiator in the development of chronic leukemia and lymphomas such as Hodgkin's disease. Farber's research demonstrated the effects of folic acid on leukemia cell growth in children with lymphoblastic leukemia: temporary remissions were induced with folic acid antagonists.[29] During World War II the focus on the isolation of penicillin and other antibiotics resulted in the discovery of cytotoxic antibiotics such as the actinomycins. Thus research on hormones, nitrogen mustard, folic acid antagonists, and antibiotics stimulated chemotherapy research in the years to come.[5]

### Cellular Effects

The purpose of chemotherapy is to disrupt the cancer cell's life cycle (Fig. 5-1). Although normal cells and cancer cells go through the same division cycle, the length of time it takes a cell to complete the cycle varies. Most chemotherapeutic agents act by modifying or interfering with deoxyribonucleic acid (DNA) synthesis; thus cells most vulnerable to cytotoxic agents are those that are actively dividing or preparing to divide. Both malignant and normal cells that are rapidly dividing are the most affected by chemotherapy. Normal, rapidly dividing cells affected by chemotherapy include bone marrow, hair follicle, gastrointestinal mucosa, skin, and gonadal cells. To allow recovery of normal cells, chemotherapy is administered in a defined cycle.

Agents may be classified by the specific mechanism of action and their interference with

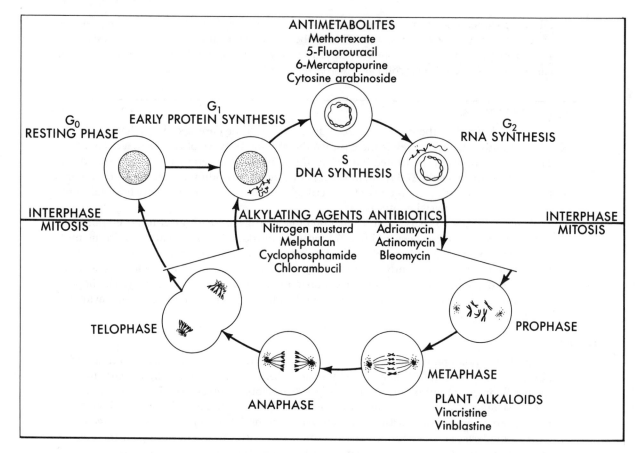

**Fig. 5-1**   Cell cycle. Drugs are identified by where they exert effects. (From Beare PG, Myers J: *Principles and practice of adult health nursing,* 1990, St Louis, Mosby–Year Book.)

cellular reproduction. Drugs specific to certain phases of the cell cyle are most effective in the treatment of malignancies with a large number of actively dividing cells. These agents are administered over a prolonged period to allow cells to reach the phase in which each drug acts. Examples of cell cycle–specific drugs include vinca alkaloids, antimetabolites, and miscellaneous agents such as asparaginase and decarbazine (Table 5-2).

*Antimetabolites* are specific to the S phase of the cell cycle. They exhibit their action by blocking enzymes necessary for DNA synthesis or become incorporated into the DNA and ribonucleic acid (RNA), which results in disruption of cell replication.

*Vinca alkaloids* are specific to the M stage of the cell cycle. They exert a cytotoxic effect by binding to microtubular proteins needed for the formation of the mitotic spindle in metaphase. The cell is unable to divide and dies.

Drugs that affect both resting and dividing cells are called cell cycle–nonspecific. These drugs harm the cell at some point in the cell cycle, with cell death occurring when the cell attempts to divide. Cell cycle–nonspecific agents tend to be more dose-dependent and are

**Table 5-2** Pharmacologic classifications of the most commonly used chemotherapeutic drugs

| Class | Major side effects and toxicities |
|---|---|
| **ALKYLATING AGENTS** | |
| Busulfan (Myleran) | Myelosuppression, nausea, vomiting |
| Carboplatin (Paraplatin) | Myelosuppression, nausea, vomiting, mild nephrotoxicity and neurotoxicity |
| Chlorambucil (Leukeran) | Myelosuppression, sterility |
| Cisplatin | Nausea, vomiting, renal damage, ototoxicity, electrolyte imbalance |
| Cyclophosphamide (Cytoxan) | Nausea, vomiting, alopecia, myelosuppression, hemorrhagic cystitis |
| Estramustine | Nausea, vomiting, gynecomastia; cardiac toxicity |
| Hexamethylmelamine (HMM, HXM) | Myelosuppression, neurotoxicity, anorexia, nausea, vomiting |
| Ifosfamide | Myelosuppression, nephrotoxicity, nausea, vomiting, phlebitis, neurotoxicity, alopecia, hemorrhagic cystitis |
| Mechlorethamine (nitrogen mustard) | Severe nausea, vomiting, extravasation, myelosuppression |
| Melphalan (Alkeran) | Nausea, vomiting may occur with high-dose myelosuppression |
| Thiophosphoramide (Thio-Tepa) | Myelosuppression, headache, fever, occasional nausea |
| **ANTIBIOTICS** | |
| Bleomycin | Fever, chills, pulmonary toxicity, hyperpigmentation, alopecia, stomatitis |
| Dactinomycin (actinomycin D, Cosmegen) | Potentiates effects of radiation therapy |
| Daunorubicin (Cerubidine, daunomycin) | Myelosuppression, alopecia, nausea, vomiting, stomatitis, red urine |
| Doxorubicin (Adriamycin) | Myelosuppression, alopecia, nausea, vomiting, diarrhea, red urine |
| Mitomycin (Mutamycin) | Myelosuppression, alopecia, nausea, vomiting, fever, stomatitis |
| Mithramycin, plicamycin, (Mithracin) | Thrombocytopenia, hepatotoxicity, nausea, vomiting, phlebitis |
| **ANTIMETABOLITES** | |
| Cytarabine (ara-C, Cytosar-U) | Potent myelosuppressant, anorexia, alopecia, nausea, vomiting, hepatotoxicity, neurotoxicity with increased dosage and intrathecal administration; conjunctivitis |
| Floxuridine (FUDR) | Myelosuppression, oral and gastrointestinal ulceration, nausea, vomiting |
| F-Fluorouracil (5-FU) | Myelosuppression, alopecia, skin rash, nausea, vomiting, ataxia, diarrhea, stomatitis |
| Hydroxyurea | Myelosuppression, stomatitis, alopecia, dysuria, nausea, vomiting, allergic reactions |

Modified from Otto S: Chemotherapy. In Otto S, editor: *Oncology nursing*, St Louis, 1991, Mosby–Year Book, pp 309–314.

*Continued.*

**Table 5-2**  Pharmacologic classifications of the most commonly used chemotherapeutic drugs—cont'd

| Class | Major side effects and toxicities |
| --- | --- |
| **ANTIMETABOLITES—cont'd** | |
| Methotrexate (Mexate) | Oral and gastrointestinal ulceration, myelosuppression, stomatitis, renal toxicity, nausea, vomiting, diarrhea |
| 6-Mercaptopurine (6-MP) | Myelosuppression, hepatotoxicity, stomatitis, anorexia |
| 6-Thioguanine (6-TG) | Myelosuppression, nausea, vomiting |
| **HORMONES** | |
| **Androgens** | |
| Fluoxymesterone (Halotestin) | Nausea, vomiting, edema, liver function abnormalities, virilization in females |
| Testosterone | Mild fluid retention; monitor blood sugar with diabetes mellitus |
| **Progestins** | |
| Megestrol acetate (Megace) | Mild fluid retention, hypercalcemia with breast cancer |
| Medroxyprogesterone acetate Provera | Mild fluid retention, hypercalcemia with breast cancer |
| Depo-Provera | Acute local hypersensitivity |
| **Estrogens** | |
| Diethylstilbestrol (DES) | Breakthrough bleeding, spotting, premenstrual-like syndrome, feminization in males |
| Conjugated estrogen (Premarin) | Breakthrough bleeding, premenstrual-like syndrome |
| Chlorotrianisene (TACE) | Increase or decrease in weight, breakthrough bleeding |
| **ANTIHORMONAL AGENTS** | |
| Aminoglutethimide (Cytadren) | Myelosuppression, dermatitis, masculinization, drowsiness, lethargy, weakness |
| Flutamide | Gynecomastia, hepatotoxicity |
| Leuprolide acetate (Lupron) | Impotence, amenorrhea, hot flashes |
| Mitotane (Lysodren) | Nausea, vomiting |
| Tamoxifen (Nolvadex) | Hot flashes, nausea, vomiting, transient bone or tumor pain |
| Zoladex | May increase bone pain, hot flashes, loss of libido, and impotence |
| **NITROSOUREAS** | |
| Carmustine (BCNU) | Myelosuppression, stomatitis, nausea, vomiting, hepatic toxicities |
| Lomustine (CCNU) | Nausea, vomiting, thrombocytopenia, myelosuppression |
| Semustine (MeCCNU) | Myelosuppression, nausea, vomiting, renal and hepatic toxicities |
| Streptozocin (Zanosar) | Mild myelosuppression, diarrhea, nausea, vomiting, chills, acute hypoglycemia |

**Table 5-2**   Pharmacologic classifications of the most commonly used chemotherapeutic drugs—cont'd

| Class | Major side effects and toxicities |
|---|---|
| **CORTICOSTEROIDS** | |
| Dexamethasone (Decadron) | Fluid-electrolyte disturbance, possible neuromusculoskeletal imbalances |
| Hydrocortisone (Solu-Cortef) | Fluid-electrolyte disturbance |
| Prednisone (Deltasone) | Fluid-electrolyte disturbance, manifestations of latent diabetes mellitus |
| Prednisolone | Similar in action to prednisone |
| **ALKALOIDS** | |
| **Vinca** | |
| Vinblastine (Velban) | Myelosuppression, stomatitis, neurotoxicity, alopecia |
| Vincristine (Oncovin) | Neurotoxicity, constipation, alopecia, stomatitis |
| Vindesine (Eldisine) | Myelosuppression, constipation, alopecia, neuropathy |
| **Podophyllin** | |
| Etoposide (VP-16) (VePesid) | Nausea, vomiting, leukopenia, anemia, alopecia, hypotension |
| Teniposide (VM-26) | Anaphylaxis, myelosuppression, severe hypotension, |
| **MISCELLANEOUS AGENTS** | |
| Asparaginase (Elspar) | Anaphylactic shock, nausea, vomiting, hyperglycemia, hepatic toxicities |
| Dacarbazine (DTIC-Dome) | Myelosuppression, venous spasm, flulike syndrome, paresthesia, pruritus |
| Levamisole | Mild gastrointestinal complaints |
| Mitoxantrone (DHAD) | Myelosuppression, diarrhea, nausea, vomiting, phlebitis, bluish discoloration of urine, alopecia |
| Procarbazine (Matulane) | Myelosuppression; avoid use of narcotics, epinephrine, antihistamines |

often given as single bolus injections. With cell cycle–nonspecific drugs, the number of cells killed is directly proportional to the amount of drug given. Examples include alkylating agents, antibiotics, nitrosureas, hormones, and corticosteroids (Table 5-2).

*Alkylating agents* are cell cycle–nonspecific. They produce breaks and cross-linking in the strands of DNA, so the cell cannot replicate. They damage DNA in both resting and dividing cells.

*Antitumor antibiotics* are cell cycle–nonspecific. They bind directly with DNA and change its configuration, thereby hindering replication. They disrupt DNA transcription and inhibit DNA and RNA synthesis.

*Hormones* are cell cycle–nonspecific. They alter the environment of the cell by affecting the cell membrane's permeability. Hormonal therapy is based on the principle that changing the hormonal environment of a cancer cell suppresses its growth.

*Antihormonal agents* neutralize the effect of or inhibit the production of natural hormones used by hormone-dependent tumors.

*Corticosteroids* provide an antiinflammatory effect on body tissues. Although the exact mechanism is unknown, corticosteroids are synergistic with some chemotherapeutic agents. They also promote a feeling of well-being and improved appetite.

*Nitrosoureas* are cell cycle–nonspecific. They are similar to the alkylating agents. DNA and RNA synthesis is inhibited. Nitrosoureas also have the ability to cross the blood-brain barrier.

*Miscellaneous agents* may be cell cycle–specific or –nonspecific or both.

## Cell Cycle

Cell cycle is the amount of time required for the cell to go from one mitosis to another.[5] Cycling cells go through four phases. The first phase is G, or the first gap. This is the stage between mitosis and the beginning of DNA synthesis, when active RNA synthesis and protein synthesis take place. The duration of the G phase may vary from 8 to 48 hours, and its duration influences the rate of cell division. Rapidly proliferating cells like those of the skin have few cells in the G phase.

As cells leave the G phase, they enter the S phase, in which DNA synthesis occurs. This phase takes 10 to 30 hours. After the S phase, the $G_2$ phase, or second-gap phase, which is a resting phase, begins. In this phase RNA and protein are synthesized for mitosis. This phase lasts 1 to 12 hours. The last phase of the cell cycle, the M phase, occurs when mitosis takes place. The M phase takes about 1 hour and involves the formation of the spindle, separation of chromosomes, and the division of the cell.

## Uses

Chemotherapy generally is used in four ways, depending on the stage of disease (see the box below). It is the primary treatment in advanced cancer for which there is no alternative

---

### USES OF CHEMOTHERAPY

**INDUCTION CHEMOTHERAPY**
Primary treatment when no alternative
  exists

**ADJUVANT CHEMOTHERAPY**
Used in conjunction with another
  treatment modality to treat
  micrometastases

**NEOADJUVANT CHEMOTHERAPY
(PRIMARY CHEMOTHERAPY)**
Used to treat patients with localized
  disease for which an alternative therapy
  is not completely effective

**COMBINATION CHEMOTHERAPY**
Administration of two or more
  chemotherapeutic drugs in the
  treatment of cancer to provide maximal
  cell kill within the range of toxicity
  tolerated by the host for each drug

treatment. *Induction chemotherapy* is a term used to describe this therapy. Selection of treatment is based on the effectiveness of the drugs in animal models. Chemotherapy given after induction therapy fails is referred to as *salvage therapy*.[9]

The second use of chemotherapy is as an adjunct after the primary tumor has been removed by an alternative method. *Adjuvant chemotherapy* is based on response rates in groups of patients with the same histologic type of advanced cancer. The determination of need for adjuvant chemotherapy is based on the risk of recurrence after local treatment alone.[9]

Chemotherapy also is used as the primary treatment for patients with localized cancer. This third use is known as *neoadjuvant chemotherapy* or primary chemotherapy.

Primary chemotherapy has the potential to decrease the size and extent of the tumor mass, which can influence the need for and effectiveness of subsequent alternative treatments. For example, chemotherapy can increase the effectiveness of a dose of radiation therapy or decrease the size of the radiation therapy field.[9]

The fourth way chemotherapy is used is as *combination chemotherapy*. The majority of cancers that can be cured with chemotherapy are cured only with combination chemotherapy.[9] A sample combination chemotherapy protocol is given in the box below. All the drugs used in combination must have activity against the cancer being treated. The minimum dose for each drug is based on the minimum effective dosage for that drug when given as a single agent. Drugs that interrupt the cell cycle at several different sites can be combined for synergistic effects. Drugs in combination should have as little cross-toxicity as possible.

Tumor cells can develop a resistance to chemotherapeutic agents. The mechanism(s) by which the drug becomes ineffective and the tumor resistant is understood for some of the agents. When drugs are combined in a treatment protocol, therefore, it is important to avoid using drugs that are rendered inactive by the same or similar mechanisms.[30]

---

### SAMPLE CHEMOTHERAPY PROTOCOL FOR BLADDER CANCER

| METHOTREXATE | | ADRIAMYCIN | |
|---|---|---|---|
| Classification | Antimetabolite | Classification | Antibiotic |
| Action | Interferes with DNA synthesis | Action | Inhibits synthesis of DNA and RNA |
| Nadir | 10 to 14 days | Nadir | 10 to 14 days |
| **VELBAN** | | **CISPLATIN** | |
| Classification | Vinca alkaloid | Classification | Alkylating agent |
| Action | Arrests mitosis | Action | Blocks DNA synthesis |
| Nadir | 5 to 9 days | Nadir | Day 20 |

## Dose Calculations

The drug dosage for a specific individual is calculated before chemotherapy is initiated. Drug doses are usually stated in terms of body surface area; therefore the dosages are calculated in milligrams per square meter ($m^2$). Because height and weight are used to determine body surface, it is important that these be measured accurately each time the dose is calculated.

## Administration Methods

The route of administration is based on the metabolism and absorption of the drug. The route of choice is that which will deliver the optimum amount of drug to the tumor without compromising organ function.

## Side Effects

Some degree of injury to normal cells occurs with the use of chemotherapeutic agents. The number of normal cells affected is determined by their rate of proliferation or cellular division. It is these rapidly proliferating tissues (bone marrow, gastrointestinal epithelium, and hair follicles) that exhibit most of the toxic effects of cytotoxic drugs (Table 5-2).

Most chemotherapeutic drugs cause some degree of bone marrow depression (myelosuppression), as evidenced by lowering counts of white blood cells, red blood cells, and platelets. A patient receiving chemotherapy usually has the lowest blood cell counts (nadir) about 7 to 14 days after treatment. The patient's blood cell counts should be monitored closely, and the patient should be taught the signs and symptoms associated with low blood cell counts. The patient must return to the clinic to have the blood cell counts measured and to ensure that the patient is not at high risk for complications associated with neutropenia, anemia, or thrombocytopenia.

## Nursing Implications

Chemotherapy can be administered as a single agent or in a multiple-agent protocol to provide maximum destruction to the malignant cells. Each drug produces specific side effects that develop, peak, and resolve within predictable time frames. When the nurse is familiar with this information, a plan of care specific for the patient with an ostomy can be developed that monitors for potential problems (such as episodes of diarrhea) and provides interventions to prevent or manage complications (such as discontinuing colostomy irrigations and wearing a drainable fecal pouch). Such prior planning and teaching offers the patient an element of control at a time when he or she may feel out of control and helps avert frantic telephone calls or clinic visits. Although all patients receiving daunorubicin or doxorubicin should be alerted that their urine may turn red, such a development in the patient with a urinary diversion could be quite alarming. Nursing implications of particular relevance to the patient with an ostomy are summarized in Table 5-3.

## RADIATION THERAPY

More than 60% of patients with cancer receive radiation therapy at some point during the illness.[39] The aim of radiotherapy may be curative or palliative. Although occasionally used alone, it more frequently is used in combination with surgery, chemotherapy, or biotherapy. Radiotherapy may be curative in treating skin cancer, carcinoma of the cervix, or Hodgkin's disease. Radiation therapy may be used on a palliative basis to provide pain relief, to prevent pathologic fractures, to prevent paralysis in the patient with spinal cord

**Table 5-3**  Management of cancer therapy complications in the patient with an ostomy

| Complication | Intervention | Rationale |
|---|---|---|
| Neutropenia, i.e., absolute neutrophil count (ANC) < 1000 cells/mm$^3$ (ANC equals percentage of neutrophils multiplied by white blood cell count [WBC]; normal WBC is 3500 to 12,000 cells/mm$^3$) | Provide gentle peristomal skin care; avoid traumatic adhesive removal<br>Do not shave peristomal skin<br>Monitor laboratory values for further decline and signs of improvement<br>Monitor peristomal skin for complications such as yeast infections, and treat accordingly<br>Perform daily head-to-toe skin assessments for potential sites for infection | Any break in skin presents potential site for infection |
| Thrombocytopenia<br>150,000 to 350,000 platelets/mm$^3$ = normal<br>< 50,000 platelets/mm$^3$ = potential risk of bleeding<br>< 20,000 platelets/mm$^3$ = risk of spontaneous bleeding<br>< 10,000 platelets/mm$^3$ = risk of hemorrhage (especially central nervous system and gastrontestinal [GI]) | Provide gentle peristomal skin care; avoid traumatic adhesive removal<br>Assess patient's pouch application and removal techniques to ensure that these are appropriate<br>Identify and eliminate any practices that may traumatize stoma (e.g., tight clothing, belt over stoma, or aspirin in the pouch)<br>Monitor for bleeding, into the pouch, and carefully ascertain source of bleeding (external mucosa or bowel lumen)<br>NOTE: Presence of blood in urine from GI conduit may represent GI or urinary tract problem<br>Stop colostomy irrigations | Gentle technique must be used to prevent traumatizing stoma or skin and inadvertently causing bleeding; friction from tight-fitting clothes and certain activities may elicit bleeding |
| Anemia<br>Less than 12g/100 ml | Reevaluate stoma care to simplify procedure and conserve energy<br>Provide assistance as necessary<br>Teach patient or significant other that pale stoma color indicates anemia<br>Encourage patient to eat well and to increase intake of iron-rich foods | Decreased oxygen-carrying capacity of blood may result in tachypnea, fatigue, and possibly confusion |

*Continued.*

**Table 5-3**    Management of cancer therapy complications in the patient with an ostomy—cont'd

| Complication | Intervention | Rationale |
|---|---|---|
| Diarrhea | Forewarn patient receiving chemotherapy and radiation to abdomen or pelvis that diarrhea may develop<br>Convert patient who wears closed pouch to use of drainable pouch<br>Discontinue colostomy irrigations once diarrhea starts; can resume irrigations 2 to 3 weeks after completion of radiation therapy and chemotherapy, if diarrhea is resolved<br>Instruct patient to modify diet to low-roughage diet once diarrhea starts<br>Encourage intake of foods that thicken stool<br>Collaborate with physician regarding use of antidiarrheals<br>Monitor for signs and symptoms of fluid and electrolyte depletion<br>Educate patient about preceding signs and symptoms | Radiation therapy and chemotherapy damage epithelial lining of GI tract, which is then sloughed in diarrheal stools; mucosal villi may atrophy temporarily and contribute to diarrhea; actions should be taken to reduce exposure of mucosal surface to irritating substances; diarrheal stools can overwhelm capacity of closed pouch, cause leakage, and require frequent changes, all of which tax patient's energy and financial resources |
| Constipation | Evaluate patient to ascertain potenial cause of constipation; *if* tumor growth is excluded, perform the following:<br>Encourage high fluid intake (1500 to 3000 ml daily)<br>Evaluate dietary habits, and encourage high-fiber diet<br>Review patient's pain control history (medication and frequency)<br>Collaborate with physician regarding the use of stool softeners<br>Evaluate colostomy irrigation technique; provide suggestions for improvement as needed | Many factors can predispose patient with cancer to constipation (dehydration, certain chemotherapeutic agents, narcotics, and tumor growth); all these factors must be evaluated before appropriate steps can be taken to relieve constipation; narcotics slow bowel transit time; although high-fiber diet and increased fluid intake create stool that is easier to pass, laxatives may also be needed (even if patient irrigates); poor colostomy irrigation technique may result in inadequate evacuation |

**Table 5-3**  Management of cancer therapy complications in the patient with an ostomy—cont'd

| Complication | Intervention | Rationale |
|---|---|---|
| Stomatitis (temporary condition usually occurring at chemotherapy nadir; may involve entire GI tract) | Provide gentle cleansing of stoma<br>Evaluate patient's stoma care techniques and dress style to identify and elminate actions that may traumatize stoma<br>Elminate use of products that may be irritating or painful (such as products that contain alcohol)<br>Avoid unneccessary manipulation of stoma, such as with digital examinations or colostomy irrigations<br>Monitor for associated complications such as candidiasis, neutropenia, and infection or erythema at mucocutaneous junction | Gentle technique must be used to prevent traumatizing stoma and inadvertently causing bleeding; friction caused by tight-fitting clothes and certain activities may elicit bleeding |
| Cystitis | Maintain proper hydration during administration of certain chemotherapeutic agents<br>Monitor for symptoms of detrusor irritability during chemotherapy regimen or radiation therapy<br>Encourage patient to reduce intake of foods and fluids known to irritate bladder (such as caffeine, fruit juices, and chocolate)<br>Rule out urinary tract infection<br>Encourage patient to maintain appropriate fluid intake<br>Collaborate with physician regarding medications used to reduce detrusor irritability (e.g., anticholinergics)<br>Identify and discontinue patient medications that may aggrevate detrusor irritability<br>Monitor for hematuria | Certain chemotherapeutic agents may produce renal insufficiency unless proper hydration is maintained; when bladder is in radiation field and during chemotherapy treatments, epithelial lining sloughs, causing bladder to become irritated and potentially to bleed; interventions to decrease detrusor irritability should be pursued |

lesions, or to reduce central nervous system symptoms caused by brain metastasis or spinal cord compression.[26] Hemorrhage, ulceration, and fungating lesions may be shrunk and sometimes eliminated by palliative radiation therapy.

Although treatment techniques and equipment may vary, the principles of radiobiology and radiation physics form the basis on which each patient's course of treatment is selected. Understanding these principles assists the nurse to support and care for the patient with cancer who is receiving radiation therapy.

## Radiation Technology

Radiation therapy uses ionizing (high-energy) radiation to interact with the atoms and molecules of tumor cells and to effect specific harmful biologic changes.[20] To understand the effect of radiation on cells, it is important to review some basic principles of radiation. Radiation is energy transmitted in the form of waves or particles. Examples include radiowaves, ultraviolet light, visible light, x rays, and gamma rays. X rays and gamma rays are types of ionizing radiation that damage the cell's DNA, causing breakage of one or both chromosomal strands. Immediate cell death may occur if the chromosomal damage is irreparable. Despite the chromosomal damage, some cells survive. The cell, however, is unable to divide and dies at the time of mitosis.[22]

The degree of cellular damage induced by ionizing radiation varies greatly. Cells that divide rapidly are more vulnerable, or radiosensitive, than are those that divide slowly. Therefore the various organ systems in the body possess differing degrees of radiosensitivity. Cells in the resting stage are less sensitive to radiation than are those involved in the active cellular division of mitosis. Poorly differentiated cells are more sensitive to radiation therapy than are well-differentiated cells. Well-oxygenated tissues are sensitive to radiation therapy because oxygen is needed to form the chemically active substances that cause the DNA breakage; poorly oxygenated cells at the center of the tumor are not as vulnerable to radiation. Thus revascularization and oxygenation of the cells at the center of the tumor after radiotherapy may allow these cells to be more vulnerable to radiotherapy.

Normal cells also are affected by the ionizing radiation, which accounts for the side effects of radiation therapy. The DNA breakage is more easily repaired in normal cells; thus treatment schedules are developed to kill as many cancer cells as possible while minimizing the damage to normal cells.

When orthovoltage x-ray equipment was used during the early years of radiotherapy, the dose that could be delivered to deep tumors was limited by normal skin tolerance rather than by damage to other structures. Skin erythema was used as a crude measurement of tissue dose.[19] Today, with the use of megavoltage equipment the maximal dose that can be delivered to deeper tissues has increased because of the skin-sparing effect of high-energy x rays. The maximum dose delivered from the cobalt-60 machines is 0.5 cm below the skin. With the linear accelerators the maximum dose may range from 1.5 to 5 cm or more below the skin, depending on the machine's energy.[28] Irradiation by linear accelerator is the treatment of choice for most cancers because it spares the skin and penetrates deeper into the patient's body than does cobalt.[33]

## Delivery Methods

The types of equipment used in radiotherapy are numerous and vary in their applications to clinical practice. Equipment may be classified according to use: external radiation, or teletherapy (treatment from a source outside the body), versus internal radiation, or

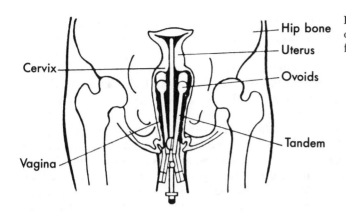

Cervix

Vagina

Hip bone

Uterus

Ovoids

Tandem

**Fig. 5-2** Intracavitary tandem and ovoids placed to provide internal radiation for cervical cancer.

brachytherapy (radiation from a source placed within the body or body cavity) (Fig. 5-2). In addition to teletherapy and brachytherapy, radiotherapy may be administered systemically by use of radioisotopes. In such cases the radioactive substance travels to the area of the body requiring treatment. Thyroid cancer frequently is treated with radioactive iodine in this way.

The use of tumor-specific antibodies that have been paired with radioactive isotopes also is being studied. These antibodies are attracted to specific antigens on certain tumor cells. They are produced in animals and injected intravenously into the patient. The radioactive isotope attached to the antibody treats the cancer.[7]

**External Radiation Therapy.** When the decision has been made to use radiotherapy, the radiation oncologist devises the treatment plan. The first steps in planning are localizing the tumor and defining the volume of tumor to be treated. A simulator is a machine that simulates the actual treatment machine. During the simulation process the tumor area is located and marked either with a temporary marker or with permanent tattoos. These marks ensure that the boundaries of the treatment areas are consistent. Anatomic areas that must be shielded from the radiation beam also are identified and protected with blocks that are constructed from lead or high-density alloys. In this way the beam of radiation reaches only specific structures. Special plastic forms or molds also may be used to help support the patient and to assist the person to maintain the necessary position during treatment. Portal films are then taken through the treatment machine to confirm the treatment field and the placement of blocks in the desired position.[20] The treatment planning usually lasts 1 to 2 hours, in contrast to the actual treatment, which lasts 2 to 5 minutes.[22]

A variety of machines are used in radiation therapy. The type of machine used depends on the tumor type, the disease stage, whether vital organs must be protected, the patient's age, and any concomitant disease.[26] The higher the energy produced by the machine, the greater the depth of penetration of the radiation beam. With higher energies the maximum effect of the radiation occurs below the skin surface. The dose to the skin is minimized or spared.

The radiation is divided into daily dosages or fractions to be given over time. This is called fractionation. With fractionation, more radiation can be given overtime to maximize its effect on the tumor while minimizing the effects on normal tissues. Normal cells can recover between treatments, but tumor cells cannot. Each treatment has a cumulative effect on the cancer.[42]

Therapeutic dosage is expressed in a unit called a gray (Gy), which refers to the dose of radiation absorbed by the tissue. The gray has replaced the rad (radiation absorbed dose); 1 Gy equals 100 rad, or 1 cGy (centigray) equals 1 rad.

**Internal Radiation Therapy.** Brachytherapy is the use of radioactive materials placed into or on the body to treat malignant disease. Brachytherapy frequently is combined with teletherapy and also may be used preoperatively and postoperatively. Radioactive isotopes for brachytherapy application are contained in a variety of forms, such as wires, ribbons, needles, grains, seeds, and capsules. The source is selected by the radiotherapist according to the site to be treated, the size of the lesion, and whether the implant is to be temporary or permanent. Intracavitary, interstitial, and metabolized are the three types. Cancers of the brain, tongue, esophagus, lung, breast, vagina, cervix, uterus, rectum, and bladder may be treated with brachytherapy and the use of intracavitary or interstitial sources. The radioactive material is encapsulated (sealed) so that no radioactive contamination of body fluids occurs. The radioactive isotopes are placed in the body by means of an afterloading technique. In the operating room the applicators are placed in or near the tumor. After the patient returns to the hospital room, the radioactive isotopes are placed within the applicator. The implant may remain in the body for 2 to 5 days.

A recent development in the United States is the use of remote afterloading brachytherapy equipment rather than manual afterloading brachytherapy. Remote afterloading precludes exposure of nursing personnel to radiation because the radioactive sources are withdrawn pneumatically into a shielded container whenever someone enters the room. As a result, time spent with the patient can focus on patient needs rather than on radiation exposure.[32]

Metabolized radiotherapy is the ingestion, instillation, or injection of radioactive materials that are absorbed by the body. An example is the ingestion of iodine-131 for thyroid cancer. When radioactive isotopes are injected or taken orally (unsealed sources), the patient, as well as bodily secretions, may be radioactive. Nursing care must follow specific radiation safety precautions.

## Radiosensitizers and Radioprotectors

The purpose of radiotherapy is to achieve maximum tumor cell kill while minimizing injury to normal tissues (referred to as the therapeutic ratio). Work to improve the therapeutic ratio has resulted in the development of certain compounds that work to increase the radiosensitivity of tumor cells or to help protect normal cells from radiation's effects. Combined-modality therapy that uses chemotherapy to enhance the antitumor effects of radiation therapy achieves greater cell kill than either therapy could achieve alone. Examples of chemotherapeutic agents that can be used as radiosensitizers include doxorubicin, 5-fluorouracil (5-FU), bleomycin, and cisplatin.[20]

The use of chemical radiosensitizing compounds to increase the effects of radiation currently is being studied. Hypoxic cell sensitizers such as metronidazole (Flagyl), misonidazole, and etanidazole damage the cell's DNA by preventing cell repair. Depending on the agent, major side effects are neurotoxicity, nausea and vomiting, and skin rashes.[22]

## Intraoperative Radiation Therapy

Intraoperative radiation therapy (IORT) combines surgery and radiation therapy in an attempt to decrease local recurrence rates for cancers that cannot be controlled by surgery or radiation therapy alone.[17] The IORT usually is a single, high-dose fraction (1000 to 4000 cGy) delivered to the exposed tumor during the surgical procedure using specialized lucite applicators. This procedure maximizes the dose to the tumor while minimizing the radiation to normal tissues. Locally advanced abdominal malignancies are the primary indications for IORT. Cancers treated with IORT in clinical trials include gastric, pancreatic, colorectal, bladder, cervical, and retroperitoneal sarcomas. The advantage of IORT in the treatment of these malignancies is twofold. First, tumor control can be obtained when local spread is so extensive that surgical resection is an inadequate approach. Second, IORT applies radiation directly to the tumor, thereby reducing injury to surrounding tissue and potentially reducing morbidity. Additionally, because the damage to surrounding tissue and capillaries is reduced with IORT, the negative sequelae of combination surgery and IORT may be fewer than those associated with the combination of surgery and external radiation therapy.[24]

Clinical information regarding complications and side effects of IORT is limited. Nausea, vomiting, and anorexia have been reported.[17]

## Side Effects

The side effects associated with radiation therapy depend on the area treated, total dose fractionation, delivery method, and individual patient differences. The response of normal tissue to irradiation is classified as either acute or chronic. Acute changes may occur within a few weeks after the start of treatment or a few weeks after completion of therapy. Since radiation has its greatest effect on rapidly dividing cells, the epithelial tissues such as mucous membranes and the skin are most susceptible to its effects. Examples of acute skin changes include erythema, permanent tanning, telangiectasia, dry desquamation, and pruritus; with continued therapy, moist desquamation can occur. Loss of sweat and sebaceous glands causes drying of the skin.

Chronic or late changes may occur several months or years later. Examples of chronic skin changes include atrophy, loss of elasticity, fibrosis, induration of the subcutaneous tissues, and tissue necrosis. Damage to endothelial and connective tissue contributes to these chronic reactions.

The new skin that develops after radiation damage is thin and never achieves normal thickness because of changes in dermal circulation.[33] Capillaries in the treatment field are narrowed and may be obliterated by the radiation. This is termed *radiation endarteritis*. Early changes are believed to be temporary, whereas late effects are more permanent.[38]

## Nursing Implications

The effects of radiotherapy to the abdomen and pelvis are primarily associated with changes in the gastrointestinal tract and damage to the skin and underlying tissue within the treatment port. Acute effects of pelvic and abdominal radiation may include mucosal injury to the stoma and acute enteritis, causing diarrhea.

Diarrhea in the patient receiving pelvic or abdominal radiation therapy results from damage to the intestinal villi and mucosa, specifically, epithelial cell death, reduction in the villi length, and a resultant decrease in the absorptive capacity of the bowel.[22] Interventions to manage the diarrhea once it develops include dietary modification, antidiarrheals, and discontinuation of colostomy irrigations. Although diarrhea is often acute and temporary (developing after 8 to 12 treatments), it also may be permanent.

Mucosal damage to the stoma can occur when the stomal is located within the treatment field. Ulcerations, sloughing, or the development of white areas resembling thrush can develop. When located within the treatment field, stomal mucosa must be protected from friction and trauma, for example, rubbing against the pouch film. Lubricants such as baby oil can be inserted into the pouch to lubricate the walls of the pouch and prevent trauma. If the patient wears only a gauze pad over the stoma, a Vaseline gauze covering should be placed over the stoma. Occassionally a mucous fistula that is within the radiation field produces significant amounts of mucus and may necessitate pouching.

When the stoma is located within the treatment field, the nurse should collaborate with the radiation oncologist to ascertain whether the pouch should remain in place or be removed during the treatment. Historically it was believed that the pouch would alter the depth of penetration of the x rays and might intensify the dose of radiation to the skin (referred to as a bolus effect). With the improved treatment machines and thinner pouch material, however, this bolus effect to the skin is believed by many experts to be minuscule.

If the pouch is to be removed during the treatment, the nurse should reevaluate the patient's pouching system. Nonadhesive pouching systems such as karaya ring pouches secured with belts or the nonadhesive ostomy system (VPI, Spencer, Indiana) should be considered. These systems accomplish two goals: elimination of adhesives in the treatment field and control of the costs of frequent pouch changes. After completion of the radiation treatments and recovery of the skin, the patient often can resume the previously used pouching system.

Whenever the stoma site is within the treatment field (whether the pouch is worn or not during treatments), the nurse must reevaluate the patient's pouching system and technique for pouch application and removal. Gentle skin cleansing, gentle adhesives, and gentle adhesive removal technique are imperative to prevent additional trauma to the skin. It generally is advisable to avoid soaps, solvents, cements, sealants, pastes, and powders unless essential. These products are potentially harmful because they may be difficult to remove from the skin and increase the risk of epidermal damage. In addition, many of these products contain alcohol and contribute to the epidermal dessication typical of radiation. Finally, these products may contain substances that can create an irritant dermatitis when applied to radiosensitive skin. Products containing bismuth, zinc, or other heavy metals must be avoided because these substances scatter radiation and create a bolus effect to the skin. Hard faceplates, belts, and hardware also must be avoided because of the potential bolus effects.[37] The box on p. 183 summarizes stomal and peristomal skin care that is appropriate when the stoma is located within the radiation field.

Radiation endarteritis persists after radiation therapy is completed. Overtime, however, collateral circulation develops. Because surgery inherently involves dissection of capillaries, an element of ischemia is induced; therefore surgical procedures conducted within irradiated skin further impair tissue perfusion. Incisions should be monitored closely for complications such as dehiscence (for example, a mucocutaneous separation can occur at the base of a newly constructed stoma). Plates 23 and 24 provide examples of compromised perfusion after surgical manipulation of irradiated tissue.

Acute and chronic effects of radiation on the gastrointestinal and integumentary systems pose difficulties with nutrition, fluid balance, and ostomy care. Many patients have

---

### CARE OF STOMA AND PERISTOMAL SKIN LOCATED WITHIN THE RADIATION FIELD

1. Empty pouch before treatment
2. Lift tail of pouch out of treatment field (if possible),
3. Cleanse skin with soft cloth and tap water.
4. Use a *dab* technique to cleanse and dry the skin; *do not* rub skin in radiation field.
5. *No* soaps, perfumes, deodorants should come in contact with the irradiated skin.
6. Avoid using unnecessary products in pouching system.
7. Avoid using products containing zinc, bismuth, or heavy metals during therapy.
8. Protect stomal mucosa from trauma between daily radiation treatments (for example, rubbing against the pouch film) by inserting lubricant in the pouch or placing Vaseline gauze over the stoma if currently not pouching stoma.
9. Encourage patient to trim nails to prevent creating breaks in the skin if the irradiated tissue is scratched accidentally.
10. Use pouch covers to absorb moisture trapped between skin and pouch.
11. Avoid sun exposure to irradiated area (during treatment *and* once treatments are completed).
12. Consult with radiation therapist for any peristomal skin complications that develop during treatment.

---

lethargy, malaise, anorexia, nausea and vomiting, and diarrhea. Most of these symptoms are self-limiting but may add to the emotional trauma of cancer and the rigors of treatment.

## HYPERTHERMIA

Hyperthermia, or the use of heat (greater than 41° C), has been used to treat locally advanced tumors and small, superficial metastatic nodules. Malignant cells are believed to be more heat-sensitive than normal cells. Tumor cells lack the ability to repair DNA damaged by heat. They also lack the capacity for heat dissipation found in normal cells. Heat increases the metabolic rate of tumor cells and thus the need for oxygen, which the tumor blood supply cannot meet. Heat also inhibits the repair of radiation damage, thereby increasing the radiation effect. Local heat can also increase permeability of the tumor cell membrane to allow chemotherapeutic penetration of the drug. The number of treatments depends on the location and size of the tumor.

Hyperthermia can be applied locally, perfused regionally as a heated solution through a part of the body, or applied to the whole body to treat widespread disease. Side effects associated with hyperthermia include local discomfort or pain and skin reactions ranging from erythema to thermal burns and blisters.

## BIOTHERAPY

Biotherapy is the treatment with agents derived from biologic sources that affect biologic responses.[34] Known as biologic response modifiers (BRMs), these agents make up the fourth type of cancer treatment. As their name suggests, BRMs boost the body's response to tumor cells and other foreign substances, so BRMs fight the cancer indirectly. Immunotherapy actually is a subcategory of BRM therapies.[40]

## History

In the late 1800s a New York City surgeon, William Coley, described tumor regressions in patients with bacterial infections. Coley used live bacteria and, later, filtered toxins known as *Coley's toxins*, to induce an infectious response in patients with cancer.[27] In 1975 Carswell named the substance tumor necrosis factor.[8]

In 1957 interferon was identified by Issacs and Lindean at the National Institute of Medical Research in London.[13] They discovered that cells exposed to a virus produced a protein that interfered with assaults by the virus.[13] In a 1960 Flash Gordon comic strip by Dan Berry, interferon injections were used to save the lives of spacemen infected with an extraterrestrial virus.[41]

The application of immunotherapy in cancer therapy has been used only since the 1960s, when many clinical trials of bacterial agents, bacille Calmette-Guérin (BCG) and Corynebacterium parvum, were begun. In the early 1970s, human alpha-interferon was produced in sufficient amounts for clinical research.[13] In 1975 the clinical trials were expanded with funding from the National Cancer Institute and, later, the American Cancer Society. In 1979 Taniquchi produced beta-interferon, which was followed by alpha-interferon subtypes and gamma-interferon.[16] In 1986 alpha-interferon received approval from the Food and Drug Administration (FDA) for use in hairy cell leukemia. In 1989 the FDA approved alpha-interferon for clinical use in acquired immunodeficiency syndrome (AIDS)–related Kaposi's sarcoma.[23]

## Immune Response

The immune response begins when a nonself cell enters the body. All organisms and cells carry proteins on their surface called *antigens*. Antigens facilitate the recognition of self and nonself cells by the immune system.

The immune response has two major components. The cellular response produces lymphocytes capable of destroying tumor cells on contact. When stimulated by an antigen, these lymphocytes (T cells) are released into the bloodstream. The T cells destroy cancer cells on contact and also release cytotoxins that damage the cell membrane, eventually resulting in lysis or death of the malignant cell.

The second component of the immune system is activation of lymphocytes (B cells) for antibody production. When stimulated by antigens, B cells differentiate into plasma cells, which are the major source of antibody production.

At present the normal immune response can "handle" only a limited number of cancer cells, up to 10 million. At between 10 million and 100 million cancer cells the effectiveness of the immune response is limited. After a growth to 100 million cells the immune response is incapable of preventing further growth; thus BRMs cannot be used as the primary mode of cancer therapy at this time.[36]

## Biologic Response Modifiers in the Treatment of Cancer

Because of the recent advances in recombinant DNA technology, BRMs are now produced in large quantities in laboratories and are available for cancer therapy. BRMs contribute either indirectly or directly to the host's immune system, promoting an antitumor response. These agents produce their effects by stimulating the host's natural defense mechanism (active immunity) or by administering immunologically active natural substances (passive immunity). For example, the interferons perform dual functions, stimulating natural killer cells and macrophages and inhibiting tumor cell growth.

Depending on the BRM, one or more therapeutic effects may be seen: (1) regulation or promotion of the immune response, or both, (2) direct antitumor or cytotoxic activity, and (3) interference with the ability of tumor cells to metastasize, differentiate, or mature.[1]

Agents used in biotherapy include cytokines (interferon, interleukin, tumor necrosis factor, and colony-stimulating factors), monoclonal antibodies (MAbs), immunologically active cells (lymphokine-activated killer [LAK] cells), tumor-infiltrating lymphocytes (TIL), and miscellaneous agents such as BCG.

## Side Effects

Common side effects of the BRMs are listed in the box below. The most common side effect is an influenza-like syndrome that includes fever, chills, myalgias, headache and fatigue. Approaches to managing this syndrome include altering the time or dose of treatment, administering medications to help control the symptoms, and providing comfort measures. Fatigue occurs in almost everyone receiving BRMs. Altering treatment times and spacing activities may help with fatigue. The side effects are limited to the duration of treatment. Combination therapy with radiation therapy or chemotherapy may magnify the toxicities more than if the biotherapy alone were used.

---

### COMMON SIDE EFFECTS OF BIOLOGIC RESPONSE MODIFIERS

**INFLUENZA-LIKE SYNDROME**
Fever
Chills
Myalgias and arthralgias
Headache
Fatigue

**GASTROINTESTINAL**
Nausea
Vomiting
Diarrhea
Anorexia
Xerostomia
Mucositis
Taste alterations

**NEUROLOGIC**
Mild confusion
Poor concentration
Somnolence
Irritability
Impaired memory
Sleep disturbances
Psychoses

**CARDIOPULMONARY**
Tachycardia/tachypnea
Pallor
Cyanosis
Hypotension (orthostatic)
Edema

**INTEGUMENTARY**
Erythematous rash
Facial flushing
Dryness
Pruritus
Desquamation

**RENAL AND HEPATIC**
Increased levels of blood urea nitrogen
 (BUN) and creatinine
Elevated findings in liver function studies

**HEMATOLOGIC**
Neutropenia
Thrombocytopenia
Anemia

## BONE MARROW TRANSPLANTATION

Conventional treatment of cancer may involve surgery, chemotherapy, radiation therapy, or a combination of these to destroy all cancer cells. Chemotherapy and radiation therapy doses are limited because of toxicity to the bone marrow. Many believe that if bone marrow toxicity could be eliminated, chemotherapy doses could be increased to levels that would cure the patient of the malignancy. If the patient's own bone marrow or that of a compatible donor can be introduced into the body and engrafted, chemotherapy doses higher than those conventionally used are possible. This is the idea behind bone marrow transplantation (BMT).[11]

### Indications

Bone marrow transplantation may be used in a variety of hematologic and nonhematologic malignancies and diseases. Donor availability, age, performance status (ability to perform activities of daily living), and patient goals are evaluated when considering BMT. BMT may be indicated for the following diseases: acute nonlymphocytic leukemia, acute lymphocytic leukemia, chronic myelogenous leukemia, lymphomas, miscellaneous hematologic conditions (multiple myeloma, myelodysplastic syndrome, and aplastic anemia), and some solid tumors (for example, breast cancer).

### Classification

There are three types of marrow transplantations: autologous, syngeneic, and allogeneic. The type of transplantation undertaken depends on the disease being treated and the availability of tissue-matched (histocompatible) donors.

*Autologous* BMT uses the patient's own bone marrow. Such a transplantation is relatively straightforward because the recipient's autologous marrow is guaranteed to be a "perfect match." For this transplantation to be undertaken, however, it is essential that the marrow not be obviously contaminated with tumor cells. For this reason the autologous marrow harvest is usually performed only when the patient is in complete remission. Nonetheless, the relapse rate after autologous transplantation is relatively high. It is thought that this relapse may be due to occult contamination of the marrow with cancer cells; therefore strategies to cleanse, or purge, the collected marrow could be beneficial. Laboratory treatments of the harvested marrow, such as with antitumor antibodies or chemotherapy, are being actively investigated at many transplantation centers.

An ideal source of "perfectly matched" bone marrow is an identical twin, a *syngeneic* transplantation. Unlike with the autologous transplantation, the identical twin's marrow is not contaminated with tumor, so purging is unnecessary. Realistically, however, only a few people who are candidates for BMT have identical twins. Even with syngeneic transplantation, the risk of relapse is high. Because these relapses cannot be attributed to reinfusion of tumor cells, it must be that tumor cells in many instances survive the chemotherapy or radiotherapy, or both, that is intended to destroy them.

The third type of marrow transplantation is the *allogeneic* transplantation. In this situation the donor of marrow is typically a sibling or an unrelated volunteer. In either case the donor must be highly tissue-matched with the recipient. Between two siblings the likelihood of a suitable match is only 25%; parents, half-siblings, and cousins are almost never matched closely enough to donate marrow. Because many persons have more than one sibling, the actual number of allogeneic candidates who have sibling donors is between 30% and 40%: the majority do not have family donors. For these individuals the only alternative

## SKIN MANIFESTATIONS OF GRAFT-VERSUS-HOST DISEASE

| | |
|---|---|
| Punctate, erythematous rash on palms and hands | Lichenifications |
| Lichen planus | Loss of skin elasticity |
| Generalized erythema | Contractures |
| Moist desquamation | Dermal indurations |
| Blisters | Ulcerations |
| Secondary infection | Alopecia |
| Sclerotic appearance | Multisystem involvement similar to |
| Pigmentation changes | collagen vascular disease |

is an unrelated, volunteer donor. Marrow donor registeries in the United States and several other countries exist for the primary purpose of locating matched, unrelated bone marrow donors.

Allogeneic transplantation is more difficult than either autologous or syngeneic transplantation because the donor marrow is never perfectly matched with the recipient. This inherent mismatch increases the possibility that the donor marrow will be rejected. The reverse situation, however, is more common. That is, T-lymphocytes within the donor marrow may attack (reject) the marrow of the recipient. This condition, which occurs in 30% to 80% of allogeneic transplantations, is termed graft-versus-host disease (GVHD). The primary target organs of GVHD are the skin, liver, and gastrointestinal tract. Symptoms are nonspecific and reflect dysfunction of these organ systems. Manifestations may include skin rash, pruritus, desquamation, abnormal results from liver function tests, jaundice, malaise, nausea, vomiting, anorexia, diarrhea, and weight loss.[2,10,11]

Graft-versus-host disease may develop soon after engraftment; it is then termed *acute* GVHD. When the disease develops more than 100 days after transplantation, it is termed *chronic* GVHD. The mechanisms of both types of GVHD are different. Although manifestations are different, some symptoms may be similar because the same organs are involved (see the box above). Medications such as cyclosporin A, antithymocyte globulin and corticosteroids are used to prevent and treat GVHD.

The benefit of the allogeneic transplantation is a lower risk of relapse. This benefit occurs because the donor marrow apparently can eradicate small numbers of tumor cells that survive the pretransplantation therapy. A direct correlation has been observed between the severity of GVHD and the likelihood that residual tumor cells will be eradicated. However, it remains unknown whether the cells in the donor marrow that cause GVHD are, in fact, the same cells that reduce the relapse risk. If the GVHD-causing cells in the donor marrow inoculum could be separated from the tumoricidal population, both the safety and efficacy of allogeneic transplantation would likely improve.

### Donation Process

Bone marrow is aspirated through hollow needles from easily accessible locations known to contain high concentrations of marrow cells. These are predominantly the iliac crests and, occasionally, the sternum. The bone marrow that is removed from these sites is mostly blood (by volume) but also contains many marrow stem cells, which are precursors to red blood cells, leukocytes, and platelets. The volume of blood and bone marrow required for transplantation depends on the concentration of cells present in the marrow and the recipient's size. Generally, about 100 needle insertions and 0.5 to 1.5 liters of mixed blood and bone marrow are needed. The bone marrow donation is performed in the operating room; general anesthesia is administered. When necessary, bone marrow can be stored in a frozen state. Autologous marrow is always stored for at least several days while the recipient receives pretransplantation therapy. The freezing procedure requires specialized equipment and careful processing of the marrow. Frozen marrow is stable for years.

### Transplantation Process

Patients usually have some type of pretransplantation therapy or conditioning. Conditioning regimens involve high-dose chemotherapy, radiation therapy (total body irradiation), and biotherapy either in isolation or in combination. The specific disease, as well as disease status, dictates the regimen used. Patients should be monitored for reactions to the conditioning regimens, which typically include nausea, vomiting, mucositis, hemorrhagic cystitis, diarrhea, and dermatologic reactions.[10] These complications can range in severity from minimal to life threatening.

Bone marrow transplantation itself is an intravenous infusion of the donor bone marrow and occurs in the hospital room. The bone marrow cells enter the bloodstream and eventually migrate to the patient's bone marrow, where the infused marrow "engrafts." This process of engraftment may require 15 to 25 days and is apparent when increased numbers of white blood cells are observed in the circulating blood. The period after the infusion of

---

### DERMATOLOGIC EFFECTS OF TOTAL BODY IRRADIATION

| | |
|---|---|
| Erythema | Dystrophic nails |
| Hair loss (regrows in 2 to 3 months) | Dryness and loss of sweat and sebaceous |
| Desquamation | glands |
| Hyperpigmentation | |

---

### SKIN CARE AFTER GRAFT-VERSUS-HOST DISEASE

| | |
|---|---|
| Avoid chemical irritants in skin care products (soaps, lotions, creams, shampoos, and cosmetics). | Eat a nutritious diet. |
| Shave with an electric razor. | Use hypoallergenic cosmetics. |
| Use a sunscreen with a sun protective factor (SPF) of 15 or greater when exposed to the sun. | Bathe in lukewarm water using a mild, nondeodorant soap. |
| | Wear loose clothing. |
| | Dust cornstarch lightly into skin folds. |

bone marrow and before engraftment is a time for many potential problems such as infection, renal failure, hepatic failure, respiratory failure, bleeding, and graft rejection.[2,10,11]

## Nursing Implications

The patient receiving BMT for the treatment of any type of disease process has significant physical, biologic, psychologic, and financial hurdles to overcome. Additionally, the nurse caring for such patients must include the family in providing care and education.

With regard to the patient with an ostomy who will have a BMT or has had a BMT, an important focus of care must be skin integrity. Collaboration with the patient's transplantation physician, dermatologist, and oncology or transplantation clinical nurse specialist is critical. Any dermatitis in the peristomal field must be carefully evaluated for possible GVHD. The nurse should also be familiar with the patient's pretransplantation conditioning regimen because total-body irradiation also affects the skin (see the box on p. 188, *top*). Skin care products recommended in the pouching system must be selected cautiously, following the general guidelines discussed for irradiated skin. The box on p. 188, *bottom*, lists care considerations for the skin after BMT and particularly after GVHD.

## SUMMARY

The term *cancer* refers to more than 200 diseases that have in common the production of abnormal cells. Effective management of the many malignant disorders requires a multimodal approach incorporating surgery, chemotherapy, radiotherapy, and biotherapy.

Surgery is the oldest treatment for cancer and involves removal of the tumor for cure or palliation. Chemotherapy interrupts the malignant cell's growth and replication. Radiotherapy destroys or interrupts the growth of the rapidly reproducing malignant cells. Biotherapy influences the patient's biologic response to the malignant cells. To provide the best possible therapy, all members of the health team, including the ET nurse, need to understand the principles of cancer therapy and the management of problems associated with each therapy.

## SELF-EVALUATION
### QUESTIONS

1. Ostomy surgery frequently results from which of the following malignancies:
   a. Bladder and ovary
   b. Bladder, cervical, and colon
   c. Cervical, urethra, and lung
   d. Prostate and liver
2. Identify a type of reconstructive surgery that may be used when the patient has a pelvic exenteration.
3. A palliative surgical procedure for cancer is performed:
   a. To improve the quality of life
   b. To prolong life
   c. As part of a research treatment plan
   d. None of the above
4. Classifications of chemotherapeutic agents are:
   a. Alkylating, antibiotics, and hormones
   b. Alkylating, beta-blockers, and hormones
   c. Alkylating, antibiotics, and narcotics
   d. Alkylating, antibiotics, and antihistamines
5. Vinca alkaloids are selected to interfere with which cell cycle phase?
   a. DNA synthesis
   b. RNA synthesis
   c. Cell division
   d. Resting phase
6. Describe the side effects of bone marrow depression that may influence nursing care of the patient with a stoma.
7. Identify three methods of radiation therapy that may be selected for a patient with a malignancy.
8. When an ostomy is within a radiation field, skin and ostomy products containing bismuth and zinc should be avoided because:
   a. These products cause diarrhea
   b. They enhance pouch adherence
   c. These products may cause an increase in the dose of radiation to the skin
   d. All of the above
9. The purpose of intraoperative radiation is:
   a. To control tumor metastasis
   b. To decrease local recurrence
   c. To avoid the skin damage of external radiation
   d. To increase the blood supply to adjacent tissues
10. Biologic response modifiers are used as a cancer treatment:
    a. To provide palliative therapy
    b. To enhance the effects of radiation
    c. To stimulate the host's natural defense mechanisms
    d. To identify the precise location of the malignancy

11. Autologous bone marrow transplantation is the use of:
    a. An unrelated donor
    b. A patient's sibling as the donor
    c. The patient's identical twin as a donor
    d. The patient's bone marrow
12. Explain the potential cause of diarrhea in a patient with an ostomy who is receiving radiation therapy.
13. The patient with an ostomy who is receiving cancer treatment that results in bone marrow depression needs to be monitored for:
    a. Neutropenia
    b. Thrombocytopenia
    c. Anemia
    d. All of the above

# SELF-EVALUATION

## ANSWERS

1. **b.** Bladder, cervical, and colon
2. A pelvic exenteration is an extensive surgery involving removal of the bladder, female organs, vagina, and sigmoid colon. Reconstructive surgery may be performed to create a neovagina by using gracilis myocutaneous flaps from each thigh.
3. **a.** To improve the quality of life
4. **a.** Alkylating, antibiotics, and hormones
5. **c.** Cell division
6. Bone marrow depression results in neutropenia and the potential for infection with the mucosa as a portal of entry; thus careful cleansing and manipulation are required to prevent damage. Thrombyctopenia can result, and excessive bleeding is a potential. Anemia that accompanies reduced oxygentation to the cells results in pale mucosa and patient fatigue in initiating self-care.
7. Radiation therapy may be administered (1) by external beam, (2) by internal, sealed sources such as wires and seeds, (3) intraoperatively, and (4) by radioisotope
8. **c.** These products may cause an increase in the dose to the skin
9. **b.** To decrease local recurrence
10. **c.** To stimulate the host's natural defense mechanisms
11. **d.** The patient's bone marrow
12. Radiation therapy may damage the intestinal villi, thus reducing the absorptive surface and capacity of the intestine.
13. **d.** All of the above

# REFERENCES

1. Abernathy E: Biotherapy: an introductory overview, *Oncol Nurs Forum* 14(suppl 6):13, 1987.
2. Beatty PB et al: Probability of finding HLA-matched unrelated marrow donors, *Transplantation* 45:714, 1988.
3. Boring CC et al: Cancer statistics 1991, *CA* 41(1):19, 1991.
4. Brown HG: The twenty-first century and the control of cancer? *Oncol Nurs Forum* 17:497, 1990.
5. Brown JK, Hogan CM: Chemotherapy. In Groenwald SL et al, editors: *Cancer nursing principles and practice*, Boston, 1990, Jones & Bartlett.
6. Brown JM: Hypoxic cell radiosensitizers: where next? *Int J Radiat Oncol Biol Phys* 16:987, 1989.
7. Bucholtz JD: Radiolabeled antibody therapy, *Semin Oncol Nurs* 3:67, 1987.
8. Currie GA, Basham C: Activated macrophages release a factor which lyses malignant cells but not normal cells, *J Exp Med* 142:1600, 1975.
9. DeVita VT: Principles of chemotherapy. In DeVita VT, Hellman S, Rosenberg SA, editors: *Cancer: principles and practice of oncology*, Philadelphia, 1989, JB Lippincott.
10. Ford R, Eisenberg S: Bone marrow transplant: recent advances and nursing implications, *Nurs Clin North Am* 25:405, 1990.
11. Freedman SE: An overview of bone marrow transplantation, *Semin Oncol Nurs* 4(1):3, 1988.
12. Gershenson DM, Smith DB: Enteric diversions. In Smith DB, Johnson DE, editors: *Ostomy care and the cancer patient: surgical and clinical considerations*, Orlando, Fla, 1986, Grune & Stratton.
13. Goldstein D, Laszlo J: Interferon therapy in cancer: from Imaginon to interferon, *Cancer Res* 46:4315, 1986.
14. Gullatte MM, Graves T: Advances in antineoplastic therapy, *Oncol Nurs Forum* 17:867, 1990.
15. Gurganus ES, Morris JE: Pelvic exenteration: the challenge of rehabilitation in a patient with multiple psychosocial problems, *J Enterostom Ther* 18(2):52, 1991.
16. Hahn MB, Jassak PF: Nursing management of patients receiving interferon, *Semin Oncol Nurs* 4:95, 1988.
17. Haibeck SV: Intraoperative radiation therapy, *Oncol Nurs Forum* 15:143, 1988.
18. Hampton B: Management of a patient following pelvic exenteration, *Semin Oncol Nurs* 2:281, 1986.
19. Hassey K, Rose C: Altered skin integrity in patients receiving radiation therapy, *Oncol Nurs Forum* 9:44, 1982.
20. Hilderly L: Radiotherapy. In Groenwald SL et al, editors: *Cancer nursing principles and practice*, Boston, 1987, Jones & Bartlett.
21. Huggins C, Hodges CV: Studies on prostatic cancer. I. The effect of castratins, of estrogen and of androgen injection on serum phosphatases in metastatic carcinoma of the prostate, *Cancer Res* 1:293, 1941.
22. Iwamoto R: Principles of radiation therapy. In Otto SE, editor: *Oncology nursing*, St Louis, 1991, Mosby–Year Book.
23. Jassak PF: Biotherapy. In Groenwald SL et al, editors: *Cancer nursing principles and practice*, Boston, 1990, Jones & Bartlett.
24. Kinsella TJ, Sindelae WF: Intraoperative radiation therapy. In DeVita VT, Hellman S, and Rosenberg SA, editors: *Cancer: principles and practice of oncology*, Philadelphia, 1985, JB Lippincott.
25. Koness RJ, Verzeridis M, Wanebo H: Major ablative surgery. In Moosa AR, Schimpff S, Robson M, editors: *Comprehensive textbook of oncology*, Baltimore, 1991, Williams & Wilkins.
26. Lewis F, LeVita M: Understanding radiotherapy, *Cancer Nurs* 11:174, 1988.
27. Mayer DK: Biotherapy: recent advances and nursing implications, *Nurs Clin North Am* 25:291, 1990.
28. McGowan K: Radiation therapy: saving your patient's skin, *RN* 52:24, 1989.
29. Meili L: Leukemia. In Otto SE, editor: *Oncology nursing*, St Louis, 1991, Mosby–Year Book.
30. Otto SE: Chemotherapy. In Otto SE, editor: *Oncology nursing*, St Louis, 1991, Mosby–Year Book.
31. Pfeifer KA: Surgery. In Otto SE, editor: *Oncology nursing*, St Louis, 1991, Mosby–Year Book.
32. Ratliff C: Brachytherapy revolution: the Selectron[137] CS unit, *Nurs News Today* 2(5):9, 1990.
33. Ratliff C: Impaired skin integrity related to radiation therapy, *J Enterostom Ther* 17(5):193, 1990.

34. Reiger PT: Biotherapy. In Otto SE, editor: *Oncology nursing,* St Louis, 1991, Mosby–Year Book.

35. Rosenberg AG: Principles and problems of cancer therapy, *J Enterostom Ther* 18(2):45, 1991.

36. Schneider SM et al: Cancer. In Long BC, Phipps WJ, editors: *Medical-surgical nursing: a nursing process approach,* St Louis, 1989, Mosby–Year Book.

37. Smith DB, Johnson DE: Preface. In Smith DB, Johnson DE, editors: *Ostomy care and the cancer patient: surgical and clinical considerations,* Orlando, Fla, 1986, Grune & Stratton.

38. Strohl RA: Radiation skin reactions, *Progressions: Developments in Ostomy and Wound Care* 1:3, 1989.

39. Strohl RA: Radiation therapy: recent advances and nursing implications, *Nurs Clin North Am* 25:329, 1990.

40. Suppers VJ, McClamrock EA: Biologicals in cancer treatment: future effects on nursing practice, *Oncol Nurs Forum* 12(3):27, 1985.

41. Toufexis A, Jecius A: The big *if* in cancer, *Time,* March 31, 1980, p 60.

42. Volker D: Neoplasia. In Beare PG, Myers JL, editors: *Principles and practice of adult health nursing,* St Louis, 1990, Mosby–Year Book.

43. Watson PG: Meeting the needs of patients undergoing ostomy surgery, *J Enterostom Ther* 12(4):121, 1985.

# 6

# Anatomy and Physiology of the Genitourinary Tract

SALLY J. IRRGANG

To effectively manage the care of the patient with a urinary diversion, the nurse needs to be knowledgeable about the structure and function of the urinary tract. Pathologic conditions of the urinary tract alter normal anatomy and function. This chapter reviews the anatomy and physiology of the genitourinary tract to lay the foundation for understanding the pathologic changes, surgical interventions, and nursing needs of patients with urinary diversions.

## URINARY TRACT

The urinary tract is composed of the kidneys, ureters, bladder, and urethra. Discussion of the male urinary system also includes the male reproductive organs: prostate, scrotum, testes, epididymis, vas deferens, spermatic cord, seminal vesicles, and penis. The female reproductive system is mentioned in this chapter in terms of location only, not structure or function.

The urinary tract is commonly divided into two areas: the upper and the lower urinary tracts (Fig. 6-1). The upper urinary tract includes the kidneys and ureters, and the lower tract comprises the bladder and urethra. Although diseases of the urinary system, such as

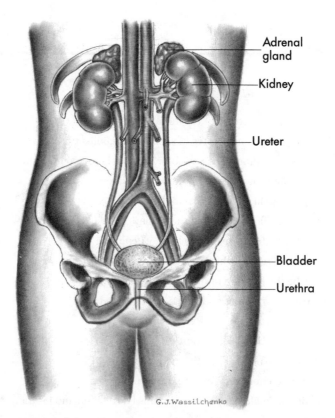

G.J.Wassilchenko

**Fig. 6-1** Components of the urinary system. (From Thompson JM et al: *Clinical nursing,* ed 2, St Louis, 1990, Mosby–Year Book.)

pyelonephritis, may be limited to the upper tract, because the urinary tract is contiguous, any pathologic condition of the lower tract often has an impact on the upper tract. For example, calculi often affect primarily the upper tract; however, if a calculus travels down the ureter and lodges in the urethra, more than one portion of the urinary tract will be affected.

## Upper Tract

### Kidneys

*Structure.* In the adult the kidney is a reddish-brown, bean-shaped organ. The average size of the kidney is 12 cm in length, 6 cm in width, 3 cm in depth, and 100 to 125 g in weight. Comparatively, as a percentage of total body weight, a newborn infant's kidney weighs approximately three times that of an adult.

Kidneys are retroperitoneal structures (located outside the peritoneum in a posterior position) on either side of the vertebral column, with their upper border at the level of the twelfth thoracic vertebrae and the lower border at the third lumbar vertebrae. Because of the liver, the position of the right kidney usually is 1.5 to 2 cm lower than the left. Adipose tissue encapsulates the kidneys to cushion them from trauma during activity.

The kidneys lie in close anatomic position to several organs. The adrenal glands rest atop each kidney. Other abdominal structures with which the kidneys are in contact include the liver, spleen, stomach, duodenum, colon, and small bowel.

The kidneys are supported anatomically by the renal pedicle, perirenal adipose tissue, abdominal muscle tone, and the sheer bulk of abdominal organs.[2] The kidneys normally move slightly with each respiration.

The medial aspect of each kidney has a depression that is referred to as *sinus:* the entrance to this sinus is the renal hilum. Blood vessels, nerves, lymphatics, and the ureters enter the kidney through the renal hilum.

The mass of the kidney comprises two distinct regions: the medulla and the cortex (Fig. 6-2). The medulla, the inner, darker area of the kidney, is composed of 8 to 12 conical renal pyramids, which house the duct system. The base of these pyramids faces the surface of the kidney; the apex of the pyramids, or renal papillae, extends toward the renal pelvis. The renal cortex forms a pale shell around the medulla. The cortex is composed of microscopic glomeruli that are the filtration units of the kidney.

The renal pelvis is a funnel-shaped structure located partially inside the renal sinus, with a capacity of approximately 5 ml. Structurally the renal pelvis consists of two or three major calices, which subdivide into a total of 8 to 14 minor calices per kidney. Minor calices then join to create the renal pelvis, which eventually tapers to form the ureter (Fig. 6-2).

Blood is delivered directly to the kidney from the aorta via the renal arteries. Approximately 20% of the cardiac output, or 1200 ml of blood, is processed by the kidneys every minute; this volume is about 20 times greater than that of any other organ. Each kidney has a renal vein that empties into the inferior vena cava. Because the inferior vena cava is located to the right of the midline, the left renal vein is longer than the right.

*Function.* The functions of the kidneys include excretion of wastes and regulation of acid-base balance and fluid-electrolyte balance. Wastes that are excreted by the kidney include water and nitrogenous products. Nitrogenous wastes are by-products of protein metabolism and are excreted primarily in the forms of uric acid, creatinine, and urea.[4,6] Regulation of acid-base balance and fluid and electrolytes occurs as the plasma passes through the kidney's filtration system. Normally the pH of urine is maintained between 4.5 and 8.0.[6]

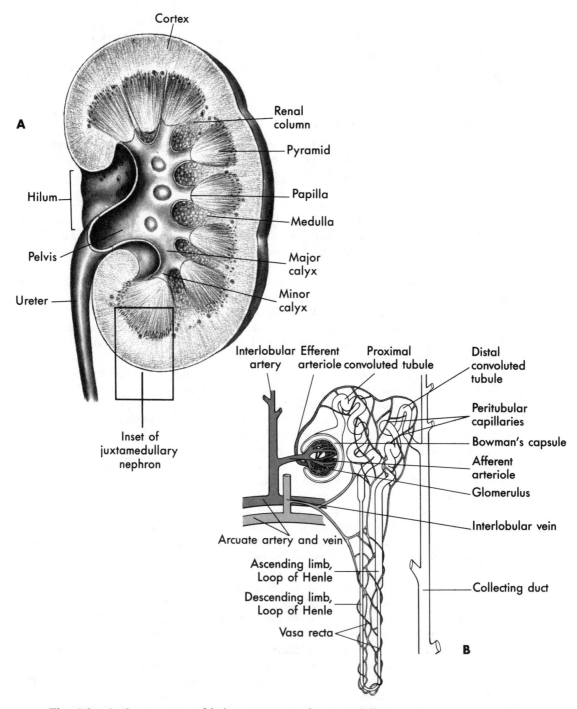

**Fig. 6-2**  **A,** Cross-section of kidney. **B,** Inset of juxtamedullary nephron structure. (**A** from Thompson JM et al: *Clinical nursing,* ed 2, St Louis, 1990, Mosby–Year Book. **B** from Seeley RR et al: *Anatomy and physiology,* St Louis, 1989, Mosby–Year Book.)

### Nephron

*Function.* The primary function of the nephron includes the removal of waste substances from the blood and the regulation of water and electrolyte concentration of body fluids. Within the nephron the continuous process of urine production includes filtration, reabsorption, and secretion.

*Structure.* Each kidney contains more than 1 million tubular nephrons, the functional unit of the kidney. Nephrons extend from the cortex through the outer medulla into the inner medulla (Fig. 6-2). Structures contained within the nephron are the glomerulus (a closely knit group of capillaries), Bowman's capsule (which surrounds the glomerulus), and the renal tubule.

*Filtrate formation.* Glomerular filtrate is created when blood flows from afferent arterioles into the glomerulus, where the capillary pressure within the glomerulus forces plasma through the filtering membrane into the capsule and then into the renal tubule. Glomerular filtrate contains the same substance as blood plasma except that it lacks a significant amount of proteins. In an average adult the glomerular filtration rate for the nephrons is about 125 ml/min, or 180 L/24 hr. Typical volume of urinary output per day, however, is considerably less: between 1 and 1.5 L. Thus it is obvious that the majority of filtrate (nearly 99%) is reabsorbed via the tubules into the blood.[4]

Blood pressure directly affects urinary output. For example, low blood pressure is directly correlated with low urinary output. The impact of high arterial pressures on renal filtration, however, is not as direct because of a process called *autoregulation*. This process prevents pressure in the glomerulus from rising at the same pace as arterial pressure, thus blunting the effect.[4]

Various changes occur as filtrate passes through the renal tubule before it is excreted as urine. Changes in the filtrate are primarily the result of tubular reabsorption: a process by which substances are transported out of the filtrate, through the epithelium of the renal tubule, and into the bloodstream via the peritubular capillary. Tubular reabsorption extracts water, electrolytes, hormones, vitamins, and other substances out of the filtrate as it goes through the tubule. Because proteins such as urea, nitrates, creatinine, phosphates, and sulfates are large molecules, they are reabsorbed into the bloodstream less easily. These substances are reabsorbed in each segment of the renal tubule by different modes of transport. For example, glucose and amino acids are reabsorbed by active transport; water is reabsorbed by osmosis; and proteins are reabsorbed by pinocytosis. Tubular reabsorption occurs throughout the renal tubule, although most of it occurs in the proximal convoluted portion of the tubule (Fig. 6-2).

Urine is composed of substances that are not reabsorbed into the bloodstream, such as excess water, as well as substances that are secreted into the renal tubule for excretion.[1] Drugs and metabolites are excreted in this fashion. Urine is transported through the tubules, calices, and renal pelvis to the ureter.

Urine volume and concentration are influenced by two hormones: antidiuretic hormone (ADH) and aldosterone. ADH is secreted by the posterior pituitary gland and prompts reabsorption in the nephron's collecting ducts. In response, urinary volume decreases and the solute concentration increases.[4]

The adrenal glands produce aldosterone in response to a low serum sodium concentration. Within the distal renal tubule, aldosterone enhances sodium and water reabsorption while increasing potassium excretion.[4,6] Other factors that influence urine volume and concentration include water loss by the lungs and skin, disease processes, and drugs, particularly diuretics.

### Ureters

The ureter is a flexible, distensible, tubular structure whose primary function is to transport urine from the renal pelvis into the urinary bladder. Each ureter has a diameter that varies from 2 to 5 mm and is about 25 cm (10 inches) in length. Ureters enter the bladder posteriorly. Because of anatomic construction, each ureter has three narrow segments: the ureteropelvic junction that is approximately 2 mm wide, the crossing of the iliac artery that is 4 mm wide, and the ureterovesical junction (UVJ), which usually is between 2 and 4 mm wide. These narrowed areas are significant because stones, or calculi, usually lodge at one of these locations.[9]

The ureter is composed of three layers: the mucosal, muscular, and adventitia. The mucosal layer is the innermost layer and is lined with transitional epithelium. Next is the muscular layer, which is responsible for the peristaltic waves that move urine through the ureter at an average of 1 to 2 ml/min.[5] The outermost layer is the adventitia, which is fibrous and protective.

The ureters enter the bladder posteriorly at the upper, outermost points of the trigone and tunnel obliquely for 1 to 2 cm through the bladder wall. Although there is no valve preventing backflow of urine into the ureter, the contraction of the bladder muscle usually occludes the ureter during micturition. Thus, normally, reflux of urine up the urinary tract rarely occurs, and the potential for infection and urethral dilation is limited.

## Lower Tract

### Bladder

The urinary bladder is a hollow distensible muscular organ with the primary functions of storage and elimination of urine. In the continent person the bladder stores urine until a socially acceptable time to empty occurs.

*Structure.* In the adult the bladder is located within the pelvic cavity that lies behind the symphysis pubis and below the parietal peritoneum. In men the bladder is positioned against the rectum posteriorly, whereas in women it sits adjacent to the anterior vaginal wall and the lower half of the uterus. In the child the bladder is an abdominal organ and more readily palpated. In either the child or the adult a severely distended bladder can push the parietal peritoneum away from the abdominal wall and reach above the symphysis. The bladder is supported in place by three structures. The urachus, also known as the median umbilical ligament, secures the superior aspect of the bladder, whereas the levator ani muscle provides lateral support and the obturator internal muscle provides posterior support.[2,8]

The bladder is divided into the dome, the body, and the base. The base also is referred to as the *trigone;* this is the triangular area formed by the two ureteral orifices and the bladder neck, or posterior urethra. Generally the trigone remains in a fixed position, although the rest of the bladder can move and change shape. The dome or fundus is the uppermost portion of the bladder. The remaining lateral and anterior walls of the bladder are known as the body of the bladder (Fig. 6-3).

The bladder wall is divided into four layers: mucosal, submucosal, muscular, and serous.[6,9] The innermost layer, the mucosal layer, is composed of many folded, convoluted ridges called *rugae;* the trigone is an exception and has a smooth surface. The submucosal layer contains the blood supply, lymphatic vessels, and most of the nerves. The muscular layer is known as the *detrusor* and is composed of smooth muscle fibers that are interlaced in all directions and depths. The outermost layer is called the *serous layer.*[6,9]

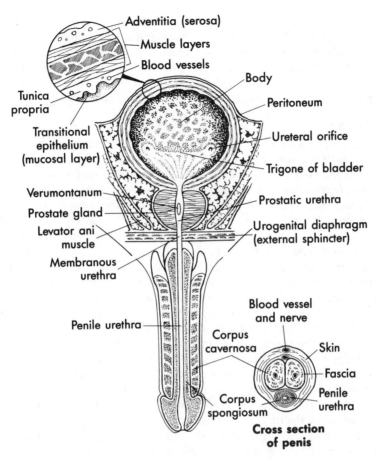

**Fig. 6-3**    Cross-section of male urinary bladder with inset of bladder wall and penis. (Modified from Broadwell DC, Jackson BS: *Principles of ostomy care*, St Louis, 1982, Mosby–Year Book.)

*Function.* One of the functions of the bladder is to serve as a low-pressure reservoir for the storage of urine. Normally, as the bladder fills with urine, the pressure within the bladder remains low at a water volume of about 5 to 10 cm.[1,5] The bladder's unique ability to adjust to increased volumes while keeping the pressure constant is termed *accommodation*. Surgical substitution of other tissue for the bladder is difficult to effect because no other tissue has this ability to accommodate. As the bladder volume approaches 250 to 350 ml of urine, bladder pressure increases to between 40 and 60 cm of water or higher, triggering the first sensation. Most persons can suppress this sensation and store 350 to 450 ml of urine comfortably. The process of suppressing bladder contractions so that pressures fall is called *inhibition*. Loss of tissue elasticity in the bladder as a result of aging may decrease the storage volume to 250 ml of urine; however, in some persons this change does not occur.[1,10]

The second function of the bladder is to empty or contract. Under normal conditions the bladder wall is highly compliant; bladder pressure remains essentially constant during filling until stretch receptors activate a series of signals that pass up through the spinal cord to the brain. If signals from the cortex do not inhibit the bladder, the pons micturition center sends signals to initiate bladder contractions. At the same time the cortex initiates relaxation of the external sphincter by means of the pudendal nerve.[11]

### Urethra

The urethra is a tubular structure that transports urine from the urinary bladder to outside the body. In men the urethra serves an additional function of providing a passageway for seminal fluid. Differences exist in male and female urethral structure.

*Female structure.* The female urethra measures approximately 4 cm (1½ inches) in length and exits from the bladder base under the symphysis. The anterior aspect of the urethra is anchored to the posteroinferior surface of the symphysis pubis by the pubourethral ligaments, which stabilizes the bladder neck and proximal urethra in the intraabdominal position.

The external urethral meatus, or orifice, is located anterior to the vaginal opening. Tissue changes that occur after childbirth, and occasionally with aging, may result in relocation of the urethral opening to within the vaginal vault.

The female urethra is subject to a number of factors that can trigger urinary incontinence. The angle between the bladder and the urethra—known as the posterior urethral vesicle angle—the position of the urethra, and the integrity of the pelvic floor are important for bladder control. If the pelvic floor (particularly the levator ani muscle) support is damaged, the occlusive force of these muscles on the urethral wall is diminished, resulting in increased leakage problems.[7,11] In addition, the elasticity and health of the submucosal tissues of the urethra affect continence. Normally the softness and elasticity of the inner urethral wall allow the mucosa to mold and form a watertight seal. The loss of normal tissue elasticity, diminished estrogen production, and possible resulting atrophic vaginitis, all of which occur with aging, may create leakage problems.[7]

*Male structure.* The male urethra is 18 to 20 cm in length, is S shaped, and functions as a passageway for urine and for secretions from reproductive organs. It is divided into three sections, the prostatic, membranous, and penile urethra (Fig. 6-3). The prostatic urethra is approximately 2.5 cm long and runs through the center of the prostate gland; prostatic ducts open into this segment of the urethra. The membranous urethra is about 0.5 cm long and passes through the urogenital diaphragm. The penile urethra is the longest segment of the male urethra, approximately 15 cm, and is surrounded by the corpus spongiosum penis. The urethra terminates at the external urethral meatus located at the tip of the penis. Both the length of the male urethra and its shape contribute to superior continence rates in men.

## External Sphincter

The external sphincter is a voluntary skeletal muscle contained within the urogenital diaphragm (Fig. 6-3). Tonically contracted, the external sphincter is modulated by the cortex via the pudendal nerve either to relax or to further contract.

## Internal Sphincter

The internal sphincter is a smooth muscle approximately 1 to 2 cm in length, is naturally contracted, and is located at the bladder neck or posterior urethra. The male internal sphincter is located within the prostatic and membranous urethra. In the female a specific internal sphincter muscle is not well defined in the bladder neck or proximal urethra.[3] Occlusion of the urethra develops as a result of involuntary contraction of the bladder neck and proximal urethra, which thereby prevents urine from entering the bladder neck as pressure in the bladder rises.

## Perineum

The external perineum is a diamond-shaped area that is bounded by the external genitalia to the front, the buttocks to the back, and the medial aspect of each thigh. A line drawn transversely between the ischial tuberosities divides this region into two triangles. The anterior triangle, known as the urogenital region, contains the urethra and genitals. The superficial tissue layers in this triangle are predominantly adipose tissue; the deeper tissue layers are fascia and muscle. The posterior triangle, or anal region, contains the distal anal canal. Adipose tissue and the levator ani muscle fill this wedge-shaped space.

# REPRODUCTIVE SYSTEM

## Female

The female external genitalia, or vulva, include the following structures: the mons pubis, labia majora, labia minora, clitoris, vestibular glands, and the hymen (Fig. 6-4). Because the location of the female reproductive organs is in such close proximity to the lower third of the urinary tract, symptoms of urinary tract problems can be quite similar to symptoms of disease in the reproductive organs. For example, because the uterus lies directly above the bladder, when the uterus is enlarged (i.e., with malignancy or pregnancy), bladder volume is decreased. The rectum lies posterior to the bladder and can create irritation or obstruction when distended.

## Male

The functions of the male reproductive system include production, storage, and ejaculation of sperm (Fig. 6-5). Organs of the male reproductive system include testes, epididymis, spermatic cord, seminal vesicles, prostate, penis, and scrotum.

**Testes.** The testes are ovoid structures, about 5 cm in length and 3 cm in diameter. They are suspended by the spermatic cord within the cavity of the scrotum. Each testis is enclosed by a capsule composed of a tough white membrane called the *tunica albuginea*, which contains 600 to 1200 seminiferous tubules that are approximately 60 cm long; the combined length of these tubules is nearly a mile. The seminiferous tubules are lined with germinal epithelium, where sperm is produced, and with Leydig's cells. Leydig's cells are responsible for production of testosterone. The seminiferous tubules converge at one end of the testes to form ducts, which then converge as they enter the epididymis.

**Epididymis.** The epididymis is a sausage-shaped structure approximately 5 cm in length, which lies on top of the posterolateral surface of the testes. The epididymis is divided into three parts, the head, the body, and the tail. The tail is filled with a single, thin coiled tube approximately 6 m in length. The primary function of this structure is transport of sperm. The vas deferens leads from the epididymis to the prostate.

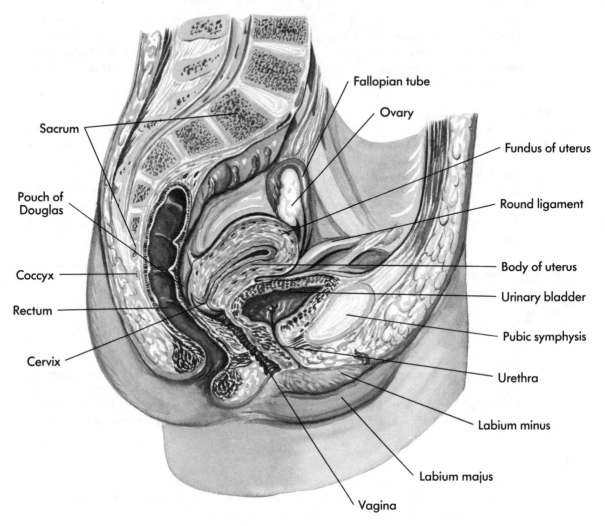

**Fig. 6-4**   Cross-section of female pelvis demonstrating proximity of reproductive organs to urinary bladder. (Adapted from Thibodeau GA: *Anthony's textbook of anatomy and physiology,* ed 13, St Louis, 1990, Mosby–Year Book.)

**Vas Deferens.** The vas deferens is a firm, muscular cylindric tube, approximately 35 cm in length, that extends from the tail of the epididymis to the prostate. The vas deferens, along with a duct of the seminal vesicle, creates the ejaculatory duct that opens into the prostatic urethra.

**Spermatic Cord.** The two spermatic cords feed and physically support the testes. They extend from the internal inguinal ring to the testicle. Each is covered by fascia and carries the blood, lymphatics, nerves, and vas deferens to the structures and tissues within the testicles.

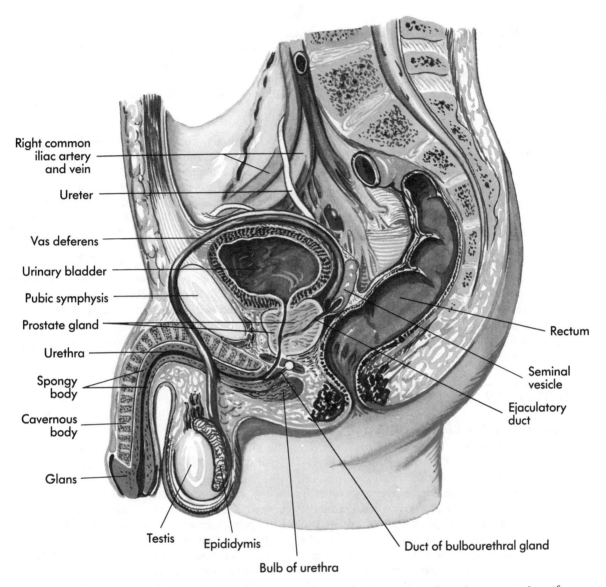

Right common
iliac artery
and vein

Ureter

Vas deferens

Urinary bladder

Pubic symphysis

Prostate gland

Urethra

Spongy
body

Cavernous
body

Glans

Testis   Epididymis

Bulb of urethra

Rectum

Seminal
vesicle

Ejaculatory
duct

Duct of bulbourethral gland

**Fig. 6-5**   Cross-section of male internal reproductive organs. Inset is cross-section of penis. (Adapted from Thibodeau GA: *Anthony's textbook of anatomy and physiology*, ed 13, St Louis, 1990, Mosby–Year Book.)

**Seminal Vesicles.** The seminal vesicles are lobulated, paired organs between the bladder and the base of the prostate. The secretions of the seminal vesicles contain a variety of nutrients thought to provide energy to sperm cells. The seminal vesicles join the vas deferens to form the ejaculatory duct that enters the prostate.

**Prostate.** The prostate gland is a doughnut-shaped structure that surrounds the prostatic urethra just below the urinary bladder. Enclosed by connective tissue, it is composed of many branched tubular glands. The prostate secretes approximately 5 ml/day of a thin milky fluid with an alkaline pH. Its primary function is to neutralize the seminal fluid, which becomes acidic because of the accumulation of metabolic wastes produced by stored sperm cells. Prostatic fluid improves the motility of sperm cells and neutralizes the acidic secretions of the vagina, thus allowing more sperm cells to survive within the female reproductive tract. The prostate gland releases its secretions into the urethra as a result of smooth muscle contractions of its capsular wall.[6]

**Penis.** The penis is a flaccid organ with the capacity for erection during sexual arousal. It has three longitudinal chambers: two corpora cavernosa and one corpus spongiosum (Fig. 6-3). The corpora cavernosa are located in separate chambers on the lateral aspects of the penis. Erection occurs when the arteries that supply the penis become dilated and blood engorges the cavernous spaces within these chambers. The corpus spongiosum surrounds the penile urethra; the enlarged distal end is called the *glans penis*. The foreskin or prepuce is the loose skin that covers the glans penis.

**Scrotum.** The scrotum is a pouch of skin and subcutaneous tissue that hangs from the region behind the penis. Although its subcutaneous tissue lacks adipose tissue, the scrotal wall contains the dartos muscle, which is a layer of smooth muscle fibers. When the dartos muscle is contracted, the scrotum becomes wrinkled and is drawn up to the warmth of the trunk. Temperature regulation is a primary function of the dartos muscle. This movement and consequent temperature regulation provide safety and viability to the sperm cells stored in the scrotum.

## MICTURITION

### Micturition Reflex and Innervation

Micturition is the act of passing urine. The micturition reflex includes a sequence of events that lead to voiding in the absence of voluntary inhibition. Normal voiding involves effective bladder contraction synchronized with relaxation of the urethral sphincters. This coordinated sequence of events provides free flow of urine and prevents reflux.

In the continent person local stimuli from stretch receptors in the bladder wall stimulate an afferent signal that travels by way of the pelvic nerve to the spinal cord. Specific tracts carry the signal up the spinal cord to the pons and cortex. Voluntary control of micturition is provided by the cerebral cortex, which sends inhibitory or excitatory messages to the pons. The pontine micturition center then coordinates the neural signals so that relaxation of the external sphincter, opening of the bladder neck, and contraction of the detrusor muscle occur in a synchronized fashion.[1,3,5,10,11]

The sympathetic nerves exit the cord in the thoracic or lumbar region; sympathetic stimulation promotes bladder relaxation and bladder neck contraction. The outflow tracts for the parasympathetic nerves and the pudendal nerve are located at S2 to S4, which is known as the sacral micturition center. The parasympathetic nerves mediate bladder contraction and bladder neck relaxation; the pudendal nerve controls external sphincter function. Sensory fiber and stretch receptors originate at this level (S3 to S4).

### Voiding Process

Afferent pathways transmit the sensation of bladder distention to the spinal cord; corticospinal pathways then transmit the message to the passive micturition center and the brain. The cortex can send either inhibitory or excitatory impulses to the pons. If voiding is inhibited, sympathetic fibers are stimulated to promote bladder relaxation and the pudendal nerve mediates voluntary contraction of the external sphincter. If voiding is facilitated, the pudendal nerve mediates external sphincter relaxation and the parasympathetic pathways are stimulated to allow bladder neck relaxation and bladder contraction.

The higher centers in the cerebral cortex keep the micturition reflex partially inhibited except when an individual wishes to void. Continence is maintained by a continual tonic contraction of the bladder neck and external sphincter and by inhibiting detrusor contractions. Voiding occurs by voluntarily triggering the micturition reflex at a convenient time.

## SUMMARY

The anatomy of the genitourinary system is complex and involves many structures. In the care of patients with urologic problems, it is important to understand the anatomic location of these urinary, reproductive, and gastrointestinal structures. Such a knowledge base forms the foundation from which interventions are derived.

# SELF-EVALUATION

## QUESTIONS

1. The structures of the urinary tract include the following:
   a. Kidneys, ureters, bladder, and urethra
   b. Kidneys, epididymis, bladder, and urethra
   c. Kidneys, epididymis, prostate, and bladder
   d. Kidneys and bladder
2. Divisions of the urinary tract include:
   a. Upper
   b. Middle
   c. Lower
   d. *a* and *c*
3. The functions of the kidney include:
   a. Absorption and reproduction
   b. Only regulation of electrolytes
   c. Urine storage and waste excretion
   d. Acid-base regulation and waste excretion
4. The blood supply to the kidney is via the:
   a. Pulmonary artery
   b. Superior mesenteric artery
   c. Renal artery
   d. Celiac artery
5. The functional unit of the kidney is the:
   a. Glomerulus
   b. Nephron
   c. Renal tubule
   d. Renal vein
6. The hormones that influence urine volume are:
   a. Antidiuretic hormone and adrenaline
   b. Antidiuretic hormone and insulin
   c. Aldosterone and adrenaline
   d. Aldosterone and antidiuretic hormone
7. Urinary stones most commonly occur at which of the following sites?
   a. Urethral vesical junction
   b. Nephron
   c. Ureteropelvic junction
   d. Glomerulus
8. The primary functions of the bladder are:
   a. Storage and elimination of urine
   b. Secretion of aldosterone and antidiuretic hormone
   c. Blood pressure regulation and storage
   d. None of the above
9. The detrusor is a:
   a. Smooth, voluntary muscle
   b. Striated, voluntary muscle
   c. Smooth, involuntary muscle
   d. Striated, involuntary muscle

10. In the normal bladder the urge to urinate is stimulated at what volume?
    a. 100 to 300 ml
    b. 300 to 500 ml
    c. 500 to 700 ml
    d. 700 to 900 ml
11. The length of the male urethra protects the individual from:
    a. Incontinence
    b. Cancer
    c. Renal stone formation
    d. All of the above
12. Continence is voluntarily controlled by the:
    a. Internal urinary sphincter
    b. Stretch receptors in the bladder
    c. Bladder trigone
    d. Cerebral cortex

# SELF-ASSESSMENT

## ANSWERS

1. **a.** Kidneys, ureters, bladder, and urethra
2. **d.** *a* and *c*
3. **d.** Acid-base regulation and waste excretion
4. **c.** Renal artery
5. **a.** Glomerulus
6. **d.** Aldosterone and antidiuretic hormone
7. **c.** Ureteropelvic junction
8. **a.** Storage and elimination of urine
9. **c.** Smooth, involuntary muscle
10. **b.** 300 to 500 ml
11. **a.** Incontinence
12. **d.** Cerebral cortex

## REFERENCES

1. Blavis JB: The neurophysiology of micturition: a clinical study of 550 patients, *J Urol* 127:958, 1982.
2. Clemente CD, editor: *Gray's anatomy of the human body*, ed 30, Philadelphia, 1984, Lea & Febiger.
3. Gosling JA: The structure of the female lower urinary tract and pelvic floor, *Urol Clin North Am* 12:207, 1985.
4. Guyton AC: *Human physiology and mechanics of disease*, ed 3, Philadelphia, 1982, WB Saunders.
5. Guyton AC: *Textbook of medical physiology*, ed 7, Philadelphia, 1985, WB Saunders.
6. Houston GR: Genitourinary system. In Broadwell DC, Jackson BS: *Principles of ostomy care*, St Louis, 1982, Mosby–Year Book.
7. Kane RL, Ouslander JG, Abrass IR: *Essentials of clinical geriatrics*, New York, 1984, McGraw-Hill.
8. Netter FH: *Atlas of human anatomy*, Summit, NJ, 1989, Ciba-Geigy Corp.
9. Smith DR: *General urology*, ed 11, Los Altos, Calif, 1984, Lange Medical Publications.
10. Wein AJ: Physiology of micturition, *Clin Geriatr Med* 2(4):689, 1986.
11. Wheeler JS, Peters MJ: Anatomy and physiology related to voiding. In Doughty D, editor: *Urinary and fecal incontinence: nursing management*, St Louis, 1991, Mosby–Year Book.

REFERENCES

# 7 Pathophysiology and Diagnostic Tests of the Genitourinary Tract

KEN McCALLA

## OBJECTIVES

1. Describe the abnormality in the embryologic process that results in exstrophy, prune-belly syndrome, and myelomeningocele.

2. Describe the urologic complications associated with prune-belly syndrome and myelomeningocele.

3. State the treatment objective for managing myelomeningocele and at least four treatment options.

4. Identify the potential urologic complications associated with ureteropelvic junction obstruction, megaureter, and vesicoureteral reflux.

5. Distinguish among the symptoms associated with urethral cancer, prostate cancer, and bladder cancer.

6. Distinguish among the clinical manifestations of posterior urethral valves, megaureter, ureteropelvic junction obstruction, and vesicoureteral reflux.

7. Identify at least five variables that place a patient at risk for the development of bladder cancer.

8. Distinguish between grading and staging bladder tumors, giving examples of how the depth of tumor penetration in the bladder is described.

9. State the preferred medical and surgical management approach for the following diseases: bladder cancer, chronic pyelonephritis, spinal cord injury, traumatic ureteral injury, male urethral injuries, palliation for pelvic cancer, and prune-belly syndrome.

10. Describe the three factors that increase the potential for development of a urinary tract infection.

11. State the most common type of bladder cancer.

12. Distinguish between acute pyelonephritis and chronic pyelonephritis, addressing clinical manifestations, pathogenesis, diagnostic test(s), and treatment.

13. State the three common sites where ureteral stones commonly lodge.

The nurse who cares for patients with ostomies provides more than technical care: these patients also need information about the disease process and supportive counseling.

Many different types of pathologic processes can precipitate the need for a temporary or permanent urinary diversion. Diseases include congenital disorders, neoplasms, traumatic injuries, and inflammatory disorders. To manage the care of the patient with an ostomy, the nurse must be familiar with the underlying disease process, medical-surgical management, and complications—the issues discussed in this chapter.

## CONGENITAL DISORDERS

### Exstrophy

Exstrophy is a complex congenital disorder that develops in utero during the first trimester. During embryologic development the genitourinary (GU) tract and the gastrointestinal (GI) empty into one organ tract within the fetus known as the *cloaca* (Fig. 7-1). The fetal tissue that comprises the cloaca, the GI tract, and the GU tract is known as *mesoderm*. Normally as the fetus matures, the cloaca divides into the urogenital sinus and the rectum. Exstrophy results when the mesoderm fails to advance and thus impedes separation and maturation of the cloaca. Although the pathophysiologic process is not clearly understood, it appears that because the mesoderm fails to advance and close the midline, the cloaca may actually rupture through the thin, fragile body wall that is called the *ectoderm*.[32]

Several types of exstrophy exist. Type is determined by the stage of fetal development at the time of cloacal rupture. Types of exstrophy include cloacal exstrophy, bladder exstro-

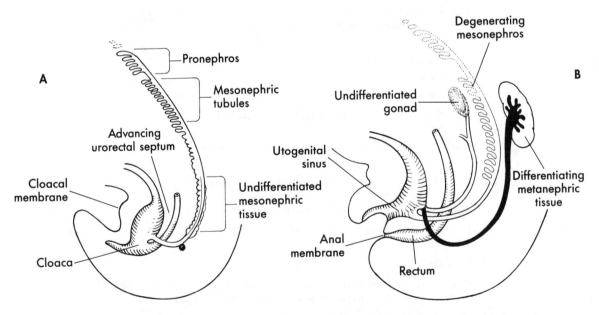

**Fig. 7-1**   Embryologic development of urogenital region. **A,** Cloaca is reservoir for rudimentary GU and GI structures. Advancing cloacal membrane divides cloaca into GU and GI tract. **B,** Migration of rectum posteriorly is complete, and anal membrane is present.

phy, and male and female epispadias, although reports cite several variants of these manifestations.[4,32]

**Cloacal Exstrophy.** The anomaly of cloacal exstrophy is one of the most severe forms of congenital disorders. It is rare: it occurs only in 1/200,000 births.[8,32] This defect occurs early in fetal growth. Structurally the urorectal septum fails to develop within the cloaca; thus the cloaca does not divide into the GI and the GU components. Because the midline abdominal wall also fails to close, the bladder and cecum are exteriorized through the abdominal wall. Therefore cloacal exstrophy is characterized by (1) an exstrophied cecum that is centrally positioned; (2) an exstrophied and divided bladder (hemibladder) that lies on both sides of the cecum; (3) a blind end to the distal bowel (hindgut), which creates an internal obstruction; (4) fusion of the mucosal borders of the cecum and hemibladders; (5) fusion of the mucosa to the skin; and (6) a separation of the pubic symphysis. In males the phallus and scrotum are bifid (divided); in females the clitoris is divided.

Surgical management of this severe disorder has not even been attempted until recently; most infants died of sepsis or short-bowel syndrome. Currently if the neonate is expected to survive the anomalies and complications, correction is accomplished through a staged surgical approach. In the absence of other life-threatening anomalies, initially the infant requires diversion of the fecal stream to prevent urosepsis. Subsequent procedures include bladder reconstruction.[15] Because of severe deformities of the phallus, most baby boys have gender reassignments and are reared as girls.

**Bladder Exstrophy.** Bladder exstrophy is the more common type of exstrophy and occurs in 1/10,000 to 1/50,000 births; the male to female ratio is 2:1.[15] Bladder exstrophy is much more likely to occur in a family with a history of bladder exstrophy. Bladder exstrophy occurs later in the fetal development process than does cloacal exstrophy: it occurs *after* the septum has divided the cloaca into the GI and the GU tracts. The infant is born with an exposed bladder, everted bladder mucosa, and fusion of the mucosa to the abdominal skin. Generally, babies with bladder exstrophy are full-term and robust but have a high incidence of associated anomalies such as renal, GI (e.g., imperforate anus), and skeletal defects.[15]

Treatment for bladder exstrophy has been fraught with complications; thus no one treatment has received unanimous approval. Treatment of this defect must address closure of the abdominal wall, obtaining urinary continence, preservation of renal function, and creation of functional and cosmetically acceptable genital structures.[17] Treatment of the symphysis pubis is controversial. Many physicians believe correction is not required because the separated pubic symphysis corrects itself once the child begins to walk. Others advocate bilateral osteotomy at the time of primary bladder closure to diminish the tension on the abdominal closure and to aid continence by repositioning the urethra and puborectalis muscles.[17]

Correction of the male genital defect is the most difficult surgical problem. Although the corpus cavernosum is of normal length, the phallus may be shortened because of the separation of the pubic bones. Generally these patients have a severe dorsal chordee (bent phallus). Treatment of female exstrophy is not as difficult.

Historically, bladder exstrophy was managed with urinary diversion and cystectomy (see Chapter 8 for a discussion of urinary diversions). In fact the first ureterosigmoidostomy was performed for bladder exstrophy in 1852.[17] Ureterosigmoidostomies, however, are associated with many complications, including pyelonephritis, renal calculi, metabolic abnormalities, and neoplasms. Although refinement in the surgical technique for construct-

---

**STAGED RECONSTRUCTION OF EXSTROPHY OF THE BLADDER (APPROXIMATE AGE OF PATIENT AT EACH STAGE INDICATED)**

| | | |
|---|---|---|
| Exstrophic bladder suitable for primary closure | Exstrophic bladder not suitable for primary closure or as an alternative to primary closure | |
| ↓ | ↓ | ↓ |
| Primary closure of bladder with or without bilateral ileac osteostomies (neonatal or at presentation) | Nonrefluxing colonic conduit and excision of exstrophic bladder with penile lengthening (6 mo) | Nonrefluxing colonic conduit (1 yr) |
| ↓ | ↓ | ↓ |
| Bladder neck reconstruction, bilateral ureteral reimplantation with or without augmentation cystoplasty (3 yr) | Internal diversion of colon conduit (4 to 5 yr) | Penile elongation (1½ yr) |
| | ↓ | ↓ |
| ↓ | Urethroplasty (puberty or age 6 to 7 yr) | Urethrovesical tubularization (2 yr) |
| Penile lengthening with single stage or multistage urethroplasty (4 yr) | | ↓ |
| | | Anastomosis of colonic conduit to urethrovesical tube (2½ yr) |
| | | ↓ |
| | | Closure of cutaneous stoma (3 yr) |

From Misrobian HGF: Exstrophy of the bladder. In King LR, editor: *Urologic surgery in neonates and young infants*, Philadelphia, 1989, WB Saunders.

ing a ureterosigmoidostomy (e.g., tunneling ureters into the colon to prevent reflux) helped decrease some of these complications, many problems have persisted. These problems make the ureterosigmoidostomy an undesirable urinary diversion.

Because of the many complications associated with the ureterosigmoidostomy, several alternative procedures for urinary diversion have been developed. These include trigonosigmoidostomy (in which the trigone itself is removed en bloc and placed in the sigmoid bowel), isolated rectal pouches that were pulled through the anal sphincter just proximal to the rectum, and finally, the ileal conduit. The ileal conduit was considered the ideal treatment for patients with bladder exstrophy because far fewer complications occurred than with ureterosigmoidostomies. For example, the incidence of pyelonephritis was much less, and the metabolic abnormalities that followed ureterosigmoidostomies did not affect ileal conduits. However, as the life expectancy for children with bladder exstrophy began to normalize, long-term complications indicated that the ileal conduit was not the optimal procedure.[17]

Present-day treatment of patients with exstrophy involves a team approach, with the goals being to obtain normal sexual and urologic function. Surgery is performed as a staged procedure, as shown in the box above. The bladder is closed within 72 hours of birth, and a suprapubic tube is left indwelling for approximately 2 weeks. After surgery the patient may be placed in modified Bryant's traction for 3 to 4 weeks to allow healing of the anterior pelvic ring.[28] As the bladder matures, it gains volume, so when the child is 3 to 5 years of age, the bladder neck and urethra can be reconstructed and the ureters reimplanted to correct the vesicoureteral reflux. Within 1 year of bladder neck reconstruction, if the child's condition is satisfactory, baby boys receive urethroplasty and penile shaft lengthening.[17]

**Epispadias.** Exstrophy can be limited to only the failure of the pelvis to close (diastasis of the pubic symphysis); that is, the bladder has closed normally. This situation results in an epispadias, a milder form of exstrophy. The urethra opens on the dorsal side of the penis in males. In females the urethra opens anteriorly to the normal position and also is characterized by a bifid clitoris and separation of labia. Epispadias in both sexes requires reconstructive surgery, although such operations are more complex in males because of the accompanying shortened penis similar to the condition that occurs with bladder exstrophy.[17]

## Posterior Urethral Valves

**Pathophysiology.** Posterior urethral valves are the most common form of bladder outlet obstruction in infant boys.[9,10] Urethral valves are embryologic remnants of the fusion point between the mesonephric duct (which becomes the ejaculatory duct) and the urogenital sinus (which becomes the bladder and prostate) (Fig. 7-1). When these membranes fail to regress, the mucosal folds that remain distal to the verumontanum are referred to as *urethral valves*. Severity (extent) of these valves varies and influences the effect on renal function and surgical repair technique.[4]

Posterior urethral valves cause varying degrees of obstruction.[29] The obstruction may be so complete as to lead to oligohydramnios (lack of amniotic fluid) and renal dysplasia, which results in fetal death.[21] In less severe cases an abdominal mass, a fluid and electrolyte disorder, and a urinary tract infection develop after birth. Chronic obstruction can lead to bladder abnormalities (trabeculation and bladder wall hypertrophy) and elevated bladder pressures that can produce dilation of the proximal urinary tract (kidneys and ureters).[9]

**Clinical Manifestations.** Urethral valves are the most common cause of neonatal ascites. Physical examination may reveal a distended bladder and bilateral flank masses. A weak or dribbling urinary stream also may be present. Significant obstructive uropathy occurs in one half of all children. Because the newborn no longer benefits from exchange with the placenta, a metabolic acidosis can develop quickly and requires prompt treatment.

Diagnosis of posterior urethral valves usually is accomplished with a voiding cystourethrogram. Although the use of cystoscopy also can be helpful in diagnosing posterior urethral valves, care must be taken for two reasons. First, the valves usually are visualized only when there is antegrade flow of irrigation out of the bladder. When the irrigation is flowing into the bladder from the cystoscope in a retrograde fashion, the valves tend to close and are not visualized. Second, the urethra in the newborn boy can be damaged easily by the cytoscope, resulting in urethral strictures later in life.

**Management.** Treatment initially requires catheter drainage of the bladder, which can reverse metabolic abnormalities quickly. After stabilization, primary resection of the valves can be performed if the male infant has a normal-sized urethra; however, if the infant is too small (less than 5 pounds), a vesicostomy may be performed so that the bladder empties under low pressure.[9]

Because highly dilated ureters drain into the bladder poorly even after correction of the obstruction, a supravesicle diversion sometimes is preferred for dilated upper tracts.[21]

When the child is approximately 2 years old, the valves are resected and the ureterostomies can be closed. Occasionally the most appropriate form of diversion is a pyelostomy; the highly dilated renal pelvis is anastomosed to the skin. Again, once the child is large enough for the valves to be treated, the pyelostomy can be closed.

Posterior urethral valves may exist with other complications such as ureterovesical junction (UVJ) obstruction and vesicoureteral reflux.[13] In UVJ obstruction the highly dilated and tortuous ureters often drain poorly into a highly trabeculated bladder and may require correction. Vesicoureteral reflux occurs in 40% to 60% of patients with posterior urethral valves.[9] After the valves have been treated, reflux ceases in about one fourth of the cases. Treatment of the remaining patients must be individualized.

## Prune-Belly Syndrome

**Pathophysiology.** Prune-belly syndrome is a rare condition that occurs in 1/35,000 to 1/50,000 live births.[39] It occurs almost exclusively in boys; however, rarely a girl can be affected. Infants with prune-belly syndrome are born with a congenital absence, deficiency, or hypoplasia of abdominal wall musculature so that the belly actually looks like a prune. The abdominal wall is quite thin, and many creases and wrinkles are present (see Plate 24). Patients have large hypotonic bladders; dilated, tortuous ureters; and bilateral undescended testicles.

The cause of the syndrome is unknown. Oligohydramnios (insufficient amniotic fluid) usually is present. Because urine is the major component of amniotic fluid, the coexistence of oligohydramnios and urinary abnormalities probably is related to the cause.

**Clinical Manifestations.** Although the kidneys may be normal, they usually are dysplastic and hydronephrotic.[40] The ureters tend to be dilated and tortuous; bilateral vesicoureteral reflux usually is present because of the absence of muscle bundles in the ureters.[41] Typically the prostate is hypoplastic, but the urethra and penis are normal. The testicles usually are undescended and generally are found in the abdomen. At this time there are no documented cases of fertility.

Patients with prune-belly syndrome may have other abnormalities, including limb defects, intestinal malrotation, and congenital heart defects (such as ventricular septal defect and tetralogy of Fallot).[40] Pulmonary complications such as pulmonary hypoplasia or inadequate lung development are common and may be incompatible with life. In less severely affected patients, the absence of abdominal wall musculature alone leads to decreased cough reflex and increased incidence of upper respiratory tract infection.

**Management.** Historically many infants with prune-belly syndrome had a poor prognosis and died of urinary sepsis. Modern treatment has improved the prognosis. Urologic evaluation of the newborn with prune-belly syndrome includes an intravenous pyelogram (IVP) and usually a voiding cystourethrogram; most children have vesicoureteral reflux or obstruction.[41] Serum creatinine levels must be followed and any urinary tract infections closely monitored.

Lifelong conservative follow-up is adequate for some patients, whereas others may require surgical treatment. In the event of recurrent infections or renal function deterioration, a vesicostomy may be warranted.[39] Vesicostomies usually are temporary; as the child grows and the bladder descends into the pelvis, closure generally is required.

A ureterostomy or pyelostomy is performed if obstruction at the ureterovesical junction exists. With a ureterostomy a dilated ureter is secured to the skin for drainage. The dilated renal pelvis also can be exteriorized to create a pyelostomy; however, the ureterostomy is preferred. Both surgical procedures are temporary measures that provide urinary drainage until more extensive reconstruction can be carried out. Treatment of the dilated ureter is controversial; most patients require extensive ureteral tapering and reimplantation to establish better drainage and to prevent infection.

The testicles usually are brought down into the scrotum; this is a difficult procedure in these patients. Plication of the abdominal wall provides better abdominal support and improves appearance. Advances in the evaluation and treatment of prune-belly syndrome have enhanced longevity and quality of life for these patients.

## Myelomeningocele

**Pathophysiology.** Myelomeningocele occurs when the vertebral arches fail to fuse in the midline and thus fail to encase the spinal cord in its usual position. Depending on the degree of severity, this failure to encase the spinal cord allows the cord to protrude out of the spinal column. A variety of musculoskeletal and neurologic defects may accompany this anomaly.

Myelomeningocele has been recorded throughout history; the earliest documented cases occurred 12,000 years ago in Morocco.[26] Archaeologists have used myelomeningocele to assess the degree of advancement of civilizations. Myelomeningocele in the skeletons of older children or adults is interpreted as indicating that the society had advanced to the point of caring for their disabled citizens.

*Spina bifida* often is used interchangeably with the term myelomeningocele; however, spina bifida describes only the defect in the vertebral arch of the spine. The two types of spina bifida are spina bifida occulta and spina bifida cystica. Spina bifida occulta occurs as a normal variant in 5% of the population and usually is merely an incidental finding on roentgenogram.[26] In spina bifida occulta the spinal cord does not protrude through the bony defect. In contrast, in spina bifida cystica the meninges herniate out through the defect in the spinal column (meningocele), or the meninges and cord protrude through the defect (myelomeningocele). Myelomeningocele is the more severe abnormality and also is the most common form of spina bifida cystica.[26] For all practical purposes, however, the terms spina bifida, myelomeningocele, and myelodysplasia are used interchangeably.

The incidence of myelomeningocele is approximately 1/1000 live births.[19,26] This defect can now be predicted prenatally by measuring the mother's blood level of serum alpha-fetoprotein (AFP), a glycoprotein normally present in amniotic fluid. During embryologic development, myelomeningocele develops when the neural tube fails to close, thus releasing increased amounts of AFP into the amniotic fluid. By 16 to 18 weeks' gestation, elevated serum AFP levels suggest that the fetus is at high risk for the neural tube defect.

**Clinical Manifestations.** Myelomeningocele is readily visible. Anomalies associated with myelomeningocele include an increased incidence of undescended testicles in male babies (up to 25 times higher than the normal incidence) and congenital renal abnormalities.[26] Exstrophy also is more common than in the general population.

Significant hydrocephalus is present in one fourth of these children at birth; another one third have a milder form of hydrocephalus.[26] Hydrocephalus occurs as a result of brainstem herniation through the foramen magnum. The initial treatment for patients with myelomeningocele involves closure of the spinal cord defect within 24 hours after birth, followed shortly by ventricular peritoneal shunt (if hydrocephalus is present). This shunt allows the cerebral spinal fluid to drain from the ventricles within the brain into the peritoneal cavity under low pressure. As the child grows, however, the spinal cord can be strictured by scar tissue, resulting in a tethered cord. This condition ultimately may contribute to sensorimotor loss to the legs and can further compromise bowel and bladder function.

**Management.** Children with myelomeningocele require long-term urologic management. Although intravenous pyelogram (IVP) results are normal in approximately 80% of children with myelomeningocele at birth, 50% demonstrate decreased renal function by the age of 5 years if the condition is left untreated.[1,19,26] Therefore the long-term goals of urologic management are to maintain renal function and to promote urinary continence.

Patients with myelomeningocele are at risk for hydronephrosis and for dilation of the upper urinary tract (calices, renal pelvis, and ureters). These complications occur as a result of detrusor-sphincter dyssynergia and high intravesical pressures. (Detrusor-sphincter dyssynergia refers to the uncoordinated voiding pattern that can develop in these patients; because of nerve damage the urethral sphincter fails to relax when the bladder contracts.) This uncoordinated voiding pattern can produce urinary stasis, high residual levels, and high intravesical pressures. The result is predisposition to urinary tract infection, hydronephrosis, and upper tract deterioration. Vesicoureteral reflux also is common in these children, as is incontinence (resulting from loss of neural pathways).

Management involves careful evaluation of the kidneys and bladder by means of periodic IVPs or renal ultrasound, voiding cystograms, and urodynamic evaluations. Intermittent catheterization, the Credé maneuver, artificial urinary sphincters, ileal conduit, and bladder augmentation are all management options to be considered.

When the bladder does not empty effectively, the Credé maneuver can be used to enhance emptying. Intermittent catheterization, however, is a more effective method of emptying the bladder. With use of clean technique, a catheter is inserted into the bladder at regular intervals to keep it empty. If it is not practical for parents to perform intermittent catheterization on their infant, a vesicostomy may be necessary.

Approximately 90% of children with untreated myelomeningocele will be incontinent.[26] By means of intermittent catheterization, continence, which is particularly desirable as the child reaches school age, can be achieved to an acceptable degree in approximately 50% to 60% of the children with myelomeningocele.[19,26] Pharmacologic treatment can improve this degree by relaxing the smooth muscle of the bladder wall, which allows the bladder to fill under low pressure; intermittent catheterization is then used to empty the bladder.[19]

Because of loss of sphincter control, some children are incontinent and have a constant dribble of urine despite a relaxed, compliant bladder. Satisfactory continence can be achieved by increasing the bladder outlet resistance with (1) an artificial urinary sphincter, (2) periurethral injections of Teflon or collagen, or (3) a rectus fascial sling.[19]

The artificial urinary sphincter is a mechanical device that is surgically implanted. It consists of a urethral cuff that is wrapped around the urethra, a reservoir balloon that is implanted in the abdominal cavity, and a control pump located in the scrotum or labia. Sterile radiopaque fluid is used to fill the cuff; this process maintains constant pressure on the urethra, which closes the urethra and prevents leakage. The control pump is used to divert fluid from the urethral cuff into the reservoir; deflation of the cuff permits voiding or catheterization.

Recently, periurethral injections of Teflon or collagen have been used to increase urethral resistance. This procedure can be performed much more easily than artificial urinary sphincter implantation.

The third option, the rectus fascial sling, involves the removal of a piece of the abdominal rectus fascia, which is then secured around the urethra and to the abdominal rectus fascia; thus a urethral "sling" is created, which also increases bladder outlet resistance.

Until recently the ileal conduit urinary diversion was believed to be the most satisfactory method of urinary management for children with myelomeningocele. It seemed to provide a method of continence that, although not ideal, would allow the kidney to drain under low pressure. In the mid-1970s, however, reports of upper tract deterioration began to occur. Statistics indicate that between 40% and 90% of the children treated with an ileal conduit began to show upper tract deterioration such as progressive pyelonephritic scarring.[26]

Urinary undiversion is increasingly common because of the long-term renal complications associated with an ileal conduit and because of the intolerance, especially in teenagers, of a stoma. An undiversion usually involves reimplantation of the ureters in a nonrefluxing fashion into a patch of large bowel that is then sewn onto the bladder augmentation. These individuals then perform intermittent catheterization to empty the bladder. The patient who also has sphincteral incontinence may require an artificial sphincter, periurethral injections of Teflon or collagen, or a rectus fascial sling.

Some patients with myelomeningocele have a noncompliant or "Christmas tree" bladder, so-named because of the radiologic appearance of a small, trabeculated, triangular-shaped bladder. Urodynamic evaluation reveals that the bladder fills only under very high pressures. These patients benefit from an augmentation cystoplasty, a surgical procedure in which the bladder is divided in half and a segment of bowel (usually sigmoid) applied. The bladder can then fill under low pressures. Some of these patients require intermittent catheterization to empty the bladder.

## Ureteropelvic Junction Obstruction

Ureteropelvic junction obstruction (see Fig. 8-1) is the most common congenital abnormality of the ureter. It occurs more frequently in males than in females, with a ratio of about 5:2.[12] It is more common in the left ureter; only about 10% to 15% of cases are bilateral.[4]

Although the cause is unclear, a dysplastic segment of ureter at this junction often is found.[23] Kinking and angulation of the ureter are present at the ureteropelvic junction, as well as abnormal peristalsis. The ureter may have a high insertion into the renal pelvis or may be obstructed by the crossing of an aberrant renal artery supplying the lower pole of the kidney.[12,20]

Clinical findings are related to the age of the patient. Many cases are being diagnosed prenatally by ultrasound. Most cases, however, manifest with an abdominal mass in infancy. Children usually have abdominal pain, vomiting, and infections. Adults classically have flank pain after consuming large volumes of fluids.[4,12]

The diagnosis is made by means of an IVP or, in some cases, a diuretic renogram. Treatment requires surgical correction of the obstructed segment. The most common procedure is a dismembered pyeloplasty, which involves a flank incision, excision of the affected segment, and creation of a funnel-shaped ureter. Newer techniques require percutaneous nephrostomy and incising of the narrowed segment through a special scope inside the renal pelvis. A percutaneous universal stent usually is left in place, which passes through the kidney and into the ureter, with the pigtail end in the bladder.

Regardless of which procedure is used, complications occur if strictures develop in the repaired segment. Placement of a percutaneous nephrostomy usually is required. Generally these procedures have good results.

## Megaureter

Megaureter, which is more common in males than in females, generally occurs bilaterally.[12] The cause appears to be an abnormality in the function of muscle fibers in the distal ureter, and the result is a failure to propel urine down the ureter. Obstruction of the ureters seldom is found; it is the absence of peristalsis that produces a functional obstruction in the segment involved. Because megaureter typically is the result of obstruction at the ureterovesicle junction, proximal ureters become dilated (see Fig. 8-3). Ureteropelvic junction obstruction does not create megaureter inasmuch as the obstruction is in the proximal portion of the ureter; a dilated renal pelvis often is discovered with ureteropelvic junction obstruction.

Clinical symptoms include fever, abdominal pain, and hematuria. Stones may be present as a result of urinary stasis. A diagnosis is made by means of an IVP; classic findings include a dilated distal ureter, less dilated proximal ureter, and near-normal renal pelvis and calices.[22]

Surgery usually is required for treatment. Because the ureter tends to be wide, it must be tapered and reimplanted into the bladder. Results generally are good, but close follow-up is essential to rule out reobstruction.

## Vesicoureteral Reflux

The flow of urine from the ureter into the bladder should be one way. This is accomplished through a complex valve mechanism in which the ureter enters the posterior bladder wall at an oblique angle and travels through the wall of the bladder until it exits into the bladder at the ureteral orifice. Reflux of urine from the bladder into the ureter can occur if any part of this system breaks down. For example, loss of neurologic control to the bladder allows reflux. If the ureter does not pass through the bladder wall obliquely or with sufficient distance, reflux can result. The most common cause is an abnormality of the trigonal muscle in the bladder, which allows reflux to occur.

Vesicoureteral reflux is dangerous because it damages the kidney by means of the following mechanisms: (1) pyelonephritis, which allows infected urine in the bladder to reach the kidney, and (2) hydronephrosis, in which the higher pressure in the bladder is transmitted to the kidney.

Pyelonephritis always should raise suspicion about reflux. In the later stages, renal pain during voiding and symptomless bacteruria associated with uremia and hypertension can occur.

Diagnosis of vesicoureteral reflux is made with a voiding cystogram or sometimes a radionucleotide cystogram, which shows dye in the bladder refluxing back up toward the kidney.[3]

A child with low-grade reflux in which the upper tracts appear fairly normal has a good chance of outgrowing reflux.[22] Continuous daily antibiotic prophylaxis is required to prevent urinary tract infection, pyelonephritis, and scarring. Spontaneous cessation of reflux has been reported in 60% to 85% of nondilated ureters and in 25% to 40% of dilated ureters.[3] Thus surgical correction can be avoided. Ureteral reimplantation usually is required for patients with upper tract changes, with breakthrough infections during a course of antibiotics, or with ureteral orifice configuration in which resolution does not occur. Two other indications for surgery are duplicated systems in which reflux does not resolve and ectopic ureteral orifices in which the ureters enter the urinary tract at some point other than the trigone. Surgery usually is 90% successful in correcting reflux.

Patients with severe reflux may require either a temporary or a permanent urinary diversion. If the patient has a small, contracted bladder and it is unlikely that a successful reimplantation can be performed, a permanent urinary diversion may be necessary. A temporary urinary diversion may be required until the bladder fully develops and gives the upper tract time to decompress. A loop of dilated ureter can be brought out to the skin (see Fig. 8-2) or the dilated renal collecting system itself can be brought out to the skin as a temporary pyelostomy. Definitive treatment can then be performed when the child is physically and psychologically ready.

## NEOPLASMS

### Urethral Cancer

Urethral cancer is a rare carcinoma that occurs more commonly in women than in men, is more common in white than in black persons, and is more common in the fifth and sixth

---

### URETHRAL CANCER STAGING

**STAGE O**
In situ (tumor limited to mucosa)

**STAGE A**
Tumor does not extend beyond the submucosa.

**STAGE B**
Female—Tumor infiltrates periurethral muscle.
Male—Tumor infiltrates periurethral muscle but not beyond corpus spongiosum or prostate.

**STAGE C**
Male—Direct extension of tumor into tissue beyond corpus spongiosum or beyond prostatic capsule

**STAGE $C_1$**
Female—Tumor infiltrates the muscular wall of the vagina.

**STAGE $C_2$**
Female—Tumor infiltrates the muscular wall of the vagina and invades the vaginal mucosa.

**STAGE $C_3$**
Female—Tumor infiltrates other adjacent structures such as the bladder, labia, or clitoris.

**STAGE $D_1$**
Metastasis to inguinal lymph nodes

**STAGE $D_2$**
Metastasis to pelvic lymph nodes below bifurcation of aorta

**STAGE $D_3$**
Metastasis to pelvic lymph nodes above bifurcation of aorta

**STAGE $D_4$**
Metastasis to distant organs

---

Modified from Hopkins SC, Grabstaed H: Benign and malignant tumors of the male and female urethra. In Walsh PC et al, editors: *Campbell's urology*, vol 2, ed 5, Philadelphia, 1986, WB Saunders.

decades of life.[16,18] With only 600 accumulated cases of male urethral cancer in the literature, it is extremely rare.[16] The most common tumor of the female urethra is squamous cell,
second most common is adenocarcinoma, and third is transitional cell carcinoma (TCC).[18]
Male urethral carcinomas are predominately of the following types: squamous cell, transitional cell, and adenocarcinoma.[16] A staging system for urethral cancer is listed in the box
on p. 223.

**Female.** The primary symptom of urethral cancer in the female is urethral bleeding or
spotting; dysuria, frequency, and obstruction also may develop. Extensive lesions may penetrate the vagina. Urinalysis may reveal red blood cells, white blood cells, and positive urine
cytologic findings. Physical examination may show a cancerous mass at the urethral meatus
that grossly mimics urethral caruncle. Biopsy of all suspect lesions is warranted.

Treatment is based on the stage and location of the lesion. A distally located superficial
lesion (for example, a lesion at the urethral meatus) may require a simple excision, whereas
more extensive tumors (stages B and C) located in the proximal urethra necessitate a radical cystectomy with urethrectomy.

The tumors are divided into anterior and posterior lesions, with a much better prognosis for anterior lesions. Posterior lesions and lesions involving the entire urethra indicate a
poor prognosis. These patients usually are treated with an anterior exenteration, which
involves removing the bladder, urethra, vaginal cuff around the urethra, cervix, uterus, fal-
lopian tubes, and ovaries; 5-year survival ranges from 10% to 20%.[16] External beam irradiation also may be included in the treatment regimen.

Distal anterior urethral lesions signify a much better prognosis than do posterior
lesions, if complete surgical excision can be achieved. Cure rates approach 90% when
lymph nodes are not involved.[16]

**Male.** Most tumors of the male urethra occur in the bulbous or bulbomembranous
urethra, with the remaining tumors occurring in the distal urethra. Chronic urinary tract
infections or chronic urethral inflammation are believed to contribute to the neoplastic
process.[16]

Symptoms of obstruction (dysuria, decreased size and caliber of stream) or hematuria
develop in most men with urethral cancer. Physical examination may reveal a tender, firm
mass in the anterior urethra or perineum; in advanced cases, erosion of the tumor through
to the scrotum and perineum can occur. Cystoscopy and biopsy generally provide the diagnosis.

Treatment again depends on the location and extent of cancer. Distal tumors can be
managed by local excision or a distal urethrectomy. Superficial distal lesions can be cured
by transurethral resection. Removal of the penis, testicle, and scrotum with perineal ure-
throstomy is advocated for more extensive distal tumors. Although lymph drains from the
distal urethra to the inguinal nodes, prophylactic lymph node dissections do not alter the
course of the disease. Local recurrence is the most common cause of treatment failure; 60%
cure rates are reported when adequate margins are possible.[16,18]

Proximal urethral cancers in the bulbous or bulbomembranous urethra may require
surgical removal of the penis, scrotum, testicles, entire urethra, prostate, and bladder; an
ileal conduit is necessary. Patients usually die of local recurrence, and 5-year survival is
poor at 13%.[16]

## Prostate Cancer

Although prostate cancer typically does not require a urinary diversion, it is discussed here because pathologic processes may manifest that are best managed with a urinary diversion (such as a percutaneous nephrostomy or ileal conduit). For example, ureteral or bladder outlet obstruction may occur initially, or complications after the treatment of the prostate cancer may develop later.

The incidence of prostate cancer has increased recently, which may be the result of better detection.[5] Prostate cancer, which ranks third among cancer deaths in men, accounts for 10% of all cancer deaths. The incidence of prostate cancer is 50% higher in black than in white men; blacks also tend to be diagnosed at a higher stage of disease initially. In contrast, Native Americans, Orientals, and Hispanics have a much lower incidence of prostate cancer than do white men. Occult prostate cancer has been reported in as many as 40% of patients older than 75 years of age.[33]

**Etiology.** It is theorized that the development of prostate cancer is related to hormone levels. The fact that prostate cancer does not occur in eunuchs lends credence to this theory. Environmental factors (e.g., automobile exhaust fumes and fertilizer) and infections may play a role in prostate cancer; however, these findings have not singled out a specific element that leads to the development of prostate cancer. Prostate cancer is not believed to be related to benign prostatic hypertrophy.

Initially prostate cancer spreads locally into the trigone and ureters, obstructing the ureters. Rectal involvement is rare. Once prostate cancer penetrates the capsule, distant spread occurs by the vascular or venous routes to the nearby obturator nodes and to the bone. Bony metastases are the most common form of hematogenous spread.

Prostate cancer, as with most cancers, produces few symptoms early in the course of the disease. It usually is found when a prostate nodule is palpated during a digital rectal examination. Such a nodule shows positive cancer findings in 50% of the cases.[5] A biopsy, commonly transrectal or transperineal, confirms the diagnosis of prostate cancer. Prostate cancer also can be diagnosed in men receiving a transurethral prostatectomy for presumably benign prostatic hypertrophy.

**Grading.** Basically tumors are graded according to histologic appearance (i.e., cell patterns and architecture). The grading of prostate cancers, however, is difficult because generally more than one cell pattern exists within one tumor. Thus many cancer centers have developed their own grading systems. A more widely accepted grading system, the Gleason grading system, considers the most prevalent cell type along with the second most prevalent type; these grades are totaled to obtain the Gleason histologic score, which ranges from 2 to 10.[5] Generally the higher the grade, the worse the prognosis.

**Staging.** Staging is performed to determine the extent of the disease. The box on p. 226 lists the staging system for prostate cancer.

Several tumor markers are used to assist the staging of prostate cancer and to monitor the status of the disease. Prostatic acid phosphatase (PAP) is released into the serum from a prostate malignancy; elevated serum levels of PAP directly reflect the extent of the cancer. PAP level is a less accurate indicator when the tumor is confined and not metastasized. Prostate-specific antigen is another biochemical marker level; because it appears to be vol-

---

## TUMOR STAGING FOR PROSTATE CANCER

**STAGE A**

**Incidental finding**
$A_1$: Focal tumor present in less than 5% of gland
$A_2$: Diffuse tumor involves more than 5% of the gland

**STAGE B**

**Confined to prostate**
$B_1$: Small discrete nodule palpated on rectal examination; tumor is less than 2 cm or limited to one lobe
$B_2$: Tumor is more than 2 cm in diameter, induration present, or tumor present in both lobes

**STAGE C**

**Penetration of prostatic capsule**
$C_1$: Minimal extracapsular extension; no invasion of seminal vesicles
$C_2$: Extensive extracapsular extension, producing bladder outlet or ureteral obstruction

**STAGE D**

**Metastasis to lymph node or bone**

---

ume-dependent, it also reflects tumor burden. It is more sensitive, however, than prostatic acid phosphatase for detection of new or relapsing prostate cancer and is useful in monitoring response to prostate cancer therapy.[18]

Bone scans are sensitive tests for detecting bony metastases (stage D); the radiopharmaceutic agent, usually technetium-99m methylene diphosphonate, is taken up in all areas of increased bone turnover. Computed tomography (CT) scans are not effective in evaluating the spread of prostate cancer. Although the CT scan can detect enlarged lymph nodes, it cannot identify them as malignant; in addition, nodes may be enlarged in reaction to either the prostate biopsy or the transurethral resection of the prostate.

Staging of prostate cancer is further clarified during prostatectomy. Pelvic lymph nodes are removed and examined, providing the most accurate method of assessing for metastasis. If nodes show positive findings, some surgeons may elect to terminate the procedure, whereas others may proceed with a radical prostatectomy.

**Management.** Prostate cancer is managed with several modalities (transurethral resection of the prostate or radical prostatectomy; interstitial irradiation or external beam irradiation, or a combination; chemotherapy; and hormone manipulation), depending on the extent of the tumor. When the tumor is believed to be confined to the prostate and the patient is in reasonably good health, removal of the entire prostate gland, seminal vesicles, and ejaculatory ducts can be curative. Patients with stage $A_2$, $B_1$, or $B_2$ prostate cancer are considered the best candidates for this procedure, with a 50% to 75% 15-year tumor-free survival reported.[5]

Adjuvant treatment with radiation is warranted when a tumor is found in the seminal vesicles at the time of the radical prostatectomy (stage C). Hormone manipulation or irradiation in conjunction with radical prostatectomy can give 15-year survival rates of 11% to 28%.[5] The 15-year survival rate in patients with stage C disease that is not treated with hormone manipulation or radiation is unknown because most reports note the use of adjuvant therapy.

When disease has spread beyond the pelvic lymph nodes to bones or other organs, a cure is not possible; however, hormone manipulation with bilateral orchiectomy or luteinizing hormone–releasing hormone agonist can delay the onset of symptoms from the metastatic disease. In fact, *immediate* hormonal manipulation in patients with stage D disease can significantly delay the spread of the disease.[5] Once metastasis with symptoms has occurred, palliation of metastatic symptoms can be obtained with hormonal treatment or radiation therapy to the sites causing the symptoms. Chemotherapy has not proved to be beneficial in treating prostate cancer.

## Bladder Cancer

The incidence of bladder cancer is approximately 45,000 new diagnoses per year.[34] It occurs more frequently in men, with nearly a 3:1 ratio.[7,34] The incidence of bladder cancer increases with age: 20 cases per 100,000 per year for persons older than 40 years of age. The risk of bladder cancer is two to three times greater for individuals living in highly industrialized urban areas such as the Northeast.[34]

**Etiology.** Several events precede the development of a true malignancy.[7,18] In the first of two important phases, initiation, a biochemical lesion is introduced into a normal cell's deoxyribonucleic acid (DNA). This represents a neoplastic transformation that damages the DNA; at this phase, however, cancer has not yet developed. The second phase, promotion, must occur. Promotion is the replication of these neoplastic transformations until they become fixed. Both initiation and promotion are reversible until the tumor actually develops. These two phases, which must occur over and over until the tumor actually develops, create a process that can take years.

Repeated exposure to several risk factors increases the risk for bladder cancer. In 1895 bladder cancer was found to develop in workers exposed to aniline dye. In most cases a long latency period—years, sometimes decades—passed before the cancer actually appeared, and the causative agent was found to be 2-beta-naphthalene. Many aromatic amines have since been found to cause bladder cancer. Epidemiologists estimate that exposure in high-risk industries accounts for 18% to 34% of all bladder cancers in men. The highest risk occurs between 40 and 50 years after exposure to the industrial carcinogen.

Cigarettes play an even greater role in the development of bladder cancer. As many as 50% of bladder cancers can be attributed to cigarette smoking.[18] Smoking one to two packs of cigarettes per day doubles the risk of bladder cancer, and smoking more than two packs per day triples the risk.[7] The incidence of bladder cancer in women has been increasing, which likely reflects the fact that more women are smoking. The etiologic agents in cigarette smoke probably are 2-naphthylamine and nitrosamine.

Cyclamates were taken off the market after they were deemed carcinogenic. Bladder cancer developed in mice who were fed cyclamates at doses 500 to 700 times that of human consumption. Although saccharine and aspartame have not been found to cause bladder cancer in humans,[7] it may be advisable for patients with recurrent tumors to avoid consumption of all artificial sweeteners because they may act as promoting agents.[18]

In some countries schistosomiasis is another factor that causes bladder cancer. *Schistosoma* organisms have complicated life cycles, in which a type of snail is used as one of their intermediate hosts before infecting humans. The infection starts from contact with contaminated water. The cercaria penetrates human skin, matures in the bloodstream, and lays eggs or ova in the muscle wall of the bladder and intestine. Eventually the eggs are passed out of the body in urine or feces, where they spend several cycles as a miracidium and then as a sporocyst in the snail before becoming a cercaria ready to infect humans again. The irritation of the ova in the bladder wall causes squamous cell carcinoma. In Egypt 70% of bladder cancers are squamous cell carcinoma.[7]

Chronic irritation in the bladder also leads to squamous cell cancers. For example, patients with neurogenic bladders and indwelling Foley catheters have a greater incidence of squamous cell carcinoma. Similarly, pyocystis (a collection of purulent material in the bladder) and a higher incidence of squamous cell cancer occur in patients with a urinary diversion in which the bladder has been retained.[7]

Phenacetin taken in large doses (more than 2 kg during a 15-year period) also causes a higher incidence of bladder cancer, usually TCC. These patients also are more subject to TCC of the renal pelvis and ureters.[7]

Another agent associated with TCC of the bladder is cyclophosphamide, which is used to treat patients with rheumatoid arthritis and systemic lupus erythematosus. A shorter latency period is observed with cyclophosphamide (6 to 13 years) than with phenacetin.[7] Some viruses found in the tissues of cancerous bladders are believed to play a causative role. The incidence of TCC in patients with cervical cancer who are undergoing pelvic radiation has been found to be two to four times greater than in the normal population.[7]

Finally, genetic predisposition may play a larger role in bladder cancer than is currently known. Reports of bladder cancer in several members of the same family have been cited.

**Types and Behavior.** The majority of bladder tumors arise from epithelial cells. The histologic distribution is 92% transitional cell, 7% squamous cell, and 1% to 2% adenocarcinoma.[17]

*Epithelial atypia* and *dysplasia* are terms for lesions that have been found to have a higher chance than normal mucosa of progressing to malignancy. No reliable predictor can identify which dysplasia will progress.

Cystitis cystica and cystitis glandularis are lesions in the bladder mucosa that resemble a water blister but do not have a higher than normal incidence of progressing to a cancer.

Common terminology used to describe the penetration of bladder tumors include carcinoma in situ, superficial bladder cancer, superficially invasive bladder cancer, and muscle-invasive bladder cancer. Carcinoma in situ is a noninvasive cancer at initial diagnosis. It has been described as having two forms. One form is dysplastic and can progress to invasion and metastasis in approximately 50% to 75% of cases. The second form, however, is less invasive and seems to pose little immediate threat.[7]

A superficial bladder tumor does not invade the lamina propria, the basement membrane that divides the epithelium of the transitional cells from the deeper layers. The majority of all bladder cancers are superficial bladder cancers. In fact, 70% of TCCs are noninvasive (i.e., the cancer is confined to the superficial layers of the bladder). When the tumor penetrates the lamina propria but not the detrusor, it is a superficially invasive cancer. A cancer that penetrates the bladder muscle is an invasive or a muscle-invasive cancer. Tumors confined to the mucosa have a 3% chance of progressing to muscle invasion, whereas the risk of muscle invasion by those tumors that penetrate the basement membrane is 24%.[7]

Bladder tumors have a predictable pattern of behavior. They recur much more frequently than they invade the layers of the bladder. Although the majority of superficial tumors recur, the tumors usually recur in the same stage and grade as the original tumor.[7] The recurrence rate of solitary superficial lesions is 67%; when the cancer develops as multiple lesions, up to 90% recur. Solid tumors are more likely to invade the muscle deeply and metastasize early; papillary tumors are less likely to metastasize than are solid tumors.

**Classification.** Bladder tumors are classified according to stage and grade. Although tumor grade and tumor stage are separate entities, the use of two classification systems provides more complete information regarding the severity of the tumor. For example, patients with a grade I tumor that is mucosally confined have a 75% chance of being disease-free at 12 months. When this tumor is a grade III, this percentage decreases to 55%.[7]

*Staging* describes the depth of tumor penetration through the bladder wall layers. Bladder cancer has been staged by means of several different methods. Marshall's staging system and the Union International Coutre le Cancer (UICC) classification are the two most commonly used systems. Table 7-1 compares these two staging systems. Fig. 7-2 provides a diagram of the depth of tumor penetration according to the Marshall staging system. Tumor, node, and metastasis (TNM) classification also is used.

Patients with muscle-invasive bladder cancers have a 20% to 40% 5-year survival rate when the lesion appears treatable.[18] Patients with an inoperable bladder cancer have less

**Table 7-1**   Classification of bladder cancer

| Marshall | UICC | Description |
|---|---|---|
| Stage O | 1a $T_{IS}$ | Tumor is limited to the mucosa, including both papillary cancer and carcinoma in situ |
| Stage A | $T_1$ | Lesions have invaded lamina propria but not muscle of bladder wall |
| Stage $B_1$ | $T_2$ | Neoplasms have penetrated less than halfway through muscle wall |
| Stage $B_2$ | $T_{3a}$ | Tumors have invaded muscle wall to a depth greater than halfway but are still confined to the muscularis |
| Stage C | $T_{3b}$ | Neoplasms have invaded perivesical fat |
| Stage $D_1$ | $T_{4a}$ | Malignant disease extends beyond the limits of the bladder and perivesical fat but still is confined to the pelvis either at or below the level of the sacral promontory; included are tumors invading contiguous organs |
| | $T_{4b}$ | Tumors involving pelvic wall or rectus muscles below the level of the umbilicus, or lymph node metastasis below the bifurcation of the common iliac artery |
| Stage $D_2$ | | Tumors have metastasized to distant organs or lymph nodes above sacral promontory (bifurcation of the common iliac artery) or are external to the inguinal ligament |

*UICC,* Union International Coutre le Cancer.

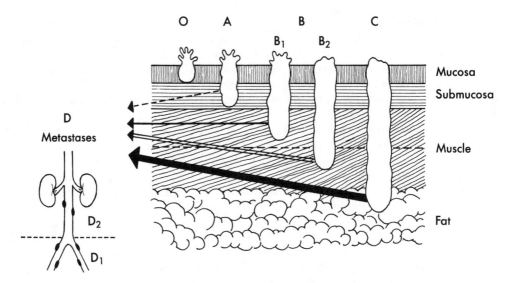

**Fig. 7-2**   Diagram of penetration of bladder tumors as staged by Marshall staging system. Arrows indicate potential for metastasis.

than a 3% 1-year survival rate. Treatment generally requires radical cystectomy with some type of urinary diversion; failures most often are the result of distant metastases at the time of the cystectomy.

*Grade* is the microscopic appearance of the cells and their orientation toward each other. For example, a low-grade tumor has a fairly close resemblance to the original cell type. As the grade of the tumor increases, the cells have less resemblance to the original mucosa and lose their orientation toward each other. Grading of bladder tumors is important in predicting recurrence.

Bladder cancers generally are graded from I to III, depending on the histologic appearance (see the box on p. 231). Grade I tumors are less aggressive and less likely to recur rapidly; grade III tumors are more aggressive. Well-differentiated, grade I tumors indicate approximately a 65% 3-year survival period, whereas a poorly differentiated tumor suggests a 20% to 30% chance of 3-year survival.[7]

**Diagnosis.** Hematuria, either gross or microscopic, is present in up to 80% of patients with bladder cancer.[18] Although the hallmark of bladder cancer is gross and painless hematuria, the amount of hematuria does not correlate with the stage or grade of the tumor. Vesicle irritability, dysuria, and frequency also may exist, especially in patients with carcinoma in situ.

Cystoscopic examination is essential when hematuria occurs, inasmuch as the majority of bladder tumors are identified with this procedure. The cystoscope, a lighted, rigid or flexible hollow instrument, is passed through the urethra into the bladder with the patient under local anesthesia, thus allowing visualization of the bladder mucosa. Typically this examination is an office procedure; if, however, a tumor is found, a transurethral resection of the bladder tumor is necessary. In this procedure, which often requires a general or

## GRADING SCALE FOR BLADDER CANCER

**GRADE I**
Tumors have the least degree of cellular
   anaplasia compatible with the diagnosis
   of a malignancy.

**GRADE III**
Tumors have the most severe degree of
   cellular anaplasia.

**GRADE II**
Tumors are intermediate between those of
   grades I and III.

spinal anesthesia, the entire tumor usually is removed, allowing determination of tumor stage and grade.

Although IVP is used to reveal large bladder tumors, a cystoscopic examination is still the gold standard for evaluating the bladder. The IVP is used in patients with hematuria because the test provides a good evaluation of the upper tracts; this area can then be eliminated as a source of the patient's symptoms.[18]

Diagnostic tests such as urine cytology and flow cytometry are conducted to closely examine the cells in the urine. Urine cytology spins the urine to permit microscopic analysis of the cells. Because cancerous cells have a characteristic appearance, urine cytology is especially effective in diagnosing carcinoma in situ. Flow cytometry, in which the cell's DNA is analyzed by means of specialized equipment, is becoming more useful in diagnosing low-grade lesions and even in predicting tumor aggressiveness.

CT scans can identify tumors but usually are used for staging rather than for diagnosing. Lymph node involvement and gross tumor invasion also can be determined with this test.

**Management of Superficial Bladder Tumor.** Transurethral resection of bladder tumors still is the standard treatment for most bladder tumors. Patients with low-grade, mucosally confined tumors can expect almost a normal life expectancy. Further treatment depends on pathologic findings of the resected specimen. If the tumor is carcinoma in situ, invades the lamina propria, or recurs rapidly at a higher grade, then intravesical chemotherapy should be considered.

Chemotherapeutic agents most commonly used are thiotepa, mitomycin, doxorubicin, or bacille Calmette-Guérin (BCG). BCG is the initial treatment of choice for carcinoma in situ and also is effective in preventing tumor recurrences in other types of bladder cancers. A usual chemotherapy schedule involves instilling the agent by catheter and then having the patient void 2 hours later. This procedure is repeated weekly for 4 to 6 weeks and then monthly for several months.

**Management of Muscle-Invasive Bladder Tumor.** Patients with muscle-invasive bladder cancer generally have a rapidly progressive tumor. Only 40% to 50% have a 5-year survival rate, even with a radical cystectomy.[18] Approximately 8% of patients with muscle invasion may be treated with a partial cystectomy if the tumor meets strict criteria: distant from the bladder neck and trigone and penetration limited to the superficial muscle.

Radical cystectomy with a urinary diversion usually is the treatment of choice for muscle-invasive bladder cancer; this procedure may be performed with a continent reservoir.

Radiation therapy has proved to be inferior to the radical cystectomy in the treatment of bladder cancer; the 5-year survival rate for radiation therapy is 20% to 39%. For a period of time, preoperative radiation was believed to be beneficial; however, further studies have failed to confirm this belief.[18]

**Management of Metastatic Bladder Cancer.** Metastatic bladder cancer limited to the pelvis ($T_{3b}$ to $T_{4a}$ and $T_{4b}$) responds poorly to radical cystectomy alone. When the cancer has spread to the prostate, vagina, cervix, uterus, or rectum, the 5-year survival is 10% to 15% at best.[18] Traditional treatment has been radiation treatment alone, which has failed to improve the survival rate. Chemotherapy with combination drugs is improving survival. For example, methotrexate, vinblastine, doxorubicin, and cisplatin (MVAC) therapy has completely eradicated some tumors and has resulted in long-term survival for other patients.[18]

Patients with stage $D_2$ metastatic disease have a poor prognosis, with 5-year survival rate approaching zero. For these patients palliation is the appropriate treatment.[18]

**Management of Palliation.** Metastatic cancer of the bladder, prostate, and other pelvic organs may require a palliative urinary diversion. Despite realization that a metastatic or aggressive cancer may be impossible to cure, control of the debilitating problems often associated with the local disease can be worthwhile. For example, a locally invasive bladder cancer may precipitate a vesicovaginal fistula, causing a constant leak of urine from the vagina. The resultant problems of skin breakdown, odor, and discomfort can make the patient's remaining time miserable. A urinary diversion (with or without a radical cystectomy) often benefits these patients.

Malignancies that obstruct the ureters also can be managed with some type of urinary diversion. For example, prostate cancer can spread locally into the bladder and trigone to cause an internal ureteral obstruction, whereas external ureteral compression may complicate other pelvic malignancies. Typically the placement of ureteral stents either prevent obstruction or facilitate drainage in the patient who already has a ureteral obstruction. Ureteral stents are small silicone tubes that are kept in proper placement from the renal pelvis to the bladder with a preformed coil at either end of the stent. Stents usually are passed cystoscopically into the ureteral orifices. When it is not possible to pass the stent through the urethra (such as with prostate cancer), a percutaneous nephrostomy is performed to facilitate the passage of the stent from the kidney down to the bladder. An internal stent can then be left in place and changed periodically.

Occasionally, an internal stent cannot be passed and the percutaneous nephrostomy becomes the only way to drain the urine. This is far from a perfect method of drainage and presents a difficult challenge for the patient, family, and health care providers.

Bleeding as a complication associated with bladder cancer also may precipitate the need for a palliative urinary diversion. Commonly this bleeding responds to conservative measures of hemostasis such as intravesical aluminum irrigations or silver nitrate instillation. An emergency cystectomy and urinary diversion can be lifesaving when the hemorrhaging is uncontrolled. Even when silver nitrate effectively stops hemorrhaging, however, the silver nitrate can cause severe bladder fibrosis, thus decreasing bladder capacity and function. Because Foley catheterization does not relieve the patient's symptoms, a urinary diversion (with or without a cystectomy) often is beneficial.

## Extensive Pelvic Malignancy

Locally advanced cancers in the pelvis, such as advanced gynecologic and rectal malignancies in addition to rhabdomyosarcomas, sometimes are treated with a total pelvic exenteration. This procedure requires removal of all organs in the pelvis, including the bladder, the rectum, and all gynecologic organs. Thus the patient is left with a urinary and a fecal stoma. The urinary diversion can be created by use of ileum, colon, or jejunum.

## Rhabdomyosarcoma

Rhabdomyosarcoma is a cancer arising from embryonic tissue that differentiates into striated skeletal muscle and fibrous tissue.[25] A disease that occurs in children, it has two peak incidence periods: 2 to 6 years of age and 15 to 19 years of age.[11] Approximately 20% of cases develop in the GU region (bladder, prostate, testicles, vagina, perineal area, and uterus), and the rest may develop in the extremities or head and neck.[25] Although rare (8% of all solid cancers of childhood are rhabdomyosarcoma), it is the most common *soft tissue sarcoma* in children, comprising 50% of all soft tissue childhood sarcomas.[11,35] It also is the most common cancer of the bladder, prostate, and vagina in children.

Rhabdomyosarcoma has a white, fleshy, vascular appearance and is categorized on histologic examination as embryonal, botryoid, pleomorphic, and alveolar. The most common of these are embryonal and botryoid. Rhabdomyosarcoma of the botryoid type has the appearance of a cluster of grapes and develops on mucosal surfaces of hollow organs such as the bladder or the vagina.[35]

Treatment of this neoplasm has improved markedly recently with the advent of combination therapy (surgery, chemotherapy, and radiation therapy). Traditionally, because this tumor is widely infiltrative into surrounding tissue, therapy required removal of all pelvic organs to obtain wide margins. Now, by a combination of chemotherapy and radiation therapy, excision of the tumor bulk can be undertaken, often leaving the bladder and other pelvic organs intact. A subsequent operation can be performed at a later date to assess the effectiveness of tumor shrinkage after chemotherapy or radiation therapy, or both; residual tumor can then be removed at that time.[11,35] This treatment fails in some patients, who then require cystectomy with a urinary diversion.

## TRAUMA

Trauma may require different types of urinary diversions. The type of diversion performed is contingent on the level of the trauma within the urinary tract. Trauma and associated complications may necessitate a percutaneous nephrostomy or even an ileal conduit.

## Renal Pelvic Injuries

Patients with a ureteropelvic junction obstruction and children who have had extensive flexion extension of the torso are prone to injury of the renal collecting system. Flexion extension injuries in children can result in disruption of the ureteropelvic junction, which is diagnosed by use of IVP or CT scan; treatment usually requires an open surgical repair, with the temporary placement of a percutaneous nephrostomy tube. Unfortunately, patients with a ureteropelvic junction obstruction are prone to rupture with mild trauma, which also may necessitate an open repair with percutaneous nephrostomy.

## Ureteral Injury

Ureteral injuries as the sole injury are rare and usually occur only with multiorgan trauma. A gunshot wound or stab wound is the most common traumatic cause for ureteral injuries. The diagnosis is made with an IVP, and repair is performed through an open procedure, depending on associated injuries. A ureteral stent usually is placed and may be brought out through the kidney as a percutaneous nephrostomy.

Iatrogenic ureteral injury occurs much more commonly than do traumatic injuries. This injury can happen in the course of surgical procedures in close proximity to ureters such as occurs in urologic and gynecologic procedures or in kidney stone procedures.[14]

Diagnosis usually is made at the time of the injury, and a simple repair can be made. If a ureteral injury is not diagnosed immediately, diagnosis becomes more difficult and may require an IVP, a CT scan, or a retrograde ureteropyelogram. Treatment often requires a percutaneous nephrostomy. Ureteral injury that involves a ureterovaginal or ureterocutaneous fistula also may be simply treated with a percutaneous nephrostomy. When the ureter has not been completely severed or ligated, this type of diversion of the urine allows the fistula to heal.

## Bladder Injuries

Bladder injuries may result from trauma (blunt and penetrating). Penetrating trauma includes gunshot wounds and injuries from knives or other sharp instruments. Blunt trauma can cause bladder rupture by compression injury that usually ruptures the dome of the bladder or by perforation from the bony fragments of a pelvic fracture. Diagnosis of bladder injuries requires a high incidence of suspicion because symptoms are so subtle. Gross hematuria almost always is found. A cystogram is essential to demonstrate the integrity of the bladder wall. Extravasation of dye is consistent with a ruptured bladder; the extravasation also reveals whether the rupture is intraperitoneal or extraperitoneal. An intraperitoneal rupture or a grossly contaminated wound warrants an open surgical repair. When the bladder has ruptured extraperitoneally and there are no signs of infection, an indwelling Foley catheter often is sufficient treatment.[6]

## Urethral Injuries

**Female.** Injuries to the female urethra occur most commonly during childbirth but can occur during any vaginal procedure, especially after pelvic radiation therapy. Repair usually involves a primary closure over a Foley catheter but may require a suprapubic cystostomy for diversion.

**Male.** Injuries to the male urethra are more common and more complicated than are female urethral injuries. Management depends on the anatomic location of the injury. Injuries that involve the proximal urethra (the membranous urethra to the bladder) are called *posterior urethral injuries*. Injuries that occur from the bulbous urethra to the meatus are called *anterior urethral injuries*. Posterior urethral injuries occur during blunt trauma and pelvic fractures. The anterior urethra is prone to straddle injuries (i.e., falling and hitting a board in the straddle position, which crushes the urethra against the pubic bone) and injuries that occur when a penis fractures during sexual intercourse.

Diagnosis of posterior urethral injuries is made with a strong index of suspicion; a drop of blood that appears at the urethral meatus may be the single most important sign.[29,30] A retrograde urethrogram may show either a complete or a partial disruption of the urethra. If a partial posterior urethra injury is found, treatment with a suprapubic cystostomy usually suffices. Controversy exists concerning the treatment of complete posterior urethral disruption. Some authors suggest that if a suprapubic tube is left indwelling and a formal repair is completed 3 to 6 months later, the incidence of incontinence and impotence is reduced.[29,30] Others argue that if a catheter can be passed by one of several different methods, the urethra will heal and an extensive surgery is avoided. Almost all these patients, regardless of which treatment is elected, initially have a suprapubic tube. It is conceivable that complications eventually could warrant some type of urinary conduit if all else fails.

Anterior urethral injuries usually require primary repair over a catheter, but a suprapubic tube also may be needed in this case. Depending on the extent of the injury, the suprapubic tube can be left indwelling until the damaged tissue heals and permanent repair is performed.

## Neurogenic Bladder

Many different neural injuries can create a neurogenic bladder dysfunction. Lesions above the sacral micturition center (S2-4) create a spastic bladder. Brain-stem lesions (dementia, vascular accidents, encephalitis, and multiple sclerosis), Parkinson's disease, and spinal cord injury above the S2-4 level all precipitate the spastic neurogenic bladder. Typical spastic bladder characteristics include reduced capacity, involuntary bladder contractions, high intravesical voiding pressures, and bladder wall hypertrophy.

Injury at or below the sacral micturition center (such as spinal cord injury or myelomeningocele) create a flaccid or atonic bladder. Neuropathies (such as those associated with diabetes mellitus) and radical pelvic surgical procedures (such as a low anterior resection) also may be complicated with a flaccid bladder. Characteristics include large bladder capacity, no voluntary bladder contractions, low intravesical pressure, mild bladder-wall hypertrophy, and decreased external sphincter tone.

Of these different situations the neurogenic bladder caused by a spinal cord injury is most likely to be managed with various forms of urinary diversions. Because complications from the urinary tract sometimes cause the greatest morbidity and mortality in the patient with a spinal cord injury, the urologist often becomes the prominent physician. Management of the neurogenic bladder in these patients is difficult and depends on the patient's preference, bladder capacity, the condition of the kidneys and ureters, and the level of the spinal cord injury. Patients manage to empty the bladder by the Credé or Valsalva maneuver, intermittent catheterization, urethral catheter, suprapubic tube, a urinary conduit, or continent diversion.

Patients with cervical injuries often lack the manual dexterity to perform intermittent catheterization, so continuous drainage by means of a urethral catheter, a suprapubic tube, or a urinary conduit is the most appropriate option. When the spinal cord injury is located in the lumbar or thoracic region, the patient may have sufficient manual motor control to perform intermittent catheterization (if the bladder is of sufficient capacity). With sufficient bladder capacity, trigger techniques can be used to stimulate bladder emptying.[38] Anticholinergics may be used to enhance bladder capacity. This type of bladder management program is ideal when bladder pressures remain low and no hyperreflexia exists.[2] It also may be best suited for male patients. At times, especially if the bladder is contracted, an elective external sphincterotomy (interruption of the external sphincter), in conjunction with the mandatory use of a condom catheter, may be desirable for managing the spastic bladder.

Female patients with spinal cord injuries may be unable to perform intermittent catheterization, despite their degree of manual dexterity. Although a skilled caregiver often can provide this care for the patient, this alternative is not always feasible when the patient is active (e.g., working or attending school).

When intermittent catheterization is not desirable, a suprapubic tube becomes necessary. This type of diversion works quite satisfactorily for a short time. However, problems such as recurrent stone formation in the tube and leakage around the catheter may develop. Eventually a urinary conduit or continent reservoir may be necessary.

Complications to which the patient with a spinal cord injury is vulnerable include renal stones, bladder stones, cystitis, pyelonephritis, and autonomic dysreflexia. Stones may develop through a process of bone demineralization as a consequence of the patient's immobility; these most commonly are composed of calcium phosphate.[38] Stones also may form in the bladder on catheters and foreign bodies such as hair introduced into the bladder during intermittent catheterization. Struvite stones (magnesium ammonium phosphate stones that form in the kidney in association with chronic urinary tract infections) have an increased incidence in patients with a neurogenic bladder.[37]

Because the bladder of most patients with spinal cord injury is colonized with one or more organisms (because of many of the factors already mentioned), cystitis also is a common problem. Pyelonephritis can develop as a result of ascending infections from the colonized bladder, as well as from dyssynergic voiding. Dyssynergic voiding—that is, bladder contraction while the sphincter remains contracted—creates high bladder pressures. This increased pressure causes reflux of urine and bacteria into the ureters and kidneys, so hydronephrosis and pyelonephritis develop.

Finally, autonomic dysreflexia occurs in patients with injuries from the cervical spine to the T10 level; autonomic dysreflexia does not occur in the patients with lumbar cord injuries. Autonomic dysreflexia is triggered by bladder overdistention and occurs because the lesion is above the sympathetic outflow from the spinal cord. The patient has severe hypertension, sweating, bradycardia, and headache. Treatment of autonomic dysreflexia requires immediate bladder drainage.

Currently there is no ideal method of urinary diversion for the patient with spinal cord injury; complications develop with and without a diversion. Neurostimulation of sacral nerve roots is being met with some success: patients perform near-normal voiding. This treatment involves neurostimulation of sacral nerve roots and may be the treatment of choice in the future, but further investigation is, of course, necessary.

## INFLAMMATORY DISORDERS

Several types of inflammatory processes can require diversion of the urinary tract. These include urinary tract infection, acute pyelonephritis, xanthogranulomatous pyelonephritis, renal abscess, acute cystitis, retroperitoneal fibrosis, pelvic mass, radiation cystitis, and urethral strictures.

In addition to these disorders, chronic indwelling Foley catheters often trigger an inflammatory response within the bladder. Some patients who are unable to perform intermittent catheterization (such as patients with multiple sclerosis or cervical spinal cord injury) may benefit from long-term indwelling Foley catheters. Complications associated with long-term catheter drainage include recurrent cystitis, urethritis, prostatitis, and urethral erosion.

## Urinary Tract infection

Urinary tract infection (UTI) develops in four ways: ascending infection, hematogenous spread, lymphatogenous spread, and direct extension.[27,31] In the female, ascending infections are common; this is because the female urethra is short and there is a tendency for bacteria, which have colonized the female vestibule, to ascend the urethra and cause a bladder infection. Bacterial colonization of the vagina occurs from rectal contamination and from sexual intercourse. Nuns who are abstinent have a much lower incidence of UTI than do age-matched, sexually active women.[27,31]

Patients with urinary conduits are even more susceptible to ascending UTI for the following reasons: there is no urethra to protect the urine; the urine usually remains colonized; and the ureteroileal anastomosis is freely refluxing.

Hematogenous spread refers to the spread of infection from the blood to the urinary tract or from the urinary tract to the blood. Obstruction usually facilitates this spread, but it most commonly occurs from the urinary tract to the blood.

Lymphatogenous spread, or infection of the urinary tract from the lymph channel, is rare and may be more of a theoretic route of spread than an actual route of spread.

Direct extension of an abscess or an infection present in another organ can occur. Parapelvic abscesses, retroperitoneal abscesses, and GI fistulas can all infect the urinary tract by direct extension.

Many factors influence the development of a UTI: host susceptibility, bacterial virulence, and host defenses.[27] For example, a urinary diversion of any kind increases a person's risk for a UTI because of the loss of the urethral barrier to bacterial invasion. Any condition resulting in obstruction and stasis or urine also renders the host more susceptible (such as ureteropelvic junction obstruction). Finally, the refluxing of urine that occurs with vesicoureteral reflux and ileal conduits also impinges on host susceptibility.

Bacterial virulence, or the ability of the bacteria to cause infections, influences the potential for the development of UTI. *Escherichia coli* is the causative organism for 90% of first-time UTI.[31] Certain types of *E. coli*, however, are more infectious than other types.

One of the characteristics that affects the virulence of bacteria is adherence; bacteria that are more adherent are more infectious. Bacterial adherence is determined partly by the presence or absence of pili, or fimbriae (tiny hairlike appendages on the bacteria that allow bacteria to adhere to mucosal surfaces).[27,36] The most virulent type of fimbriae are call P pili or P-fimbriae. These organisms tend to cause pyelonephritis rather than cystitis and can even cause pyelonephritis in patients who do not have vesicoureteral reflux.[31]

Host defenses, such as the consumption of large amounts of water and an intact glycosaminoglycan layer that lines the urinary tract, are believed to protect the body from UTI. Large amounts of fluid dilute the bacterial inoculum and, during voiding, clear the urinary tract of transient bacteria.[27] The glycosaminoglycan layer is important in preventing bacterial adherence to the urinary tract mucosa.[36]

A breakdown in any of the host defenses predisposes the patient to an infection. Obstruction, which can be caused by stenosis or stones in the ureter, kidney, urethra, or conduit, should be ruled out in the evaluation of an infection.[36] Stenosis may develop at the ureterointestinal anastomoses or at the stoma-skin level in patients with urinary diversions. Foreign bodies such as stones, nonabsorbable sutures or staples, and hair (which can be introduced during intermittent catheterization) all increase the probability of an infection because they serve as a nidus for bacterial aggregation, adherence, and proliferation.

## Acute Pyelonephritis

Acute pyelonephritis is an inflammation of the kidneys that usually affects the renal parenchyma and the renal pelvis. The causative organism is *E. coli* but also may include *Proteus, Klebsiella, Staphylococcus,* or *Streptococcus* species.[27] The kidney usually is enlarged as a result of the edema or inflammation, and microabscesses may be present throughout the kidney. The parenchyma may show extensive tissue destruction, especially in the cortex; however, the glomeruli usually are not extensively involved.

Pyelonephritis usually occurs from ascent of a lower tract infection. Women, especially those who are sexually active, are much more prone to UTI because the female urethra is short and straight. Men are much less susceptible to UTI because of the length of the male urethra and because the prostate secretes antibacterial substances.[27,31]

Patients with ileal conduits have essentially a direct tract for infections from the skin into the conduit and up both ureters, because the ileal conduit usually is made with a freely refluxing anastomosis. Considering the increased risk of infection associated with a urinary conduit, it is surprising that pyelonephritis is not more common.

The usual symptoms of acute pyelonephritis include the abrupt onset of shaking chills, high fever, and back pain; dysuria, frequency, and urgency also occur if there is associated cystitis.

Patients appear quite ill, with fevers of 38° to 40° C (101° to 104° F) and associated tachycardia. Palpation over the affected side usually causes pain; if cystitis is present, there is suprapubic pain also. Children usually have vague abdominal pain; the flank pain and tenderness are not nearly as pronounced in children as in adults.

Urinalysis usually reveals pyuria, bacteriuria, and hematuria; the hematuria may be readily apparent. Urine cultures generally grow more than 100,000 colonies per milliliter of the offending organisms. Lesser numbers, however, do not rule out infection. Serial blood cultures should be performed to rule out associated bacteremia.

An IVP may reveal decreased function of the affected kidney but almost always shows an enlarged kidney as a result of the inflammation. Although IVPs can be performed during the acute phase of the infection, voiding cystograms and cystoscopic examination, if indicated, should be delayed until the infection is cleared.

Pancreatitis and pneumonia in the lung bases can mimic pyelonephritis; appendicitis, cholecystitis, and diverticulitis must be ruled out as well.

If the appropriate diagnosis is made and treatment is begun promptly, the infection usually resolves with no scarring of the kidneys; complications rarely occur. Any obstruction must be treated to prevent the development of more serious complications. If one area of obstruction is causing the pyelonephritis, a ureteral stent or a percutaneous nephrostomy may be required.

After the diagnosis is made and blood and urine cultures are drawn, intravenous broad-spectrum antibiotics are indicated (usually ampicillin and gentamicin). After the patient has responded, the route can be switched to oral.

## Chronic Pyelonephritis

Chronic pyelonephritis is a diagnosis that is as much a radiologic diagnosis as an actual clinical entity. Chronic pyelonephritis implies a long-term kidney infection; however, this may or may not be the case. Generally, chronic pyelonephritis occurs early in childhood and is a result of vesicoureteral reflux. The kidney has cortical thinning and dilated renal calices, which suggests scarring. This damage can progress, if the reflux and infections persist, to produce a thin hydronephrotic kidney with minimal function. The severity of the scarring varies directly with the degree of reflux and infection.

After the age of four years, renal scarring rarely occurs, even in the presence of reflux with infection.[27,31] Adults seldom show scarring in the kidneys despite repeated bouts of infection. Exceptions to this are patients with obstruction, stress, underlying renal disease, or urinary diversions. Obstruction, stones, and renal disease, as well as small shrunken kidneys, can develop in patients with a urinary diversion.

Because chronic pyelonephritis is a disease based on a radiologic diagnosis, some scarring must be present before the diagnosis is made. Usually a smaller kidney is seen on the affected side, and the calices are blunted with thin parenchyma over the scarred areas. Voiding cystourethrograms usually demonstrate vesicoureteral reflux.

Patients with chronic pyelonephritis usually have no symptoms unless acutely infected, in which case they have symptoms similar to acute pyelonephritis (fever, chills, and flank pain). As with acute pyelonephritis, acute infection is documented by urine cultures positive for the offending organism. The results of blood cultures also may be positive, and the complete blood cell count may show a leukocytosis. When patients are not acutely infected, bacteriuria may not be present. Proteinuria may be present in advanced disease and indicates significant renal damage. Patients can lose renal function, depending on the duration and severity of the infection.

Careful monitoring for acute infection and prompt treatment are essential for patients with chronic pyelonephritis. Surgical correction of contributing factors, for example, ureteral reimplantation for a high-grade vesicoureteral reflux, should be employed.

## Xanthogranulomatous Pyelonephritis

Xanthogranulomatous pyelonephritis is an uncommon and chronic form most often seen in middle-aged or older patients. The hallmark of the disease is a nonfunctioning kidney, with one or more renal calculi. These patients have had a chronic infection for some time, and the kidney has essentially ceased to function.[27]

Flank pain, malaise, anorexia, and weight loss are common when symptoms first occur. The symptoms are more chronic and less severe than those that accompany acute pyelonephritis. Laboratory studies reveal leukocytosis, anemia, pyuria, and microhematuria. Urine cultures demonstrate *Proteus mirabilis* and *E. coli*. Treatment requires a nephrectomy.[31]

## Renal Abscess

Renal cortical abscesses develop primarily from hematogenous spread of *Staphylococcus aureus* infections from distant sites. Intravenous drug abusers and persons with diabetes mellitus are especially prone to the development of a renal abscess. Usually multiple small abscesses coalesce to form an abscess that may rupture into the pyelocaliceal system.

Manifestations include flank pain, fever, and chills. A complete blood cell count usually shows a marked leukocytosis with a left shift, and blood cultures may show positive findings. Urinalysis is positive for pyuria only if the abscess has ruptured into the collecting system.

A bulge or renal mass may be seen on plain abdominal film, or the kidney may simply look enlarged. Depending on the size of the abscess, a space-occupying lesion may appear on the IVP. CT scans probably are the most accurate study to diagnose a renal abscess, and CT-guided aspiration can confirm the pathologic condition.

In the early stages, appropriate antibiotics alone may provide adequate treatment of the abscess. If clinical symptoms do not improve, drainage by either percutaneous or open drainage may be necessary.

## Acute Cystitis

Acute cystitis usually is caused by an ascending infection from the urethra and occurs much more commonly in women than in men. *E. coli* is the most common organism.[31] Viral infections of the urinary tract are rare in adults; however, adenovirus may cause a hemorrhagic cystitis in girls.

Irritative voiding symptoms such as frequency, urgency, and dysuria usually occur, but fevers and flank pain are rare. The onset of hematuria frequently follows sexual intercourse; thus acute cystitis has been called "honeymoon cystitis."

Although a urinalysis reveals pyuria (that is, bacteria and leukocytes in the urine), the serum white blood cell count usually is normal. Prominent hematuria warrants a cystoscopic examination.

Prevention is important in women. Avoiding a prolonged distended bladder is helpful, although this sometimes is difficult in the workplace. Patients with frequent infections should be instructed to void frequently, to void before and after intercourse, and to practice proper hygiene. If acute cystitis persists despite these measures, a course of low-dose antibiotics for 3 to 6 months may be effective.

Oral antibiotics usually are started when the diagnosis is confirmed by culture, and ordinarily the infection quickly resolves. Acute cystitis rarely creates long-term problems. Complications of acute cystitis occur when the infection ascends to the kidneys, which is most common in the presence of vesicoureteral reflux.

## Ureteral Stones

Stones that lodge in the ureter can precipitate ureteral obstruction and create the risk of infection proximal to the stone. Points of ureteral narrowing where stones commonly lodge are (1) at the ureteropelvic junction, (2) at the point where the ureter crosses over the iliac vessels, and (3) in the ureterovesical zone.[37] The most prudent treatment for infections proximal to an obstruction is immediate drainage. This can be achieved by means of a percutaneous nephrostomy or a ureteral stent. Once the obstruction and infection have been relieved, treatment of the ureteral stone can proceed with ureteroscopy, laser lithotripsy, extracorporeal shock wave lithotripsy, or, rarely, open surgery.

## Retroperitoneal Fibrosis

Retroperitoneal fibrosis is a disease involving the tissue that lies over the lumbar vertebrae in the retroperitoneal space. Obstruction of one or both ureters can develop. Malignant disease such as Hodgkin's disease, metastatic breast cancer, and colon cancer have been implicated as a cause of this disease. Methysergide, a medication used in the treatment of headaches, also has been implicated as a causative factor.[24] In many cases no cause can be found. In mild cases, corticosteroids may provide sufficient therapy. In most cases, however, surgery (with biopsy) to release the ureters is required.

## Pelvic Masses

The pelvis can fill with purulent material from a variety of diseases; all can cause obstruction of the ureters and may require diversion. Ruptured tuboovarian abscesses, diverticular disease (which also can create an enterovesical fistula), inadvertent surgical injury to the ureter, and a urine leak from any cause can all lead to a pelvic abscess. In addition, diverticular disease can precipitate an enterovesical fistula, whereas a urine leakage can lead to a ureterovaginal fistula (especially common after a vaginal hysterectomy if the ureter is injured or ligated). Treatment depends on the specific clinical condition; however, if an abscess has formed, a percutaneous nephrostomy allows the pelvis to heal until a definitive procedure can be performed.

## Radiation Cystitis

A number of bladder complications may develop in patients receiving pelvic radiation: bladder instability, reduced bladder capacity, or ulcerations. These ulcerations can precipitate fistula formation (e.g., vesicovaginal fistulae in women receiving radiation therapy for cervical cancer). Symptoms of radiation damage may occur immediately or months after the radiation therapy has been completed and may necessitate a urinary diversion.

## Urethral Strictures

Strictures may develop in the urethra as a result of trauma, from long-term use of indwelling urethral catheter, or, more commonly, after infections (such as gonococcal urethritis).[29] Strictures occur almost exclusively in men; the bulbous urethra is the most common location. The most common symptom is a decreased urinary stream, which usually causes the patient to seek treatment. Urinary retention, which can develop as a result of strictures, increases the risk for infection and generalized sepsis. Occasionally a periurethral abscess can occur and rupture to the skin. When this occurs in multiple areas, it results in a "watering pot perineum."

Strictures usually can be treated with urethral dilation or an internal urethrotomy to incise the stricture under direct vision through cystoscope. The patient with complications such as a periurethral abscess needs a urinary diversion in the form of a suprapubic cystostomy tube. This usually is a temporary measure until the inflammation completely resolves and the urethra is repaired.

## SUMMARY

Many different GU diseases may precipitate the need for a urinary diversion. These diseases occur at any age from infancy to older age and are not limited to malignant disease. Because of the potential negative sequelae on kidney function, GU diseases require prompt investigation and treatment and additional surveillance after treatment. The type of diversion required by the disease process is varied and depends on the level of the disease within the urinary tract, the extent of the disease, the patient's condition, and the treatment goals. The nurse who cares for patients with an ostomy or a continent diversion not only must be familiar with the various diseases addressed in this chapter but also should be able to articulate the rationale for the various treatment options for each disease.

# SELF-EVALUATION

## QUESTIONS

1. The congenital disease that results when the urogenital sinus fails to close properly is:
   a. Exstrophy
   b. Megaureter
   c. Myelomeningocele
   d. Prune-belly syndrome

2. Which of the following statements is true of bladder exstrophy?
   a. The infant is born with an everted bladder and fusion of the mucosa to the skin.
   b. Exstrophy of the cecum to a central location on the abdomen occurs.
   c. The exteriorized bladder is divided (hemibladder).
   d. The infant often has gender reassignment because of severe deformities of the phallus.

3. Prune-belly syndrome has which of the following urologic features?
   a. A contracted bladder
   b. Dilated, tortuous ureters
   c. Normal kidney size and function
   d. Trabeculation of the bladder

4. Artificial urinary sphincter is an option for managing:
   a. Myelomeningocele
   b. Posterior urethral valves
   c. Prune-belly syndrome
   d. Radiation cystitis

5. Obstruction, hematuria, and frequency are the symptoms most commonly associated with:
   a. Bladder cancer
   b. Prostate cancer
   c. Urethral cancer
   d. Ureteral cancer

6. Which of the following diseases is the most common congenital abnormality of the ureter?
   a. Ureteropelvic junction obstruction
   b. Posterior urethral valves
   c. Megaureter
   d. Vesicoureteral reflux

7. List three clinical manifestations or pathologic findings indicative of megaureter, vesicoureteral reflux, and ureteropelvic junction obstruction.

8. List five risk factors for the development of bladder cancer.

9. A superficially invasive bladder tumor is one that:
   a. Is confined to the mucosa of the bladder
   b. Is invasive of the detrusor muscle
   c. Penetrates the lamina propria but not the detrusor
   d. Penetrates the bladder serosa

10. Define tumor staging and tumor grading.

11. The most common type of bladder cancer is:
    a. Cloacogenic
    b. Squamous epithelial
    c. Transitional cell
    d. Adenocarcinoma
12. Describe the urologic management approach for patients with a spinal cord injury.
13. Radical cystectomy and ileal conduit or continent urostomy is most appropriate for which disease?
    a. Carcinoma in situ of the bladder
    b. Palliation of recurrent pelvic cancer
    c. Penetrating bladder trauma
    d. Muscle-invasive bladder cancer
14. Describe how the following affect a person's susceptibility to urinary tract infection (UTI): ileal conduit, vesicoureteral reflux, ureteral stones, and fluid intake.
15. Which of the following statements about chronic pyelonephritis is true?
    a. The urine is always infected.
    b. Kidney damage is rare when treated promptly with antibiotics.
    c. An ileal conduit prevents chronic pyelonephritis.
    d. Reflux of urine is the common cause of chronic pyelonephritis.
16. Ureteral stones commonly lodge in which three sites?

# SELF-EVALUATION

## ANSWERS

1. **a.** Exstrophy
2. **a.** The infant is born with an everted bladder and fusion of the mucosa to the skin.
3. **b.** Dilated, tortuous ureters
4. **a.** Myelomingocele
5. **c.** Urethral cancer
6. **a.** Ureteropelvic junction obstruction
7. *Ureteropelvic junction obstruction:* kinking and angulation of the ureter; abdominal mass in the infant; pain, vomiting, and urinary tract infections
   *Megaureter:* fever, abdominal pain, and hematuria; dilated distal ureter and less dilated proximal ureter with near-normal renal pelvis
   *Vesicoureteral reflux:* pyelonephritis, renal pain on voiding, asymptomatic bacteriuria, hypertension, uremia
8. Repeated exposure to 2-beta-naphthalene.
   Cigarette smoking
   Schistosomiasis infections
   Chronic irritation of the bladder (indwelling Foley catheter or pyocystitis)
   Large doses of phenacetin and other analgesics
   Cyclophosphamide administration
   Genetic predisposition
9. **c.** Penetrates the lamina propria but not the detrusor
10. *Tumor stage* describes the depth of tumor penetration through the layers of the organ. *Tumor grade* is the microscopic appearance of the cells and their orientation toward each other.
11. **c.** Transitional cell
12. Management options include Credé and Valsalva maneuvers, intermittent catheterization, urethral catheter, suprapubic tube, urinary conduit or continent stoma. When the spinal cord injury is a high injury such as a cervical injury, limited mobility of the hands minimizes the success of techniques such as intermittent catheterization and the Credé and Valsalva maneuvers. Generally, these patients require urethral catheterization, suprapubic catheterization, or urinary conduit. Whatever management method is selected for any patient with a spinal cord injury, regular evaluation of the appropriateness and effectiveness of the intervention is imperative.
13. **d.** Muscle-invasive bladder cancer
14. *Ileal conduit* bypasses the urethra that serves as a normal barrier to bacteria; in addition, free reflux at the ureteroileal junction allows retrograde reflux of urine (and bacteria) into the ureters.
    *Vesicoureteral reflux* indicates that the normal antireflux mechanism of the vesicoureteral junction is not functioning and that, just as free reflux of urine occurs in the ureters, so, too, bacteria can migrate in a retrograde fashion.
    *Ureteral stones* serve as a nidus for bacteria to proliferate but also may occlude the ureter and cause stagnation of urine, thus rendering the host more susceptible to an infection.

*Fluid intake* is a mechanism of clearing the urinary tract of transient bacteria. When the fluid intake is decreased, the person becomes more vulnerable to urinary tract infection.

**15. d.** Reflux of urine is the common cause of chronic pyelonephritis.

**16.** The three points of ureteral narrowing where stones may form are (1) ureteropelvic junction, (2) at the point where the ureter crosses over the iliac vessels, and (3) in the ureterovesical zone.

## REFERENCES

1. Bauer SB: Urodynamic evaluation and neuromuscular dysfunction. In Kelalis PP, King LR, and Belman AB, editors: *Clinical pediatric urology*, vol. 1, ed 2, Philadelphia, 1985, WB Saunders.
2. Bauer SB, Joseph DB: Neurogenic bladder dysfunction, *Urol Clin North Am* 17:395, 1990.
3. Bellinger MF: The management of vesicoureteric reflux, *Urol Clin North Am* 12:23, 1985.
4. Belman AB, Kaplan GW, editors: *Genitourinary problems in pediatrics*, Philadelphia, 1981, WB Saunders.
5. Catalona WJ, Scott WW: Carcinoma of the prostate. In Walsh PC et al, editors: *Campbell's urology*, ed 5, Philadelphia, 1986, WB Saunders.
6. Corriere JN Jr, Sandler CM: Management of extraperitoneal bladder rupture, *Urol Clin North Am* 16:275, 1989.
7. Droller MJ: Transitional cell cancer: upper tracts and bladder. In Walsh PC et al: editors: *Campbell's urology*, ed 5, Philadelphia, 1986, WB Saunders.
8. Duckett JW, Caldemone AA: Bladder and urachus. In Kelalis PP, King LR, Belman AB, editors: *Clinical pediatric urology*, vol 2, ed 2, Philadelphia, 1985, WB Saunders.
9. Duckett JW, Snow BW: Disorders of the urethra and penis. In Walsh PC et al, editors: *Campbell's urology*, vol 2, ed 5, Philadelphia, 1986, WB Saunders.
10. Firlit CF: The urethra and Cowper's gland: congenital disorders. Urethral valves. In Kaufman JK, editor: *Current urologic therapy*, ed 2, Philadelphia, 1986, WB Saunders.
11. Freeman AI, Woods GM: Genitourinary tumors. In Ashcraft KW, editor: *Pediatric urology*, Philadelphia, 1990, WB Saunders.
12. Glassberg KI, Hackett RE, Waterhouse K: Congenital anomalies of the kidney, ureter and bladder. In Kendall AR, Karafin L: *Practice of surgery: urology*, vol 1, Philadelphia, 1981, Harper & Row.
13. Gonzales ET Jr: Alternatives in the management of posterior urethral valves, *Urol Clin North Am* 17:335, 1990.
14. Guerriero WG: Ureteral injury, *Urol Clin North Am* 16:237, 1989.
15. Hanna MK: The bladder. Congenital disorders: bladder exstrophy. In Kaufman JJ, editor: *Current urologic therapy*, ed 2, Philadelphia, 1986, WB Saunders.
16. Hopkins SC, Grabstald H: Benign and malignant tumors of the male and female urethra. In Walsh PC et al, editors: *Campbell's urology*, vol 2, ed 5, Philadelphia, 1986, WB Saunders.
17. Jeffs RD, Lepor H: Management of the exstrophy-epispadias complex and urachal anomalies. In Walsh PC et al, editors: *Campbell's urology*, vol 2, ed 5, Philadelphia, 1986, WB Saunders.
18. Johnson DE, Swanson DA, von Eschenbach AC: Tumors of the genitourinary tract. In Tanagho EA, McAninch JW, editors: *Smith's general urology*, ed 12, Norwalk, Conn, 1988, Appleton & Lange.
19. Kaplan WE: Management of myelomeningocele, *Urol Clin North Am* 12:93, 1985.
20. Kelalis PP: Ureteropelvic junction. In Kelalis PP, King LR, Belman AB, editors: *Clinical pediatric urology*, vol 1, ed 2, Philadelphia, 1985, WB Saunders.
21. King LR: Posterior urethra. In Kelalis PP, King LR, Belman AB, editors: *Clinical pediatric urology*, vol 1, ed 2, Philadelphia, 1985, WB Saunders.
22. King LR, Levitt SB: Vesicoureteral reflux, megaureter and ureteral reimplantation. In Walsh PC et al, editors: *Campbell's urology*, vol 2, ed 5, Philadelphia, 1986, WB Saunders.
23. Koff SA: Pathophysiology of ureteropelvic junction obstruction: clinical and experimental observations. *Urol Clin North Am* 17:263, 1990.
24. Kogan BA: Disorders of the ureter and ureteropelvic junction. In Tanagho EA, McAninch JW, editors: *Smith's general urology*, ed 12, Norwalk, Conn, 1988, Appleton & Lange.
25. Kramer SA: Pediatric urologic oncology, *Urol Clin North Am* 12:31, 1985.
26. Kroovand RL: Myelomeningocele. In Walsh PC et al, editors: *Campbell's urology*, vol 2, ed 5, Philadelphia, 1986, WB Saunders.
27. Kunin CM: *Detection, prevention and management of urinary tract infections*, ed 4, Philadelphia, 1987, Lea & Febiger.
28. Lepor H, Jeffs RD: The bladder. Congenital disorders: epispadias repair in male patients with classical blader exstrophy. In Kaufman JJ, editor: *Current urologic therapy*. ed 2, Philadelphia, 1986, WB Saunders.
29. McAninch JW: Disorders of the penis and male urethra. In Tanagho EA, McAninch JW, editors: *Smith's general urology*, ed 12, Norwalk, Conn, 1988, Appleton & Lange.

30. McAninch JW: Injuries to the genitourinary tract. In Tanagho EA, McAninch JW, editors: *Smith's general urology,* ed 12, Norwalk, Conn, 1988, Appleton & Lange.

31. Meares EM: Nonspecific infections of the genitourinary tract. In Tanagho EA, McAninch JW, editors: *Smith's general urology,* ed 12, Norwalk, Conn, 1988, Appleton & Lange.

32. Muecke EC: Exstrophy, epispadias, and other anomalies of the bladder. In Walsh PC et al, editors: *Campbell's urology,* vol 2, ed 5, Philadelphia, 1986, WB Saunders.

33. Neuwirth H, deKernion JB: Prostate. In Haskell CM, editor: *Cancer treatment,* ed 3, Philadelphia, 1990, WB Saunders Co.

34. Neuwirth H, Haskell CM, deKernion JB: Bladder cancer. In Haskell CM, editor: *Cancer treatment,* ed 3, Philadelphia, 1990, WB Saunders.

35. Snyder H McC III et al: Pediatric oncology. In Walsh PC et al, editors: *Campbell's urology,* vol 2, ed 5, Philadelphia, 1986, WB Saunders.

36. Sobel JD, Kaye D: Host defense mechanisms in urinary tract infections. In Schrier RW, Gottschalk CW, editors: *Disease of the kidney,* Boston, 1988, Little, Brown.

37. Spirnak JP, Resnick MI: Urinary stones. In Tanagho EA, McAninch JW, editors: *Smith's general urology,* ed 12, Norwalk, Conn, 1988, Appleton & Lange.

38. Tanagho EA, Schmidt RA: Neuropathic bladder disorders. In Tanagho EA, McAninch JW, editors: *Smith's general urology,* ed 12, Norwalk, Conn, 1988, Appleton & Lange.

39. Woodward JR: Prune-belly syndrome. In Kelalis PP, King LR, Belman AB, editors: *Clinical pediatric urology,* vol 2, ed 2, Philadelphia, 1985, WB Saunders.

40. Woodard JR, Trulock TS: The prune-belly syndrome. In Walsh PC et al, editors: *Campbell's urology,* vol 2, ed 5 Philadelphia, 1986, WB Saunders.

41. Woodard JR, Zucker I: Current management of the dilated urinary tract in prune belly syndrome, *Urol Clin North Am* 17:407, 1990.

# 8

# Genitourinary Surgical Procedures

DOROTHY B. DOUGHTY
DEBORAH J. LIGHTNER

## OBJECTIVES

1. Identify three indications for urinary diversion.

2. Differentiate between nephrostomy and cutaneous pyelostomy.

3. Identify the three most common complications after nephrostomy, and describe nursing implications.

4. Define the following terms:
   Loop ureterostomy
   End ureterostomy
   Double-barrel ureterostomy
   Transureteroureterostomy
   Ring ureterostomy
   Y ureterostomy

5. Identify two common complications associated with ureterostomy.

6. Explain the rationale for interposing a bowel segment between the ureters and the skin as is done in the construction of a ureteroenterocutaneous diversion.

7. Describe the surgical procedure for construction of an ileal conduit.

8. Identify factors that increase the risk of renal compromise after small bowel conduits, and describe the nursing implications.

9. Explain why jejunal conduits are rarely performed.

10. Differentiate between an end stoma and a Turnbull loop stoma.

11. Identify the potential benefit offered by colon conduits as compared with small-bowel conduits.

12. List four complications commonly associated with ureterosigmoidostomy.

13. Explain why vesicostomy is considered a pediatric diversion.

The normal pathway for urine elimination is from the collecting tubules within the kidney into the renal pelvis, down the ureters, and through the nonrefluxing ureterovesical junction into the bladder for temporary storage; at a convenient time the bladder empties through the urethra, and urinary elimination is complete. Urinary diversion refers to any procedure that diverts the urinary stream away from distal structures and out of the body through an alternative pathway. Urinary diversion may be accomplished at almost any level of the urinary system; diversions usually are named for the structures involved in the diversion. For example, a cutaneous ureterostomy means that the ureter has been anastomosed to the skin, and the urine is eliminated at that point. An ileal conduit is so named because a segment of ileum is used as a pathway for urinary elimination. A more complete term for this procedure is "ureteroenterocutaneous diversion," which, of course, means that the ureters have been anastomosed to a segment of small bowel, which in turn has been anastomosed to the skin. The trend in urinary diversions is toward continent procedures (see Chapter 4); many of these are named for the surgeon or the institution perfecting the procedure, such as the Kock urinary reservoir or the Indiana (ileocecal) reservoir.

A urinary diversion may be constructed on either a temporary or a permanent basis and as a tube or a tubeless diversion; tube diversions are almost always temporary, whereas tubeless diversions may be either temporary or permanent. Urinary diversion most commonly is required when disease or injury necessitates the removal of the bladder; diversion also may be performed to relieve obstructive uropathy, to promote healing of fistulous tracts involving the bladder, or as a last resort for the management of urinary incontinence.

In this chapter, commonly performed urinary diversions are described in terms of indications, surgical procedure, and common complications. A thorough understanding of the anatomic alterations involved in a particular diversion prepares the nurse to provide effective preoperative counseling and appropriate postoperative management.

## DIVERSIONS OF THE RENAL PELVIS

The most proximal diversions involve tube or tubeless diversions of the renal pelvis. Diversions at this level most commonly are performed as a result of ureteral disruption or obstruction, such as a ureteral stricture resulting from radiation therapy. These diversions usually are intended to be temporary; however, the patient who has a malignancy that obstructs the ureter or whose ureter has been severely damaged by radiation therapy may require lifelong diversion at the level of the renal pelvis.

### Nephrostomy

A nephrostomy is a tube diversion of the renal pelvis; this procedure involves insertion of a tube through the flank into the renal pelvis (Fig. 8-1). Most commonly this procedure is performed percutaneously with radiologic guidance and the patient under local anesthesia; it can also be performed as an open procedure with administration of general anesthesia. Several types of tubes may be used for nephrostomy; latex Pezzer (mushroom) or Malecot (bat wing) catheters most commonly were used in the past, whereas small-lumen silicone catheters with Luer lock adapters are in current favor. A U-shaped catheter also has been used to reduce the risk of dislodgment; this catheter has both an entry and an exit point, and the two ends are connected with a Y-connector.[5] Catheters with a coiled retention device also are available; the coil helps maintain placement within the renal pelvis.[2]

Common complications after nephrostomy tube insertion are hemorrhage, obstruction,

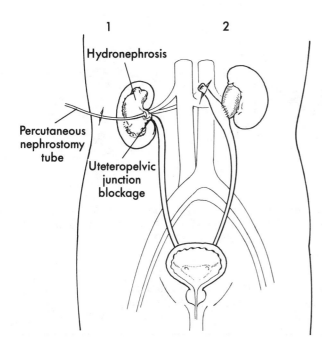

1

2

Hydronephrosis

Percutaneous
nephrostomy
tube

Uteteropelvic
junction
blockage

**Fig. 8-1** *1,* Percutaneous nephrostomy tube placed to facilitate drainage in kidney that is hydronephrotic because of ureteropelvic junction obstruction. *2,* Y ureterostomy fashioned by dividing ureter at renal pelvis; side of ureter is then anastomosed to renal pelvis, and proximal ureteral end is brought to skin surface as stoma. (Modified from Cukier J: Ureteral diversion. In Glenn J, editor: *Urologic surgery,* ed 4, Philadelphia, 1991, JB Lippincott.)

and infection.[5,7] Hemorrhage can occur because the renal parenchyma is extremely vascular; therefore close monitoring for hematuria is important after tube placement or tube exchange. Obstruction may result from mineral encrustations within the tube or from external compression or angulation of the tube. The tube should be monitored regularly for evidence of encrustation; the tubing can be rolled between the fingers to detect and dislodge any deposits. Fluid intake also is of paramount importance in preventing tube obstruction. Tube patency must be a prime concern when repositioning patients; because the renal pelvis has low capacity (5 to 10 ml), obstruction of the nephrostomy tube rapidly results in pain and infection. Nephrostomy tubes should be well secured by tape or suture in a position that promotes drainage. Pyelonephritis represents a constant threat because of the entry into the renal pelvis; in addition, many patients alternate between leg-bag drainage and bedside drainage systems, which necessitates disruption of the closed system. Prevention of infection depends on scrupulous technique and high-volume daily fluid intake.

## Cutaneous Pyelostomy

Cutaneous pyelostomy is a tubeless diversion into the renal pelvis, performed with the patient under general anesthesia. It involves an open surgical procedure in which the renal pelvis is brought to the flank and sutured to the skin.[8,11] The procedure may be used to provide effective drainage in patients with severely dilated ureters and severely compromised renal function. It is used primarily in infants, although its use is rare even in this patient population. Infection is the primary risk factor after diversion; prevention depends on adequate fluid intake and avoidance of fecal contamination. The infant's care usually is managed with diapering, although pouching may be required to deal with skin breakdown or to

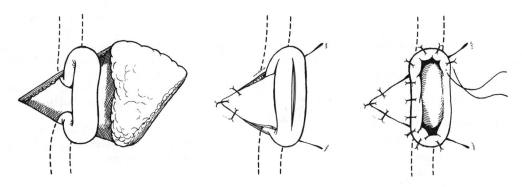

**Fig. 8-2**    Loop ureterostomy is created by elevating loop of ureter to skin surface. Triangular wedge of skin is used to stabilize loop. (Modified from Cukier J: Ureteral diversion. In Glenn J, editor: *Urologic surgery*, ed 4, Philadelphia, 1991, JB Lippincott.)

prevent contamination of the stoma with stool. Caregivers are taught to avoid immersing the stoma during bathing and to provide pouching before the child swims.

## URETERAL DIVERSIONS

The urinary stream also can be diverted at the ureteral level, a technique used when the distal ureter is obstructed or when the bladder must be removed or bypassed because of malignancy, trauma, or severe dysfunction. Ureteral diversions include ureterostomy and ureteroenterocutaneous procedures (intestinal conduits).

### Ureterostomy

Ureterostomy has been the most common approach to urinary diversion for many years and still may be the procedure of choice for the patient with ureteral dilation resulting from distal obstruction or for the patient who is a poor candidate for an intestinal conduit (ureteroenterocutaneous diversion).[3] Ureterostomy may be preferable to nephrostomy for long-term diversion because the risk of bleeding and obstruction is lower in the ureterostomy than in a tube diversion. However, limitations and complications must be considered. (1) Construction of a viable functional ureterostomy depends on the ability to mobilize the ureter enough to obtain a tension-free anastomosis to the skin without interfering with the ureter's blood supply, and (2) the ureter must be dilated enough to provide a widely patent anastomosis to the skin. If the anastomosis is under tension or there is interference with the blood supply, stomal necrosis and retraction may occur. If the ureter is too small to provide a widely patent opening at skin level, the risk of stenosis and obstruction is high.[3,8]

The ureterostomy can be constructed by means of a variety of techniques; loop and end ureterostomies are the most commonly performed, although ring and Y procedures also have been described.[3,8] A *loop ureterostomy* is constructed by mobilizing the ureter and bringing a loop of ureter to the skin surface; the loop is supported at the skin level by a full-thickness V-shaped skin flap (Fig. 8-2). The anterior wall of the ureter is then opened and sutured to the skin. An *end ureterostomy* involves division of the ureter at the most distal point possible (i.e., as close to the bladder as possible); the proximal end of the ureter is

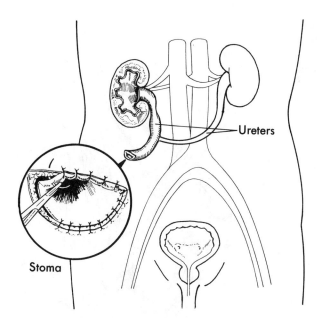

**Stoma**

**Ureters**

**Fig. 8-3** Transureteroureterostomy is created by end-to-side anastomosis of one ureter to the other. Ureter is incised or spatulated to create V-shaped lumen, which is then sutured to triangular skin defect. Spatulation is performed to fashion stoma that is less prone to stenosis. (Modified from Cukier J: Ureteral diversions. In Glenn J, editor: *Urologic surgery*, ed 4, Philadelphia, 1991, JB Lippincott.)

then brought through the abdominal wall and anastomosed to the skin. The end of the ureter may be incised to create a V-shaped defect; a matching skin flap at the cutaneous opening for the stoma is then sutured into the defect to prevent stenosis[3] (Fig. 8-3). If at all possible, the ureteral stoma is everted to create a slight "bud"; however, eversion depends on ureteral length and mobility. The distal ureter is sutured closed and left in place, unless the ureterostomy is performed in conjunction with bladder removal. Ureteral stents are left in place for 2 weeks after surgery to support the ureters and to maintain patency.

End ureterostomies may be *unilateral* or *bilateral*, depending on whether one or both kidneys are functional and on the reason for the procedure. For example, a unilateral ureterostomy may be performed in the patient who has only one functioning kidney or in the patient who has two functioning kidneys but whose disease is localized to one ureter. Bilateral ureterostomies are indicated for the patient who has two functioning kidneys and bilateral disease requiring diversion. A *transureteroureterostomy* is an alternative to bilateral ureterostomies; in this procedure, one ureter is anastomosed to the other ureter, which is then brought to the skin surface for diversion (Fig. 8-3). This procedure provides bilateral diversion with only one stoma.[3] The decision regarding the ureter to be used for stoma construction and the ureter to be anastomosed is made on an individual basis and is determined by the length, mobility, and size of the two ureters. The ureter that can be more easily brought to the surface and that provides the greater diameter for construction of an adequate opening is selected.[3]

A *ring ureterostomy* is depicted in Fig. 8-4; this procedure involves a side-to-side anastomosis between the proximal and distal ureter and the formation of a cutaneous stoma at a point midway between the two limbs of the anastomosis. This procedure provides proximal diversion while permitting urine to flow distally as well; it may be used with ureteral reconstructive procedures to maintain patency of the distal ureter and to provide diversion of the

**Fig. 8-4**   Ring ureterostomy. Proximal ureter anastomosed to distal ureter with side-to-side anastomosis; loop of ureter is exteriorized midway between site of anastomosis, and stoma is established. (From Cukier J: Ureteral diversions. In Glenn J, editor: *Urologic surgery*, ed 4, Philadelphia, 1991, JB Lippincott.)

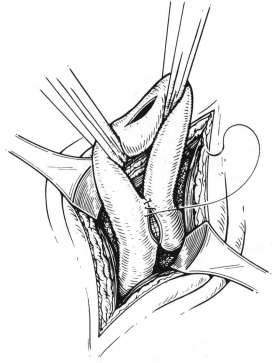

major portion of the urinary stream.[3,8] A *Y ureterostomy*, illustrated in Fig. 8-1, involves transection of the ureter at the renal pelvis; the renal pelvis is then anastomosed to a lateral incision in the ureteral wall, and the end of the ureter is brought to the skin surface as a stoma. This procedure may be performed when temporary diversion is needed; once the distal obstruction has been resolved, the segment of ureter used for stoma construction can be easily excised and closed.[3,8]

Cutaneous location of ureterostomy stomas is variable, depending on the length and mobility of the involved ureters. Ideally the ureter is mobilized sufficiently to be brought out at a premarked site visible to the patient and on a flat abdominal surface. If both ureters are diverted, the goal is to create a double-barrel ureteral stoma by bringing the longer and more mobile ureter to the opposite side, incising the most distal portion of the two ureters to permit a side-to-side anastomosis, and bringing the anastomosed ureters to the skin as one stoma. In some situations, however, ureteral stomas are located in a more lateral position because of extensive or proximal ureteral disease that dictates a more proximal diversion.

Because of the difficulty in obtaining a well-budded stoma in a good location and because of the high incidence of stenosis, ureterostomy is no longer considered the procedure of choice for diversion at the ureteral level. Stenosis is particularly common in the adult with nondilated ureters inasmuch as the thickness of the abdominal wall tends to compress the narrow ureter.[3]

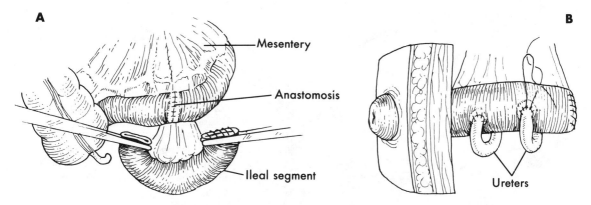

**Fig. 8-5** Surgical construction of ileal conduit. **A,** Segment of ileum is isolated with mesentery intact. Bowel continuity is reestablished; proximal ileal segment is closed. **B,** Distal end of ileal segment is brought to abdominal surface as stoma; ureters are anastomosed to ileal segment. (From Broadwell DC, Jackson BS: *Principles of ostomy care,* St Louis, 1982, Mosby–Year Book.)

## Ureteroenterocutaneous Diversions

In 1950 Bricker described use of an ileal segment interposed between the ureters and the abdominal wall as an alternative to cutaneous ureterostomy[4,9]; these diversions rapidly became the procedure of choice for diversion at the ureteral level. The ileum is the bowel segment most commonly used to construct a urinary conduit; however, almost any bowel segment can be used. The ureteroenterocutaneous diversion has two major advantages because of its use of a bowel segment: (1) it permits construction of a budded stoma in a good location, and (2) it significantly reduces the risk of stomal stenosis.

The ileal conduit is described in terms of surgical construction and potential complications, followed by a comparison with other intestinal conduits.

**Ileal Conduit.** The ileal conduit as originally described by Bricker still is the most commonly performed urinary diversion. This procedure, also known as the Bricker loop, can be summarized as follows (Fig. 8-5)[4,5,9]:

1. A segment of ileum close to the ileocecal valve is resected with its mesentery intact.
2. The proximal end of this ileal segment is closed, and the distal segment is brought to the abdominal wall as a stoma.
3. The ureters are anastomosed to the ileal segment.

The ileal segment should be of sufficient length to extend from the point of ureteroileal anastomosis to the abdominal wall without tension, but no longer; the goal is to create a short, straight passageway that drains urine freely without residual. An excessively long, redundant, or angulated conduit creates a predisposition to urinary stasis, which is associated with increased risk of urinary tract infection and electrolyte imbalance caused by urine reabsorption.[4,5,9]

The stoma can be constructed either as an end stoma or as a Turnbull loop stoma.[4,9] An end stoma is constructed by bringing the distal end of the ileal segment through the abdom-

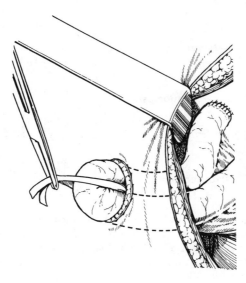

**Fig. 8-6**  Turnbull loop end stoma. Distal portion of bowel segment is brought to abdominal surface as loop. Anterior wall of bowel segment is opened and matured to form functional and nonfunctional limbs characteristic of loop stomas.

inal wall, everting it, and suturing the stoma to the dermis; the ileal segment also is secured at fascial level. Alternatively the stoma can be constructed as a Turnbull loop; this approach is particularly advantageous when the patient is obese, because the length of mesentery required to reach the skin through the abdominal wall is less with the loop approach than with an end approach. The Turnbull procedure involves closure of both ends of the ileal segment; the ileal segment is secured at fascial level, and the stoma is created by bringing the distal end of the segment to the abdominal wall in a looplike fashion. The anterior wall of the ileal segment is then opened with a transverse incision, and the stoma is matured to create a nonfunctional (usually proximal) limb and a functional (usually distal) limb[9] (Fig. 8-6). Maturation involves eversion of the bowel to expose the mucosal layer and suturing of the stoma to the dermis.

The ureters can be anastomosed to the ileal segment at the proximal end of the conduit or to the side of the conduit; each ureter can be anastomosed separately, or the ureters can be conjoined and anastomosed as a single unit.[4,9] It is important that the anastomosis be made between the mucosal layer of the bowel and the mucosal layer of the ureter to prevent anastomotic stricture. A negative aspect to ileal conduit diversion is that the ureteroileal anastomoses are freely refluxing, which means that urine can travel in either direction through the anastomosis.[4,9] If the pressure within the renal pelvis and the ureter is higher than the pressure within the conduit, urine flows freely. If, on the other hand, pressure within the conduit exceeds the pressure in the renal pelvis and the ureter, obstruction to urinary flow and possibly reflux occurs.

The ileal conduit has definite advantages over cutaneous ureterostomy procedures. The ability to construct a budded stoma on a flat abdominal plane tremendously facilitates self-care for the patient, and the ileal stoma is much less prone to stenosis than is the ureterostomy stoma. This diversion, however, is not complication-free; both early and late complications can occur. One of the most serious early complications is intrabdominal urinary leakage caused by anastomotic breakdown, which occurs in approximately 4% of the patients. Use of ureteral stents reduces the incidence of anastomotic leaks. Any leaks that do occur must be identified promptly and managed appropriately to reduce morbidity and mortality. Significant anastomotic breakdown usually requires early surgical intervention.[4]

The most significant late complication is renal deterioration; the reported incidence varies from 18% to as high as 56% and is directly related to the status of renal function at the time of diversion and the length of follow-up after diversion. The most significant etiologic factor in the development of renal damage is obstruction to urinary flow, which results in urinary stasis; stasis in turn causes predisposition to infection and stone formation.[4] Obstruction may occur as a result of an excessively long or angulated conduit, ureteroileal stenosis, or stomal stenosis; long-term surveillance with evaluations of catheterized loop residuals, routine cultures, creatinine studies, pyelography, and "loopogram" is essential for the early detection and prompt correction of any obstructive condition. (A "loopogram" involves instillation of contrast medium into the conduit through the stoma; radiologic studies are then obtained that reveal the length and direction of the conduit, the status of the upper tracts, and any obstruction to flow.) The nurse caring for these patients must be aware of the significance of obstruction in the long-term prognosis and must promptly report any evidence of poor drainage, such as loop residual urine greater than 20 ml.

Additional late complications associated with ileal conduit diversion include urinary tract infection, stone formation, and electrolyte disturbances. The incidence of pyelonephritis ranges from 10% to 20%; the incidence increases with obstruction to flow.[4] The incidence of stone formation is about 4% in adults and about 10% in children; again, the incidence is increased by obstructive conditions. Patients with ileal conduits also are at risk for serious electrolyte disturbances as a result of contact between the urine and the absorptive intestinal mucosa. The most common disturbance in patients with ileal (or colon) conduits is hyperchloremic metabolic acidosis with hypokalemia; this condition is caused by reabsorption of sodium and chloride with corresponding loss of bicarbonate and potassium.[6] The occurrence is relatively infrequent; the disturbance is more common in the patient with compromised renal function in whom urinary stasis results from a long or an angulated conduit, anastomotic strictures, stomal stenosis, or inadequate fluid intake.

The incidence of complications correlates with the length of follow-up, and patients with obstructive conditions or compromised renal function at the time of diversion are more prone to the development of complications. In addition, complications are more common in children than in adults.[4] Surgical technique and long-term follow-up must therefore focus on prevention of urinary stasis and its sequelae (infection, stone formation, and electrolyte reabsorption), which depends on maintenance of a short, straight conduit with a widely patent stomal opening, stricture-free anastomoses, and adequate daily fluid intake.

**Jejunal Conduit.** The jejunum is rarely used for conduit construction because its highly absorptive surface increases the risk of urine reabsorption and resultant electrolyte imbalances. The jejunal conduit syndrome is an electrolyte disturbance reported with use of jejunal segments. It is characterized by azotemia, hyperkalemia, hyponatremia, hypochloremia, and acidosis and occurs because the jejunal mucosa tends to reabsorb potassium and urea while secreting sodium, chloride, and water into the conduit.[5,6] This disturbance is particularly common in the patient with compromised renal function, which causes an inability to compensate by renal excretion of potassium and reabsorption of sodium.[6] Because of the potential for long-term electrolyte disturbances, the jejunum is used only when other bowel segments are unavailable, as in the case of radiation damage that affects the ileum and in diverticular disease that prohibits the use of colonic segments.

**Ileocecal Conduit.** The ileocecal segment of the bowel has been used in an attempt to create a nonrefluxing urinary diversion. In this procedure the ileocecal portion of the bowel is isolated with its mesentery intact, the ileal end of the segment is closed, the ureteroileal anastomosis is completed, and the cecal end is used to construct the stoma.[5] This means that the ureters empty into the ileal end of the segment above the ileocecal valve; the hope is that the ileocecal valve will prevent reflux and thus reduce the complication rate. In practice, however, the competence of the ileocecal valve is variable; it does not provide uniform protection against reflux. The nurse catheterizing the ileocecal conduit must prevent damage to the ileocecal valve by limiting advancement of the catheter.

**Colon Conduit.** Large bowel segments can be used to construct urinary conduits. The major advantage of a large bowel conduit is the potential to create a nonrefluxing diversion by tunneling the ureters through the thick muscular wall and the submucosal layer of the colon. Colonic segments also may be used when extensive pelvic radiation has damaged the ileum. The sigmoid colon is the most commonly used large bowel segment, although the transverse colon is a good alternative for the patient who requires proximal ureteral diversion (the ends of the transverse colon lie in the same plane as the renal pelves) or who has sigmoid disease such as diverticulosis.[4]

Colon conduits were thought to be particularly advantageous for children; the hope was that prevention of reflux would reduce the incidence of complications. These concerns are particularly important because many of these children require lifelong diversion. Although early results regarding the complication rate with colon conduits were encouraging, they were based on short-term follow-up. In a study of 41 children followed for 9 to 20 years, the complication rate rose significantly; renal deterioration occurred in 48%.[4] The advantage offered by the colon conduit is thus unclear; the one certain indication for this particular procedure is in the patient who has received extensive pelvic radiation with damage to the ileum and who requires an intestinal conduit.[4]

Intestinal conduits have provided a much more satisfactory approach to urinary diversion than do cutaneous ureterostomy procedures. Significant incidence of long-term complications, however, means that these patients require careful long-term follow-up. As noted earlier, the trend in permanent diversions is toward continent procedures (see Chapter 4); in addition to continence, these diversions provide protection from reflux.

## Ureterosigmoidostomy

The ureterosigmoidostomy procedure involves transplantation of the ureters into the intact sigmoid colon; elimination of both urine and stool is then controlled by the anal sphincter. Historically a number of attempts have been made to transplant the ureters into the intact colon, but most were discarded because of unacceptable complication rates. In 1911 Coffey described a procedure for anastomosing the ureters to the intact sigmoid through an antirefluxing submucosal tunnel.[1] Various modifications to Coffey's technique have been employed to develop a continent diversion with a low incidence of obstruction, reflux, and infection.[1] Patients for whom ureterosigmoidostomy is contraindicated include persons with compromised renal or liver function (because of an inability to compensate for the metabolic abnormalities produced by sodium, chloride, and ammonia reabsorption from the urine), those with colonic disease, and those with compromised anal sphincter function. Urinary calculi and pyelonephritis must be satisfactorily treated before this procedure is performed.

The surgical procedure can be summarized as follows:

1. The ureters are divided as close to the bladder as possible to obtain maximum ureteral length.
2. The site for anastomosis in the sigmoid colon is selected, with the goal of using the most distal site possible within the constraints posed by ureteral length and colon mobility.
3. Two nonrefluxing submucosal tunnels about 5 cm in length are created underneath the taeniae at the site for anastomoses.
4. The ureters are passed through the submucosal tunnel and anastomosed to the colonic mucosa.

Ureteral stents and a rectal drain usually are left in place for about 1 week after surgery.[1]

Early complications include anastomotic leaks and pelvic abscesses in addition to the complications usually encountered with abdominal and intestinal surgery. Any anastomotic leaks must be promptly investigated; small leaks may heal spontaneously, whereas larger leaks require immediate surgical revision.[1]

The incidence of late complications is still high, which has led many centers to abandon this procedure. Ureteral obstruction occurs in 32% to 62% of the patients, and 67% have ascending urinary tract infections. The incidence of metabolic complications (hyperchloremic metabolic acidosis with hypokalemia, ammonia reabsorption) ranges from 35% to 100% in reported studies.[1] Probably the most significant complication is an increased risk of malignancy at the anastomotic site; the risk is thought to be 100 to 500 times that of the normal population. Additional complications are tenesmus and incontinence.

This procedure, which is infrequently performed, requires that patients receive frequent, thorough, long-term follow-up, including colonoscopy or barium enema.[1]

## DIVERSION AT THE BLADDER LEVEL

Diversion at the bladder level may be indicated on either a temporary or a permanent basis for the patient with urethral obstruction or dysfunction. Diversion at this level can be accomplished by means of a cystostomy tube or vesicostomy.

Cystostomy involves percutaneous placement of a suprapubic catheter with the patient under local anesthesia. The procedure usually is used to provide immediate diversion for the patient with bladder outlet obstruction who cannot tolerate surgery and in whom urethral catheter placement is not possible.[10]

Vesicostomy is most commonly used to provide temporary bladder drainage in infants and young children; it is an ideal diversion in this group of patients because the infant's bladder is located more abdominally than is the adult bladder and the infant's care can be easily managed with diapers. Vesicostomy is performed through a small transverse incision midway between the umbilicus and the symphysis pubis; the dome of the bladder is mobilized and the wall of the bladder is secured to the rectus fascia, a small transverse incision is made in the anterior wall of the bladder, and the bladder mucosa is sutured to the abdominal skin opening. Vesicostomy in the adult is a more complex procedure and has been largely replaced by other forms of medical and surgical management.[10,11]

Complications associated with vesicostomy include peristomal dermatitis, stomal stenosis, infection, and stone formation.[10] Management must focus on instruction in daily care, adequate fluid intake, and routine surveillance for infection, stones, or stenosis. In most children the vesicostomy is closed before the child reaches the age to be toilet trained. Vesicostomy rarely is used as a permanent diversion.

## SUMMARY

The urinary stream can be diverted at the level of the renal pelvis, the ureters, or the bladder; diversion can involve use of a tube or can be tubeless; and diversion may be performed either for temporary drainage or as a permanent alternative to urethral voiding.

To date, urinary diversions have been associated with a high incidence of complications. The trend therefore is to perform fewer diversions and to replace standard diversions with continent procedures; these diversions provide a more normal "bladder substitute" in that a reservoir is created that has both an antireflux mechanism and a continence mechanism. (Continent diversions are discussed in Chapter 4.)

The key principles in managing urinary diversion include (1) selection of an appropriate diversion, based on assessment of the patient's disease and self-care abilities, (2) meticulous surgical technique, and (3) comprehensive long-term surveillance with aggressive management of any complications.

# SELF-EVALUATION

## QUESTIONS

1. Urinary diversions may be created in any area of the urinary system except the:
   a. Ureter
   b. Bladder
   c. Renal pelvis
   d. Renal parenchyma
2. List three reasons for the creation of a urinary diversion.
3. Which of the following complications can occur when a nephrostomy tube is inserted?
   a. Obstruction
   b. Infection
   c. Hemorrhage
   d. All of the above
4. Identify five types of ureterostomy urinary diversions that may be created.
5. The most frequently performed urinary diversion is a:
   a. Jejunal conduit
   b. Transverse colon conduit
   c. Ileal conduit
   d. Pyelostomy
6. The Turnbull loop technique is used to create a urinary stoma and diversion in which of the following situations?
   a. Obesity
   b. History of urinary stone formation
   c. Cancer of bladder
   d. None of the above
7. When an intestinal conduit is constructed, the ureters are anastomosed to the bowel segment at the:
   a. Proximal end or side of the conduit
   b. One ureter proximal and one ureter distal on the conduit
   c. Distal end of the conduit
   d. Urinary meatus
8. A jejunal urinary conduit may result in which of the following electrolyte disturbances?
   a. Hypokalemia only
   b. Hyperkalemia and hypercalcemia
   c. Hypokalemia, hypernatremia, and hyperchloremia
   d. Hyperkalemia, hyponatremia, and hypochloremia
9. Complications of ureterosigmoidostomy that may occur include:
   a. Hyperkalemia and hypercalcemia
   b. Hypokalemia and hypercalcemia
   c. Hyperchloremia and hypokalemia
   d. Hypochloremia and hypocalcemia
10. Identify urinary diversions that are performed at the level of the bladder.
    a. Pyelostomy and cecostomy
    b. Vesicostomy and vasectomy
    c. Cystostomy and vesicostomy
    d. Ureterostomy and pyelostomy

# SELF-EVALUATION

## ANSWERS

1. **d.** Renal parenchyma
2. These diversions may be temporary or permanent and are required when injury or disease dictates removal of the bladder, to relieve obstruction to the bladder, to relieve obstructive uropathy, or to promote healing when a fistula is present.
3. **d.** All of the above
4. End ureterostomy, loop ureterostomy, double-barrel ureterostomy, Y ureterostomy, ring ureterostomy, and transureteroureterostomy
5. **c.** Ileal conduit
6. **a.** Obesity
7. **c.** Proximal end or side of the conduit
8. **d.** Hyperkalemia, hyponatremia, hypochloremia
9. **c.** Hyperchloremia and hypokalemia
10. **c.** Cystostomy and vesicostomy

## REFERENCES

1. Arap S: Ureterosigmoidostomy. In Glenn J, editor: *Urologic surgery,* ed 4, Philadelphia, 1991, JB Lippincott.
2. Carson C: Endourology. In Glenn J, editor: *Urologic surgery,* ed 4, Philadelphia, 1991, JB Lippincott.
3. Cukier J: Ureteral diversions. In Glenn J, editor: *Urologic surgery,* ed 4, Philadelphia, 1991, JB Lippincott.
4. DeKernian JB and Mukamel E: Urinary diversion and continent reservoir. In Gillenwater J et al, editors: *Adult and pediatric urology,* vol 1, Chicago, 1987, Mosby–Year Book.
5. King A: Nursing management of stomas of the genitourinary system. In Broadwell D, Jackson B: *Principles of ostomy care,* St Louis, 1982, Mosby–Year Book.
6. McDougal W: Perioperative care. In Gillenwater J et al, editors: *Adult and pediatric urology,* vol 1, Chicago, 1987, Mosby–Year Book.
7. Munch L: Techniques of nephrostomy. In Glenn J, editor: *Urologic surgery,* ed 4, Philadelphia, 1991, JB Lippincott.
8. Parrott T: Pediatric urinary diversions. In Glenn J, editor: *Urologic surgery,* ed 4, Philadelphia, 1991, JB Lippincott.
9. Persky L: Large and small bowel urinary conduits. In Glenn J, editor: *Urologic surgery,* ed 4, Philadelphia, 1991, JB Lippincott.
10. Smith M: Cystostomy and vesicostomy. In Glenn J, editor: *Urologic surgery,* ed 4, Philadelphia, 1991, JB Lippincott.
11. Woodard J: Prune-belly syndrome. In Kelalis P, King L, Belman A, editors: *Clinical pediatric urology,* vol 2, ed 2, Philadelphia, 1985, WB Saunders.

# 9 Anatomy and Physiology of the Gastrointestinal Tract

RUTH A. BRYANT
DOROTHY B. DOUGHTY
KATHLEEN A. FITZGERALD

## OBJECTIVES

1. Define the terms *alimentary canal* and *accessory organs*.

2. Describe the four layers of the bowel wall.

3. Identify at least three functions performed by structures within the mouth.

4. Explain the role of the pharyngoesophageal and esophagogastric sphincters.

5. Describe the mechanisms that normally protect the gastric and duodenal mucosa from ulceration.

6. Describe gastric secretions in terms of volume, components, and functions.

7. Identify factors that increase and factors that decrease gastric secretion.

8. Identify factors that affect the rate of gastric emptying and nursing implications.

9. Explain the role of intrinsic factor in the prevention of pernicious anemia and implications for the patient who has had a gastrectomy.

10. Explain the relationship between the peritoneum and the mesentery.

11. Explain why the small intestine is critical to life and health.

12. Describe features of the small-bowel mucosa that serve to tremendously increase its absorptive surface.

13. Differentiate between the intrinsic and extrinsic nervous systems in terms of structures involved and impact on intestinal motility.

14. Identify the volume of fluid secreted by each of the following organs each day:
    Salivary glands
    Stomach
    Small intestine
    Pancreas
    Biliary system

15. Trace the digestive-absorptive pathway for each of the following:
    Carbohydrates
    Proteins
    Fats
    Fat-soluble vitamins

16. Describe vascular supply and venous drainage for the small intestine and the colon.

17. Describe structural characteristics and key functions of each of the following:
    Duodenum
    Jejunum
    Ileum
    Ileocecal valve
    Colon

18. Explain the role of the enterohepatic circulation.

19. Explain how the colonic mucosa differs from the small-bowel mucosa.

20. Explain why the patient with a large-bowel stoma usually has more gas and more fecal odor than the patient with a small-bowel stoma.

21. Compare the anal epithelium above and below the dentate line in terms of sensory function.

22. Describe the relationship between the external sphincter and the puborectal muscles and between the puborectal and the levator ani muscles.

23. Compare the internal and external anal sphincters in terms of function, innervation, and response to rectal distention.

24. Describe the normal defecation process.

25. Describe the exocrine functions of the pancreas.

26. Identify factors that affect the liver's rate of regeneration.

27. Explain why the liver is a common site of metastasis for gastrointestinal malignancies.

28. List key functions of the liver.

29. Explain the role of the gallbladder in digestion of fats.

---

The gastrointestinal (GI) tract plays an important role in the maintenance of life and health; it is responsible for the ingestion, digestion, and absorption of nutrients, as well as for the storage and elimination of fecal wastes. These are complex processes that involve multiple physiologic functions, for example, enzyme production and secretion, absorption via many carrier systems, peristalsis, and voluntary control of defecation. Gastrointestinal tract function also has a significant impact on fluid-electrolyte balance because large volumes of fluid are secreted into and reabsorbed from the lumen of the bowel every day during the processes of nutrient digestion and absorption (Table 9-1).

The organs within the GI tract can be divided into the alimentary canal and the accessory organs. The alimentary canal is the tube extending from mouth to anus and includes the mouth, esophagus, stomach, small intestine, colon, rectum, anal canal, and anus. Accessory

**Table 9-1**   Characteristics of gastrointestinal fluid (24-hr vol)

| Fluid | pH | Sodium (mmol) | Potassium (mmol) | Chloride (mmol) | Bicarbonate (mmol) | Volume (cc) |
|---|---|---|---|---|---|---|
| Saliva | 6.0-7.0 | 20-80 | 16-23 | 24-44 | 20-60 | 1000 |
| Gastric juice | 1.0-3.5 | 20-100 | 4-12 | 52-124 | 0 | 2000 |
| Bile | 7.8 | 120-200 | 3-12 | 80-120 | 30-50 | 800 |
| Pancreatic juice | 8.0-8.3 | 120-150 | 2-7 | 54-95 | 70-110 | 1200 |
| Intestinal juice | 7.5-8.9 | 80-130 | 12-21 | 48-116 | 23-30 | 3000 |

Modified from Givens BA, Simmons SA: *Gastroenterology in clinical nursing,* ed 4, St Louis, 1984, Mosby–Year Book and Thelan LA, Davie JK, Urden LD: *Textbook of critical care nursing: diagnosis and management,* St Louis, 1990, Mosby–Year Book.

organs are those organs located outside the alimentary canal that contribute to the ingestion and digestion of nutrients; the liver, gallbladder, and pancreas are important accessory organs (Fig. 9-1).

A clear understanding of normal anatomy and physiology provides the framework for understanding pathologic states and physiologic changes induced by surgical procedures. Thus the nurse caring for the ostomy patient must understand normal GI tract function to provide appropriate care and education for the individual with altered structure and function. This chapter addresses GI tract anatomy and physiology with an emphasis on structures and functions that are likely to be altered in the patient requiring a fecal diversion. The first section deals with the alimentary canal; each structure along the canal is discussed in terms of key structural characteristics, major functions, vascular supply, and innervation. By means of the same organizational approach the second half of the chapter deals with the accessory organs.

## ALIMENTARY CANAL

### General Structure

The histologic characteristics of the alimentary canal are essentially the same throughout its length, with minor variations, and comprise four tissue layers: the mucosa, the submucosa, the muscularis, and the serosa, or adventitia (Fig. 9-2). General characteristics of the tissue layers are described in this section; any variations are identified in the discussions concerning the various organs of the alimentary canal.

**Mucosa.** The innermost layer of the gut wall is the mucosal layer, which is composed of three distinct tissue layers: the mucous epithelium, or surface layer; the lamina propria, which is a connective tissue layer; and the muscularis mucosa, which is a thin layer of circular muscle that separates the mucosa from the submucosa. The mucosal layer has multiple mucus-secreting glands; thus it is always moist.

**Submucosa.** The second layer of the gut wall is the submucosal layer; key structures in this layer include connective tissue, blood and lymph vessels, nerve fibers, and a number of

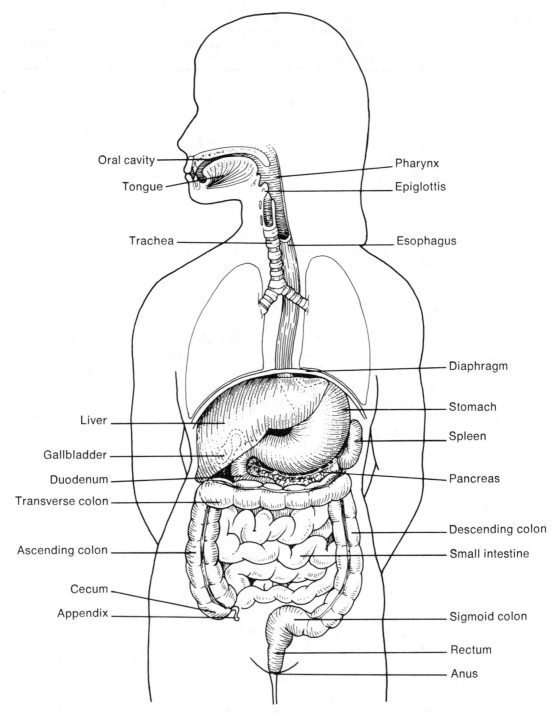

**Fig. 9-1** Anatomy of gastrointestinal system. (From Broadwell D, Jackson B: *Principles of ostomy care*, St Louis, 1982, Mosby–Year Book.)

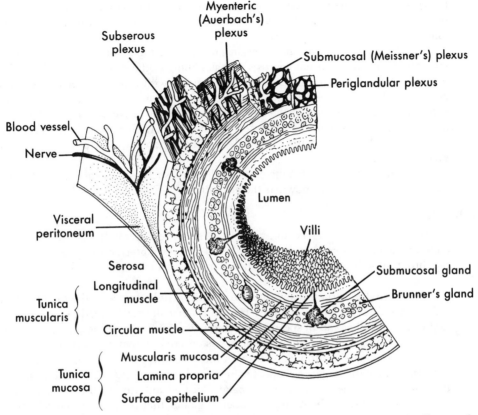

**Fig. 9-2**   Basic structure of digestive tract in cross-section. (From Broadwell D, Jackson B: *Principles of ostomy care*, St Louis, 1982, Mosby–Year Book.)

reticuloendothelial cells. The nerve fibers within the submucosal layer are known as Meissner's plexus, which is a component of the enteric nervous system.

**Muscularis.** The third layer of the gut wall is the muscularis; this layer actually consists of two layers of smooth muscle, an inner layer that is a circular muscle and an outer layer that is a longitudinal muscle. The myenteric plexus, or Auerbach's plexus, is located between these two muscle layers. The myenteric plexus and submucosal plexus are jointly known as the *intramural plexus,* or enteric nervous system. The intramural plexus contains nerve cells and nerve fibers that originate in receptors located in the mucosal surface and in the intestinal wall. These receptors are sensitive to stretch and possibly to chemical stimuli. The intramural plexus is the primary mediator for intestinal secretion and motility.[3,12]

**Serosa.** The outermost layer of the alimentary canal is known either as the *serosa* or as the *adventitia.* Structures located within the peritoneal cavity are covered by serosa, which is a connective tissue layer that in turn is covered by the visceral peritoneum. This continuity with the visceral peritoneum is a factor in the severe abdominal pain frequently experienced by patients with transmural inflammatory bowel disease; if the inflammation involves the serosa, it also may involve the peritoneum, resulting in a generalized peritonitis.

Because the serosa does not contain mucus-secreting glands, exposure to air results in inflammation, with eventual necrosis and sloughing of the serosal layer. This inflammatory response is significant to nurses caring for patients with ostomies, because stomas that are not matured (i.e., everted to expose the mucosal layer) are prone to develop serositis, which is accompanied by edema of the stoma and can result in partial or complete obstruction. Stomas that are not matured at surgery or shortly thereafter must "self-mature," a process that occurs when the inflamed serosal surfaces adhere to each other, causing a gradual eversion of the stoma.

Structures located outside the peritoneal cavity, such as the esophagus, are covered with a connective tissue layer known as the adventitia.

## Mouth

The mouth, also referred to as the oral cavity, represents the proximal end of the alimentary canal. It is bordered laterally by the cheeks, anteriorly by the lips, posteriorly by the throat, superiorly by the palate, and inferiorly by a muscular floor.

**Structure.** Key structures within the mouth include the teeth, the tongue, the hard and soft palates, and the salivary glands. The adult normally has 32 teeth, which play an important role in chewing and in speech. The tongue is a muscular organ that is covered by moist squamous epithelium; the anterior surface is covered by papillae, where the taste buds are located. The tongue is supplied with both intrinsic and extrinsic muscles, and jointly these muscles control the tongue's shape, position, and movements.[12] The palates form the *roof* of the mouth, with the *hard*, or bony, palate located anteriorly and the *soft*, or muscular, palate located posteriorly. A large number of glands that contribute to production of saliva are present in the mouth; the three largest pairs are the parotid, the submaxillary, and the sublingual glands. Saliva actually represents a combination of mucus and thin serous secretions; saliva also contains amylase, which is an enzyme capable of beginning carbohydrate digestion. Usual volume of saliva production is about 1 to 1.5 L/day.[12]

**Function.** Major functions carried out by structures within the oral cavity include speech, nutrient ingestion, initiation of digestion, and swallowing.

*Speech.* Both the tongue and the teeth play an important role in the precise formation of words required for clear speech.

*Ingestion of nutrients.* Normally nutrients are taken into the body through the mouth; disease or injury resulting in inability to eat and drink necessitates alternate routes for nutrient ingestion. The tongue provides for the sensation of taste, which is mediated by means of the taste buds present in some of the papillae. Because taste is an important stimulus to nutrient ingestion, this is an important function.

*Digestion.* Mechanical digestion of nutrients begins in the mouth with the process of chewing, or mastication, which breaks large food particles into smaller particles and thereby increases the surface available for enzymatic action. Thorough chewing of food can contribute significantly to the efficiency of the digestive process. Structures that contribute to the ability to chew are the tongue, the teeth, and the muscles of mastication.

Enzymatic digestion of carbohydrates also is initiated in the mouth by the action of salivary amylase, which can reduce polysaccharides into maltose and isomaltose. Actually only a small percentage of carbohydrates are digested in the mouth because most starches are covered with cellulose and therefore are "protected" from enzymatic action.[12]

*Swallowing.* An important function of the mouth and related structures is swallowing, which begins transport of the nutrients along the digestive pathway. Any condition that interferes with the ability to swallow places the individual at risk for nutritional compromise as a result of inadequate intake.

Swallowing is a complex act that involves the tongue, the soft palate, the muscles of the oropharynx, the upper esophageal sphincter, the epiglottis, the muscles of the esophagus, and gravity. The normal sequence of events is as follows: the tongue forms a bolus of food and pushes the bolus of food into the oropharynx; the soft palate is elevated to close the opening to the nasopharynx, and elevation of the larynx and movement of the epiglottis close the opening to the larynx; the pharyngeal muscles contract, respiration is inhibited, and the upper esophageal sphincter relaxes, which pushes food through the pharynx and into the esophagus. Movement of the bolus through the esophagus is accomplished by peristaltic waves; that is, the muscles distal to the food bolus relax while the muscles proximal to the food bolus contract and push the food along.[1,12]

Swallowing is initiated voluntarily but is completed as a reflex action; reflex activity takes over once the food bolus reaches the oropharynx. Swallowing is facilitated by the presence of saliva, which acts as a lubricant for the food particles.

Saliva also helps prevent infections of the oral cavity, because it constantly "bathes" the mouth and because it has some degree of antibacterial action.

## Esophagus

**Structure.** The esophagus, which is approximately 25 cm in length, is the muscular tube that connects the oropharynx to the stomach. The walls of the esophagus are composed of the four layers discussed earlier in this chapter, with the outer layer being adventitia as opposed to serosa. The muscular layer consists of striated (skeletal) muscle in the proximal portion of the esophagus and smooth muscle in the distal esophagus. The mucosal layer is composed of moist, stratified squamous epithelium.

The esophagus generally is divided into three sections: the upper esophagus, midesophagus, and lower esophagus. The esophagus is bounded proximally and distally by sphincter mechanisms, the upper esophageal sphincter (pharyngoesophageal), and the lower esophageal sphincter (esophagogastric); these sphincters prevent reflux from the esophagus into the oropharynx and from the stomach into the esophagus.[1,12]

**Functions.** The major functions of the esophagus include transport of food from the mouth and oropharynx into the stomach and the production of mucus. Transport of food occurs via the aforementioned swallowing mechanism. A food bolus in the oropharynx causes reduced pressure within the upper esophageal sphincter; the sphincter opens and allows the food or fluid to enter the esophagus. The bolus is moved toward the stomach by peristalsis; as the bolus approaches the lower esophageal sphincter, the sphincter relaxes to allow the food or fluid to enter the stomach. The lower esophageal sphincter relaxes only with the approach of a food bolus; at all other times it is tonically contracted to prevent reflux of gastric contents into the esophagus.[1,12]

Peristaltic waves within the esophagus are stimulated by the presence of food or fluid within the esophagus, which activates the intramural plexus; the presence of food or fluid also causes vagal stimulation, which stimulates contraction of the skeletal and smooth muscles within the esophagus.[12]

The esophageal mucosa is protected by a thick mucus that is produced in the submucosal layer and delivered through ducts to the mucosal surface.

**Blood Supply and Innervation.** Vascular supply to the esophagus derives from the esophageal branch of the thoracic aorta and from the left gastric artery, which branches from the celiac trunk of the abdominal aorta.[12] Venous drainage occurs as follows: the upper esophagus is drained by the superior vena cava, the midesophagus is drained by the azygos vein, and the lower esophagus is drained by gastric veins that empty into the portal system. The esophagus is innervated by the vagus nerve.[12]

### Abdominal Cavity and Peritoneum

Most of the organs in the gastrointestinal tract are contained in the abdominal cavity. The abdominal cavity is separated from the thoracic cavity by the diaphragm and actually is continuous with the pelvic cavity; the stomach, intestines, liver, spleen, pancreas, and kidneys are located within the abdominal cavity, and the pelvic cavity contains the urinary bladder, portions of the colon, and the internal reproductive organs.

The peritoneum is a serous membrane that lines much of the abdominal cavity and covers most of the abdominal organs. Organs located outside the peritoneum are said to be retroperitoneal. The portion of the peritoneum that lines the abdominal cavity is referred to as the *parietal* peritoneum, whereas the peritoneum that covers the abdominal organs is known as the *visceral* peritoneum. The *mesentery* is a double layer of peritoneum with a central layer of loose connective tissue; the mesentery encircles most of the small intestine and anchors it to the posterior abdominal wall. The mesentery is a vital support structure for the bowel in that it contains the blood vessels and nerve fibers that nourish and innervate the intestine. The *lesser omentum* is the name given to the mesentery that attaches the lesser curvature of the stomach to the liver and the diaphragm, and the mesentery that attaches the greater curvature of the stomach to the transverse colon and posterior abdominal wall is termed the *greater omentum*. The greater omentum is also known as the "fatty apron" because it hangs down in front of the stomach and large amounts of fat tend to accumulate in and between its double folds.[12]

### Stomach

**Structure.** The stomach is a distensible organ located in the left upper quadrant of the abdomen. Its size depends on its state of fullness; at capacity (about 1 L) the stomach is approximately 25 to 27.5 cm long and about 10.25 cm wide.[1,12]

*Histology.* The wall of the stomach consists of the four layers common to GI tract histology, with the following variations:

1. The stomach has three muscle layers rather than two; there is an inner oblique layer, in addition to the middle circular layer, and the outer longitudinal layer. This additional muscle layer, increases the stomach's ability to "churn" the gastric contents, thus contributing to mechanical digestion of nutrients.
2. The submucosal and mucosal layer are arranged in deep folds known as rugae; these folds allow for "stretching" of the gastric lining as the stomach fills with food and fluid.

3. The mucosal layer contains a large number of openings known as "gastric pits"; the gastric pits communicate with the gastric glands and provide drainage for their secretions. The gastric mucosa is covered with simple columnar epithelium.

*Regions.* The stomach can be divided into several anatomic regions. The *cardiac region* is the area of the stomach that surrounds the opening from the esophagus (gastroesophageal junction) and is so named because of its proximity to the heart. The *fundus* is the portion of the stomach that is to the left of and superior to the cardiac region. The *body* is the largest portion of the stomach; it curves toward the right, and this curve creates the lesser and greater curvatures of the stomach. The most distal area of the stomach is known as the *pyloric region* (or antral region); it lies just above the pyloric sphincter, which controls the flow of gastric contents into the duodenum.[1,12]

*Cells.* Five types of cells are found within the stomach. The surface mucous cells cover the gastric surface and line the gastric pits. The remaining four types of cells are found within the gastric glands: mucous neck cells, parietal cells, chief cells, and endocrine cells. The surface mucous cells and the mucous neck cells are responsible for secreting a viscous and alkaline mucus that coats the superficial epithelial cells of the stomach. This mucous blanket normally is about 1 to 1.5 mm in thickness and helps create a barrier against the proteolytic and acid gastric secretions. (Mucus production increases in the presence of gastric irritation.) An additional barrier to gastric contents is provided by the surface membranes of the mucosal cells and by the tight junctions found between the mucosal cells. Ulcers may result when the barrier is damaged; substances known to be "barrier breakers" include aspirin, alcohol, and bile salts, which contact the gastric mucosa when duodenal contents reflux into the stomach.[1,12]

The parietal (oxyntic) cells produce hydrochloric acid (HCl) and intrinsic factor. The low pH created by the HCl inactivates the salivary amylase and inhibits carbohydrate digestion, but it also serves to activate pepsin, which initiates protein digestion. Intrinsic factor bonds with vitamin $B_{12}$ and facilitates its absorption in the ileum. The chief cells (zymogenic cells) secrete pepsinogen, which is the precursor of the proteolytic enzyme pepsin. The endocrine cells secrete regulatory hormones that affect gastric secretion; for example, gastrin is produced in the pyloric region and is a powerful stimulant to the secretion of hydrochloric acid.[12]

**Gastric Secretion.** The total volume of gastric secretion normally is about 2 to 3 L/day. Gastric secretion is known to occur in three phases: the cephalic phase, in which the stimulus is the thought, smell, and taste of food; the gastric phase, in which the stimulus is food in the stomach; and the intestinal phase, in which the stimulus is chyme in the intestine.[12] Gastric secretion is regulated by neural phenomena and by hormonal secretion. Neural regulation involves the autonomic and central nervous systems, in addition to local reflexes coordinated by the intramural plexus. Gastric secretion also is affected by the hormones produced by secretory cells in the stomach and the duodenum; gastrin is a powerful stimulant for gastric secretion, whereas secretin, gastric inhibitory polypeptide, and cholecystokinin have an inhibitory effect.

Factors known to increase gastric secretion include pleasant thoughts, the taste and smell of food, tactile stimulation resulting from chewing and swallowing, gastric distention and partially digested proteins in the stomach, and moderate amounts of alcohol and caffeine, which explains the positive effect of caffeinated and alcoholic beverages on appetite.

Factors known to inhibit gastric secretion include distention or irritation of the duodenum, highly acidic duodenal contents, and hypertonic or hypotonic duodenal contents. Emotions also are thought to affect gastric secretions; anger and hostility have been noted to increase gastric secretion, whereas fear and depression are considered inhibiting factors.[1,3,12]

**Functions.** The stomach has several important functions:
1. It serves as a reservoir for ingested nutrients and provides controlled emptying into the duodenum.
2. It continues the digestive process begun in the mouth.
3. It contains the secretory cells for intrinsic factor.
4. It provides for limited absorption.
5. The acidity of the gastric secretions inhibits bacterial proliferation.[1,12]

*Nutrient reservoir.* The stomach serves as a reservoir for ingested nutrients and provides gradual and controlled emptying into the duodenum; this function of the stomach permits the healthy person to eat at intervals. (When the stomach is removed or by-passed, enteral feedings must be provided on a more continual basis.) A number of factors affect gastric motility and the rate of gastric emptying; these include the consistency of gastric contents, the acidity and fat content of the gastric contents, vagal stimuli, and emotional states.[1,12]

Ingested foods and fluids are retained in the stomach until they have been thoroughly mixed with the gastric secretions and converted to a semifluid material known as *chyme*. This is accomplished by means of a combination of mixing waves and peristaltic waves. Both mixing waves and peristaltic waves proceed from the proximal end of the stomach to the distal (pyloric) end; the difference is that the mixing waves are weaker and primarily act to mix the ingested contents with the gastric secretions, whereas the peristaltic waves are stronger and actively sweep the liquid chyme toward the pylorus. The more solid material, which is toward the center of the stomach, is pushed back toward the proximal end of the stomach so that it is exposed to further mixing before it reaches the pylorus. This "mixing and moving" process continues until the gastric contents have been emptied into the duodenum.[1,12]

The rate of gastric emptying is primarily determined by the pH, fat content, osmolality, consistency, and temperature of the chyme. Highly acidic chyme is delivered to the duodenum at a slower rate, which allows time for the chyme to be neutralized by pancreatic secretions and mucus production; meals with significant protein content usually result in more acidic chyme because of the increased production of HCl and pepsin. Meals with high fat content also retard gastric emptying to allow for bile secretion and fat emulsification. Hyperosmolar and hypoosmolar substances empty more slowly than do isotonic substances, and solids empty more slowly than liquids. Temperature extremes can also slow gastric emptying. Other factors that affect gastric motility include vagal stimuli, medications, pathologic states, and emotions. Vagal stimulation increases gastric motility; therefore cholinergic medications such as metoclopramide enhance gastric emptying, whereas surgical vagotomy retards gastric emptying. Narcotics commonly slow gastric motility, as do a number of pathologic conditions (e.g., hypokalemia, peritonitis, and uremia), pain, anxiety, and depression.[1]

*Digestion.* In addition to serving as a reservoir for ingested nutrients and providing controlled emptying into the duodenum, the stomach contributes to the digestive process in the following ways. Mechanical digestion is continued as ingested nutrients are mixed with gastric secretions to form a semifluid chyme. The breakdown of starches is interrupted because the acidic pH inactivates the salivary amylase; however, the acidic pH provides the needed environment for initiation of protein digestion. The HCl produced by the parietal cells converts pepsinogen to pepsin, which is a proteolytic enzyme that breaks intact protein down into peptide chains. Pepsin exhibits optimal activity at a pH of 3.0 or below.[12]

*Intrinsic factor secretion.* Another important function of the stomach is secretion of intrinsic factor. Intrinsic factor is necessary for effective absorption of vitamin $B_{12}$ (cyanocobalamin) in the ileum; if the stomach is surgically removed, lifelong parenteral administration of vitamin $B_{12}$ is required to prevent pernicious anemia.

*Absorption.* A less important function of the stomach is its capacity for limited absorption; substances that can be partially absorbed in the stomach include carbohydrates that have undergone chemical digestion in the mouth, as well as alcohol and some medications (e.g., aspirin).[3,12] The stomach's role in nutrient absorption is minimal.

A final function of the stomach is the antibacterial effect provided by the low gastric pH; the hydrochloric acid eliminates most of the ingested bacteria.[3]

**Blood Supply and Innervation.** Arterial blood is supplied to the stomach through branches of the celiac trunk; venous drainage is provided by the gastric and gastroepiploic veins, which in turn empty into the portal vein. Innervation of the stomach is autonomic, with the vagus nerves providing parasympathetic innervation and the celiac plexus providing sympathetic innervation.[1,12]

## Small Intestine

The small intestine in the adult is approximately 22 feet in length; in the newborn infant the small intestine is only 25% of its adult length and 13% of its adult diameter. The tremendous growth of the small bowel throughout the life cycle is illustrated by the fact that the infant has about 950 cm of absorptive surface, whereas the average adult has about 7600 cm.[1] The small intestine is the major organ for digestion and absorption of nutrients and as such is critical to life and health. The small intestine is divided into three anatomic and functional sections: the duodenum, the jejunum, and the ileum. Features common to all sections are described first, followed by a discussion of the individual sections.

**Histology.** The wall of the small intestine contains the four layers common to the GI tract. Several characteristics, however, are unique to the small intestine. The submucosal and mucosal layers are arranged in folds known as the *plicae circulares,* which, together with the villi, serve to significantly increase the absorptive surface. The mucosal layer is divided into three layers: the muscularis mucosa, the lamina propria, and the surface epithelium. The muscularis mucosa is a thin layer of circular muscle that separates the mucosa from the submucosa. The lamina propria layer contains the intestinal villi and crypts, as well as connective tissue, fibroblasts, reticuloendothelial cells, smooth muscle cells, and plasma cells. The surface epithelium is composed of simple epithelial cells (enterocytes) that cover the villi. The mucosal layer also contains both solitary and aggregated lymphatic nodules; the aggregated nodules are known as *Peyer's patches* and are particularly common in the ileum.[1,12]

The villi are significant structures of the mucosal layer (Fig. 9-3). They are fingerlike projections, 0.5 to 1 mm in length, that cover the mucosal surface and increase its absorptive area. Each villus contains a capillary network, a lymphatic vessel, and smooth muscle

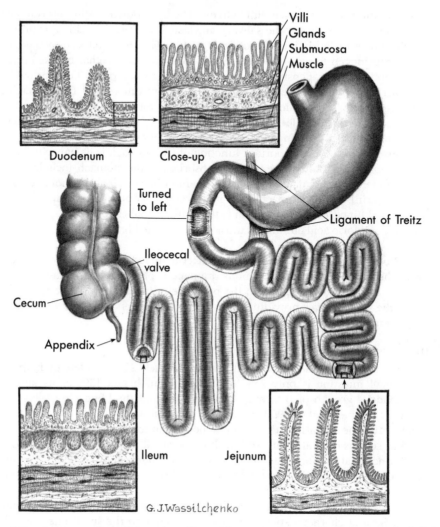

**Fig. 9-3**   Anatomy of small intestine. (From Thompson J et al: *Mosby's manual of clinical nursing,* St Louis, 1989, Mosby–Year Book.)

fibers. The villi are covered with absorptive cells that have cytoplasmic extensions known as *microvilli;* the microvilli serve to further increase the absorptive surface. The total increase in absorptive surface provided by the plicae circulares, the villi, and the microvilli is about 600-fold.[1] The microvilli form what is known as the *brush border;* the cells that make up the brush border contain many enzymes and carrier substances that facilitate the digestion and absorption of nutrients. Enzymes present in the brush border include peptidases, disaccharidases, and nucleases.[12]

The villi actually have the ability to elongate, or hypertrophy, which partially explains the phenomenon of bowel adaptation after partial bowel resection. The converse is also true; patients maintained on a regimen of nothing by mouth (NPO) for more than a few days may have temporary atrophy of the villi, with resultant loss of absorptive capacity.

**Mucosal Proliferation.** Mucosal cells are reproduced on a continuing basis in Lieberkühn's crypts, which are located at the base of the villi. These mucosal cells then migrate toward the surface of the villi, where they are sloughed into the lumen of the bowel. The average life span of the mucosal cell is about 2 to 5 days. The constant proliferation of mucosal cells provides rapid repair of any mucosal trauma.[3]

**Function.** The small intestine is the primary organ responsible for the digestion and absorption of nutrients, vitamins, minerals, fluids and electrolytes, and miscellaneous substances such as drugs. Specific functions that contribute to the digestive process include intestinal motility, intestinal secretion, and absorption.

*Motility.* Two types of contractions occur regularly in the small bowel: segmental contractions and peristaltic waves.[12] Segmental contractions are ringlike contractions that produce a back-and-forth motion that acts to mix and churn the intestinal contents and to increase exposure of the chyme to the absorptive mucosal surface. Peristaltic waves act to propel the chyme distally. When the intestine is distended, it stimulates a strong contraction that begins just behind the point of stimulus and sweeps along the intestine toward the ileocecal valve. Normally peristaltic waves occur almost continuously, propelling the chyme distally at a rate of 2 to 25 cm/min.[1]

Small-bowel motility is affected by both extrinsic and intrinsic innervation, but the intrinsic system is far more important. Extrinsic innervation is provided by sympathetic fibers, which inhibit intestinal motility, and parasympathetic fibers (vagal stimulation), which increase intestinal motility.[1] Both segmentation and peristalsis, however, can be mediated by an intact myenteric plexus even in the absence of extrinsic stimuli.[3] Motility is most affected by local factors, such as distention of the bowel wall, hypertonic or hypotonic bowel contents, highly acidic chyme, and some products of digestion. Response to these stimuli is mediated primarily by the intramural plexus; vagal stimulation is much less important in the small bowel than in the stomach.[1]

Transit time from the mouth to the colon averages 4 to 9 hours.

*Secretion.* The small intestine contains many intestinal glands known as Lieberkühn's crypts. The secretory cells of these glands (Paneth's cells) secrete as much as 3 L of extracellular fluid a day, with a pH of about 6.5 to 7.5. This fluid contains no enzymes; the enzymes needed to complete the digestive process are found in the cells of the brush border, as already described, and the watery intestinal fluid functions primarily to promote the absorptive process. In addition to the fluid secreted by the intestinal glands, large amounts of mucus are secreted by goblet cells located throughout the mucosal layer of the small intestine.[12]

*Absorption.* Nutrients undergo mechanical and chemical digestion in the mouth, stomach, and small bowel; the digestive process breaks down the complex molecules into substances that can be absorbed into the bloodstream. Absorption is then supported by the vast mucosal surface of the small intestine and by the numerous carrier systems located in the brush border of the villi.[1,12] Most nutrient absorption occurs in the proximal small bowel, reflecting the tremendous absorptive capacity of this organ; however, the ileum can take over much of the absorptive function in the event of disease or surgical resection involving the proximal small bowel. The intact bowel provides significant reserve capacity for nutrient absorption; thus segmental bowel resection usually is well tolerated. The effects of any particular resection depend on the length and function of bowel removed and the length and function of the remaining bowel.[10] For example, resection involving the ileocecal valve is more likely to result in compromised absorption than is resection of an equal length of

**Table 9-2**   Nutrient digestion and absorption

| Nutrient | Digestive enzymes | Site | | |
|---|---|---|---|---|
| | | Production | Action | Absorption |
| Carbohydrates | Amylase | Salivary glands<br>Pancreas; brush border of small intestine | Mouth<br>Small intestine | Stomach (limited)<br>Small intestine |
| | Disaccharidase (sucrase, maltase, isomaltase, lactase) | Brush border of intestine | Small intestine | |
| Proteins | Pepsin | Chief cells | Stomach | Small intestine |
| | Trypsin, chymotrypsin, carboxypeptidase | Pancreas | Small intestine | |
| | Peptidases | Brush border of intestine | Small intestine | |
| Lipids | Bile (not enzyme) | Liver | Duodenum | Small intestine |
| | Lipase | Pancreas, brush border of intestine | Small intestine | |
| | Esterase | Pancreas | Small intestine | |

bowel that does not involve the ileocecal valve. Critical bowel length—that is, the length of absorptive small bowel that is essential for absorption of adequate nutrients—is difficult to determine because of differences in measurement techniques. It has been suggested that the adult needs at least 100 to 200 cm and the infant needs at least 60 cm of absorptive small bowel; however, many factors affect an individual patient's response to massive small-bowel resection.[2,4,10]

The small intestine also plays a vital role in maintenance of fluid and electrolyte balance through its reabsorption of intraluminal fluids. The volume of fluid secreted into the small intestine may be as much as 7 to 9 L/day (Table 9-1); with the average oral intake of 2 L/day, the volume of secreted and ingested fluids may reach 11 L/day. The vast majority of this fluid is reabsorbed into the bloodstream, with less than 2 L passing through the ileocecal valve daily.[1] Any abnormal losses—for example, losses resulting from vomiting, diarrhea, or fistula drainage—may result in fluid and electrolyte imbalance. Hypokalemia, hyponatremia, and metabolic acidosis commonly occur along with fluid volume deficit because intestinal fluid is usually neutral or alkaline and contains large volumes of sodium and potassium.[1,10]

Digestion and absorption of specific nutrients are discussed in the section concerning the appropriate bowel segment (summarized in Table 9-2).

**Blood Supply and Innervation.** The superior mesenteric artery supplies blood flow for most of the small intestine, that is, the jejunum, the ileum, and the distal duodenum. The proximal duodenum (the portion above Vater's ampulla) derives its blood supply from the celiac vessels.[12] Venous drainage for the small bowel is provided by the superior mesenteric vein; the superior mesenteric vein then empties into the portal vein, which drains into the liver. This vascular arrangement provides the necessary "detoxification" of the blood that passes through the intestinal tract before it reenters the systemic circulation.[2,12] This vascular arrangement also explains the frequency of metastatic disease involving the liver in a person with a malignancy of the intestinal tract.

Innervation of the small bowel involves both an intrinsic and an extrinsic system. Intrinsic innervation is provided by the plexus located within the bowel wall, Auerbach's plexus and Meissner's plexus; intrinsic innervation is the primary stimulus for intestinal secretion and motility. Extrinsic innervation is mediated by the sympathetic and parasympathetic branches of the autonomic nervous system. Autonomic nerve fibers synapse at the level of the intramural plexus (intrinsic system) and primarily serve to modify the stimuli provided by the intrinsic nervous system. Sympathetic stimuli have an inhibitory effect on intestinal secretion and motility, whereas parasympathetic (vagal) stimuli act to stimulate secretion and motility.[1,12]

**Bacterial Counts.** Bacterial counts in the small intestine are relatively low, probably due to the bactericidal effect of the extremely low gastric pH and the usually rapid transit of small bowel contents, which limits the potential for bacterial proliferation.[3] This explains why patients with large-bowel stomas usually have more flatus than do patients with small-bowel stomas.

## Duodenum

**Structure.** The duodenum is an immobile C-shaped segment of small bowel that lies just distal to the pylorus; it is secured to the pyloric region of the stomach by Treitz's ligament, which is the dividing point between the duodenum and the jejunum[1,3,12] (Fig. 9-3). The duodenum is located retroperitoneally and lies in close proximity to the stomach, pancreas, liver, gallbladder, and transverse colon. The cystic duct from the gallbladder and the hepatic duct from the liver merge to form the common bile duct; the common bile duct and the pancreatic duct both empty into the duodenum at Vater's ampulla.[1,12] The sphincter of Oddi controls the flow of secretions through Vater's ampulla into the duodenum.

### Function

*Chyme neutralization.* The duodenum's major function is to neutralize the highly acidic gastric contents as they enter the duodenum. This process is accomplished partly by secretion of alkaline mucus by the duodenal (Brunner's) glands, which are located in the submucosal layer of the duodenum. In addition, the presence of acid chyme within the duodenum causes the release of secretin, which stimulates the pancreas to secrete fluid with a high concentration of bicarbonate ions. This highly alkaline fluid drains through the pancreatic duct into the duodenum at Vater's ampulla and plays a major role in neutralizing the acidic chyme. When the presence of fats in the duodenum stimulates delivery of bile, the alkaline bile also helps neutralize the acidic gastric contents.[1,12]

*Digestion continuation.* A second function of the duodenum is to continue the digestive process begun in the proximal alimentary canal. Fatty acids and amino acids in the duodenum stimulate the release of cholecystokinin, which causes contraction of the gallbladder and secretion of enzymatic juices by the pancreas. Bile delivered to the duodenum acts to emulsify the fats, rendering them more susceptible to enzymatic breakdown. The pancreatic juice contains a number of digestive enzymes: amylase, which continues carbohydrate digestion; lipases, which continue the digestion of lipids; and the proteolytic enzymes trypsin, chymotrypsin, and carboxypeptidase. (Actually the proteolytic enzymes are secreted in precursor form; trypsin is activated in the duodenum by enterokinase, and trypsin then activates the other proteolytic enzymes.) The higher pH in the duodenum inactivates pepsin but provides an optimal environment for pancreatic enzyme activity.[1,12]

*Absorption.* The duodenum also plays a role in absorption; substances that are absorbed in the duodenum include carbohydrates and minerals such as iron, calcium, and magnesium.

## Jejunum

The jejunum is the midportion of the small intestine; it measures about 9 feet in length and about 1 to $1\frac{1}{2}$ inches in width. The jejunum is the major organ for nutrient absorption; most of the fats, proteins, and vitamins are absorbed in this area, as well as carbohydrates not absorbed in the stomach and duodenum. The enzymes in the brush border finalize nutrient digestion, and the carrier systems facilitate absorption. The large volume of intestinal secretions also promotes nutrient absorption. The jejunum has prominent villi, consistent with its role in nutrient absorption[1,12] (Fig. 9-3).

## Ileum

The third segment of the small intestine is the ileum, which is about 12 feet long and about 1 inch wide. Although no clear demarcation exists between the jejunum and the ileum, the ileum is narrower than the jejunum and the villi are less prominent.[1,12] The ileum provides for absorption of any nutrients not absorbed by the duodenum and jejunum. The ileum also contains the only receptor sites for absorption of the intrinsic factor–vitamin $B_{12}$ complex and for bile salts; these sites are located in the terminal ileum.[1,3,12] Patients who have had significant lengths of the terminal ileum resected may require lifelong replacement with parenteral vitamin $B_{12}$ to prevent pernicious anemia; fat intolerance and weight loss also may occur in these patients. Fat intolerance results from failure to reabsorb bile salts in the terminal ileum, which retards production of bile in the liver. Normally the bile produced by the liver is concentrated in the gallbladder until gallbladder contraction is stimulated by cholecystokinin. The bile is then delivered to the duodenum, where it emulsifies the fats; the residual bile salts continue to pass through the lumen of the bowel until they reach the terminal ileum. At this point the bile salts are reabsorbed into the bloodstream and delivered back to the liver, where they are again used to produce bile. This recycling of bile salts is known as the enterohepatic circulation; it promotes bile production and therefore fat absorption.[3,12]

## Ileocecal Valve

The ileocecal valve is a one-way valve located at the junction between the ileum and the large intestine. The ileocecal valve works in conjunction with the ileocecal sphincter, a ring of smooth muscle, to regulate emptying into the large intestine and to prevent reflux of contents back into the small intestine. Normally the sphincter is partially contracted; peristaltic waves in the distal ileum cause the sphincter to relax, permitting passage of chyme into the colon. In contrast, distention of the cecum causes increased contraction of the sphincter, which protects the small bowel from reflux.[12]

The ileocecal valve and sphincter provide some delay in the passage of chyme from the small bowel into the colon; this delay factor may be critical in the patient with a short-bowel syndrome or compromised absorptive capacity because it increases the exposure of nutrients to the absorptive surface of the small bowel.[12]

## Colon

The colon is a long, distensible tube that extends from the ileocecal valve to the anus and brackets the small intestine. In the adult the colon is 5 to 6 feet in length and has a variable width of 1 to $2\frac{1}{2}$ inches. The colon is subdivided into the following segments: cecum, ascending colon, transverse colon, descending colon, sigmoid colon, rectum, and anal canal (Fig. 9-1).

**Histology.** The colon wall has the same morphologic layers as the rest of the GI tract. Several features of these layers, however, are unique to the colon. The outer layer, serosa, covers most of the colon and forms peritoneal sacs that enclose fat (epiploic appendices) and hang from the bowel.

The muscular layer (tunica muscularis) has two smooth-muscle layers (longitudinal and circular), as does the small intestine. The longitudinal muscle of the colon, however, differs from the small intestine in that it is gathered into three muscular bands, or taeniae. The taeniae coli extend from the appendix to the rectosigmoid junction; at this junction the taeniae fuse into one continuous longitudinal muscle. Each taenia traverses one of the following surfaces of the colon: the anterior surface, the posteroinferior surface, and the posterosuperior surface. Because the taeniae coli are shorter than the length of the colon, they are responsible for the colon's sacculated appearance, or haustra (Fig. 9-1). If a loop colostomy is opened parallel to the taeniae, the natural haustrations create two separate openings, one proximal and one distal; this separation provides almost complete diversion of the fecal stream.

The submucosal layer contains small arteries, veins, and lymphatic vessels and serves to attach the muscular layer to the mucosal layer. The submucosal layer has no important distinguishing features. The inner layer of the colon, the mucosa, has several features that distinguish it from the small intestine.[7] Tall, simple, columnar epithelial cells line the mucosa; because villi are not present, the colon provides no nutrient absorption. Only a few goblet cells are scattered among the epithelial cells. Lieberkühn's crypts (intestinal glands) are deeper, contain no Paneth's cells, and have more goblet cells. The muscularis mucosa is located at the base of the crypts.

**Secretions.** Colonic secretions that consist of water, mucus, potassium, and bicarbonate are produced by Lieberkühn's crypts and goblet cells. Mucus, produced by the goblet cells, serves several functions: lubrication of the fecal bolus to aid transport of the material; protection of the mucosa from injury; and binding of the fecal material together. The parasympathetic nervous system and colonic irritants (bacterial, mechanical, or chemical) stimulate mucus production; anxiety and tension decrease mucus secretion. The secretion of bicarbonate creates an alkaline fecal matter with a pH of 7.8.

**Composition of Fecal Material.** Fecal material consists primarily of bile pigments, mucus, unabsorbed minerals, undigested fats, cellulose, meat protein toxins, desquamated epithelial cells, potassium, chloride, sodium, bicarbonate, and water. Fecal composition is approximately three-fourths water (50 to 150 ml) and one-fourth solid matter. The pH of fecal matter is 6.8 to 7.8.[5,13]

Intestinal bacteria are vital to many colonic functions. Anaerobic bacteria present in the colon serve to putrefy remaining proteins and indigestible residue; to synthesize folic acid, vitamin K, nicotinic acid, riboflavin, and some B vitamins; and to convert urea salts to ammonium salts and ammonia for absorption into the portal circulation. Common bacteria include *Escherichia coli, Aerobacter aerogenes, Clostridium perfringens,* and *Lactobacillus bifidus.* The concentration of bacteria in the colon is higher in the more distal portions of the colon. These bacteria are partially responsible for the odor associated with feces, which explains why an output from a sigmoid colostomy has more odor than does output from an ileostomy.

Bacterial action also creates intestinal gas. In addition, swallowed air and diffusion from the blood contribute to intestinal gas production. Intestinal gas is composed of oxygen, nitrogen, carbon dioxide, methane, hydrogen, and trace gases. Such gas production also creates fecal odor. Because many of these gases are flammable, an effective bowel preparation before any procedure that requires cautery (such as a surgical procedure and colonoscopy) is essential to prevent explosions.

**Structure.** The cecum is the first section of colon and also is the widest segment. Measuring $2^1/2$ to 3 inches in length, the cecum contains the ileocecal valve. Distention of the cecum causes apposition of the two semilunar lips of the ileocecal valve, thus preventing reflux of cecal contents into the ileum. This antireflux mechanism, however, is somewhat incompetent.[9] The appendix arises from the posteromedial aspect of the cecum.

The ascending colon extends approximately 15 cm from the cecum to the right hepatic flexure and is slightly narrower than the cecum. Peritoneum covers the front and sides of the ascending colon but generally not the posterior surface.

After a sharp 90-degree left turn, the colon continues as the transverse colon. Approximately 45 to 50 cm in length, the transverse colon is quite mobile because it is fixed only at its two end points, the hepatic flexure and the splenic flexure. In fact, the central portion of the transverse colon can gain sufficient mobility to lie in the hypogastrium near the cecum or near the sigmoid colon. The greater omentum lies in front of the transverse colon and must be elevated to expose the colon. At the splenic flexure the transverse colon makes an acute, almost 180-degree turn downward and backward to continue as the descending colon. The left splenic flexure is slightly higher than is the right hepatic flexure.

The descending colon is 25 cm long (longer than the ascending colon) and extends from the hepatic flexure to the brim of the true pelvis. Peritoneum covers the front and both sides of the descending colon; the posterior surface does not have a peritoneal covering.

The sigmoid colon begins where the descending colon passes over the psoas muscle and continues in an S-shaped curve to the upper end of the rectum. Although the length of the sigmoid varies widely, the average is 40 cm. A loop of sigmoid bowel is present when the sigmoid colon is particularly redundant. Peritoneum completely surrounds the sigmoid colon.

The rectum is a hollow, distensible, angulated structure that begins at the termination of the sigmoid colon and is marked by the third sacral vertebra; some experts, however, use the sacral promontory as the landmark. The rectum measures 12 to 15 cm in length and follows the curve of the sacrum and coccyx before angulating sharply downward and backward. As the rectum passes through the levator ani muscle, it becomes the anal canal.

The diameter of the upper portion of the rectum is the same as that of the sigmoid colon; however, the lower part of the rectum, which is dilated to facilitate storage of fecal

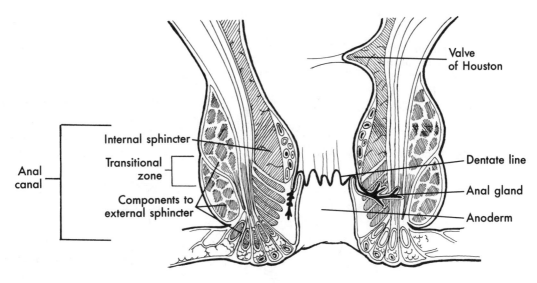

**Fig. 9-4**    Anal canal.

material, forms the rectal ampulla. The rectum has neither haustra nor epiploic appendices. The rectum, which normally is in a collapsed state, is surrounded by a continuous, strong muscular coat of longitudinal fibers formed by the merging of the taeniae coli.

The rectal mucosa forms three folds in the rectum known as the valves of Houston; two valves are located on the left, and one is on the right (Fig. 9-4). These folds consist of mucosa, muscularis mucosa, submucosa, and circular muscle. These structures serve as important landmarks and must be carefully negotiated during proctosigmoidoscopic examination.[6] An additional 5 cm of length can be obtained by straightening the rectum, as is accomplished with a low anterior anastomosis. Because the distal 7 to 8 cm of rectum is below the peritoneal reflection, it is not covered by peritoneum.

The anal canal, which is 2.5 to 3 cm in length, is the terminal portion of the colon, extending from the anorectal junction to the anal verge. The muscles surrounding the anal canal are tonically contracted, thus completely collapsing the anal canal. An angulation of approximately 60 to 105 degrees is created by the presence of the puborectalis muscle that loops around the anal canal at the anorectal junction.[11]

Midpoint in the anal canal is the dentate line (also referred to as the pectinate line) (Fig. 9-4). This is an important reference point because of the differences that exist in the tissues above and below this line. Proximal to this line, the mucosa assumes a pleated appearance known as the columns of Morgagni. These longitudinal folds are created by the narrowing of the rectum into the anal canal. Above the dentate line, the anal canal is lined with columnar epithelium, whereas squamous epithelium lines the anal canal distal to the dentate line. This transition from columnar to squamous epithelium is gradual, occurring in an area 6 to 12 mm proximal to the dentate line, known as the transition, or cloacogenic, zone.[6]

Other important differences are observed in the tissue surrounding the dentate line. The color of the epithelium changes; whereas the rectal mucosa is pink, the area proximal to the dentate line is deep purple or plum color as a result of the internal hemorrhoidal plexus.

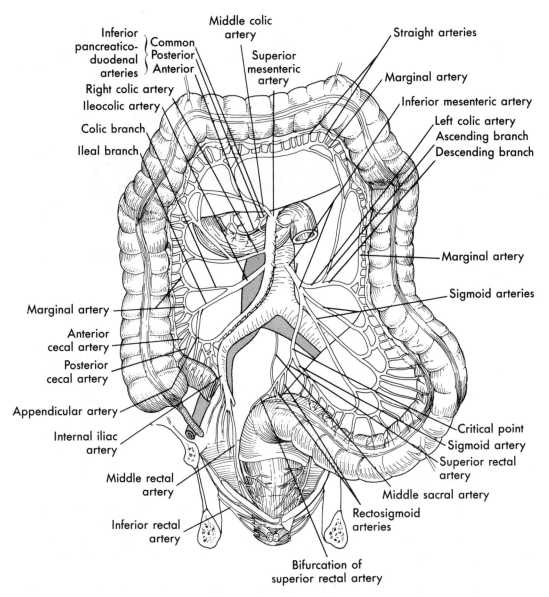

**Fig. 9-5** Blood supply to colon. (From Broadwell D, Jackson B: *Principles of ostomy care*, St Louis, 1982, Mosby–Year Book.)

Proximal to the dentate line, the epithelium is innervated with autonomic nerves; on the other hand, the submucosa distal to the dentate line contains numerous encapsulated and free sensory nerve endings. Thus, whereas the rectum is insensitive to ordinary tactile and painful stimuli, the mucosa in the distal anal canal is highly sensitive. The nerve endings in the anal canal provide differentiation among gas, liquids, and solids.[6,9] The area below the dentate line, referred to as the anoderm, resembles skin except for the absence of accessory skin structures (i.e., hair, sebaceous glands, and sweat glands).

**Blood Supply and Innervation.** The superior mesenteric artery supplies the cecum, right colon, and transverse colon up to the splenic flexure. The inferior mesenteric artery supplies the descending colon, the sigmoid colon, and the proximal portion of the rectum. The remainder of the rectum is supplied by the middle and inferior hemorrhoidal arteries, which arise from the internal iliac arteries (Fig. 9-5).

Blood is drained from the colon in a pattern similar to the arterial supply; the right colon is drained by the superior mesenteric vein, and the left colon is drained by the inferior mesenteric vein. As part of the portal system, these veins deliver the blood to the liver. The proximal portion of the rectum drains into the superior hemorrhoidal vein and into the portal system by way of the inferior mesenteric vein. The remainder of the rectum is drained by the middle and inferior hemorrhoidal vein, which flows to the iliac veins and therefore the systemic system.

The nerve supply to the colon is both parasympathetic and sympathetic and closely resembles the small bowel because it also involves an intrinsic and an extrinsic system. The intrinsic system involves the same structures as does the small bowel and mediates the secretion of mucus and colonic movement. Extrinsic innervation involves both branches of the autonomic nervous system. Parasympathetic innervation of the right colon is from the vagus nerve; the remainder of the colon receives parasympathetic innervation from branches of the sacral nerves. Parasympathetic stimulation causes increased intestinal contraction, increased mucus secretion, and relaxation of the rectal sphincter. Sympathetic fibers (splanchnic nerves) synapse in the intramural plexus and cause inhibition of the colonic muscles and secretions, as well as contraction of the rectal sphincter.

**Function.** The functions of the colon include collection, concentration, transport, and elimination of intestinal waste material. Approximately 1.5 to 2 L of intestinal contents pass through the ileocecal valve to be collected in the cecum daily. Water and electrolytes (sodium and chloride), glucose, and urea are reabsorbed from this material, thereby concentrating the contents so that only 100 to 150 ml of fluid remains to be excreted from the body.[5] Colonic motility transports fecal material through the colon by the synchronous activity of the colonic musculature. Elimination of intestinal waste then occurs at regular intervals after the occurrence of a complex set of interelated processes.

*Colonic motility.* The longitudinal and circular muscles work together to propel the fecal material through the colon (peristalsis) and to "knead" the material into a bolus (segmentation). The longitudinal muscle is primarily responsible for peristalsis, the movement of the fecal bolus through the colon. Several types of peristalsis occur. Receptive relaxation allows the cecum to fill with ileal contents; adaptive relaxation allows the fecal material to accumulate and be stored; pendulum movements (continuous back-and-forth movement of fecal material) aid absorption; and mass movement (the en masse contraction of the left colon) propels the fecal bolus into the rectum to be evacuated.[5]

Segmentation, the alternate contraction and relaxation of the haustra, is created by the circular muscle. Segmentation facilitates the grinding of food masses and fluid and electrolyte reabsorption.

Colonic motility is stimulated by hostility, anger, physical activity, colonic distention, lactose, and medications that absorb water or prevent the movement of water (e.g., bulking agents and saline cathartics). Factors that decrease colonic motility include sleep, anxiety, and fear. The average transit time from the ileocecal valve to the rectum is 24 hours or more.

*Elimination.* Feces are eliminated from the colon through the defecation process, a complex process that involves the coordination of the anal sphincters, pelvic floor muscles, and voluntary efforts.

*ANAL SPHINCTER.* The internal and external sphincters compose the anal sphincter (Fig. 9-4). Anatomically the internal sphincter is a continuation of the thick circular muscle and encircles the anal canal to a point approximately 1.5 cm distal to the dentate line. The internal sphincter, which is tonically contracted, is not under voluntary control because it is a smooth muscle. The external sphincter is a striated muscle that surrounds the anal canal. The superficial component is attached to the coccyx by an extension of the muscle fibers. The deep component of the external sphincter is not attached posteriorly; the proximal portion is continuous with the puborectalis muscle. The external sphincter is innervated through the pudendal nerve and is under voluntary control; the external sphincter also exhibits tonic continuous activity at rest. Rectal distention stimulates increased contraction of the external sphincter.[6,7,9]

These two sphincters work together. In response to rectosigmoid distention, the internal sphincter immediately relaxes while the external anal sphincter contracts. This allows the sensitive epithelium of the anal canal the opportunity to "sample" the contents to determine if the contents are air, liquid, or solid. Although the internal sphincter responds only to rectal distention, the external sphincter responds with contraction to rectal distention, increased intraabdominal pressure, anal dilation, and perianal stretch, as well as to voluntary effort. Tonic contraction of the external sphincter is inhibited by voluntary effort or by the act of micturition.[7]

*PELVIC FLOOR.* The pelvic floor comprises the levator ani muscle that forms a cone-shaped diaphragm over the perineum. Through the center of this muscle the pelvic organs exit the pelvis and enter the perineum. The levator ani muscle is divided into four components: the iliococcygeus, pubococcygeus, puborectalis, and ischiococcygeus. (The puborectalis is believed to be a part of the external sphincter structure.) These striated muscles form a sling to support the anal canal and distal rectum and alter the anorectal angle to facilitate or inhibit defecation.

*PROCESS.* Fecal material is delivered to the rectum or sigmoid rectum through mass movement. As this material is forced into the rectum and anal canal, the internal sphincter promptly relaxes while the external sphincter automatically contracts. If the individual chooses to proceed with defecation and strains to push the contents into the rectum, intrarectal pressures increase. These pressures are sufficient to overcome the external sphincter contraction. Simultaneously, the external sphincter and pelvic floor muscles relax, thus straightening the rectum and eliminating any resistance presented by Houston's valves or rectal angles. Reduced angulation is also facilitated by the squatting position. Continued relaxation of the external sphincter occurs as a result of the stimulation of the mucosa of the anal canal by the fecal material. (Other textbooks[6,11] present a more detailed discussion of the defecation process.)

## ACCESSORY ORGANS

The pancreas, the liver, and the biliary system are considered accessory organs to the digestive system. Each of these is discussed with emphasis on its role pertaining to digestion.

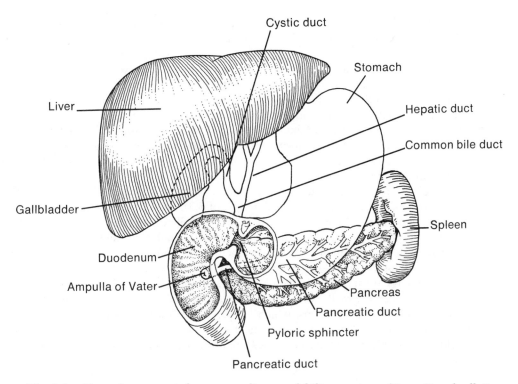

Cystic duct

Stomach

Liver

Hepatic duct

Common bile duct

Gallbladder

Spleen

Duodenum

Ampulla of Vater

Pancreas

Pancreatic duct

Pyloric sphincter

Pancreatic duct

**Fig 9-6**    Normal anatomy of pancreas, liver, and biliary system. (From Broadwell D, Jackson B: *Principles of ostomy care*, St Louis, 1982, Mosby–Year Book.)

## Pancreas

**Structure.** The pancreas is a fish-shaped, lobulated organ that weighs approximately 85 g (3 ounces); it is 10 to 22 cm long and 5 cm wide. The pancreas is divided into the head (which lies over the vena cava and rests in the C-shaped curve of the duodenum), the body (which extends horizontally across the abdomen and hides behind the stomach), and the tail (which contacts the spleen at the level of the first and second lumbar vertebrae (Fig. 9-6).

The pancreas is described as a lobulated organ because the internal structure is composed of numerous small alveoli lined with special secretory cells called *tubuloacinar cells* (tiny tubes and grapes). These cells secrete digestive enzymes also known as pancreatic secretions. Clusters of the acinar cells form an acinus, which in turn forms lobules. Connective tissue joins each lobule to form the pancreas.

Each acinus contains small ducts that empty into larger lobule ducts. The ducts within the lobules receive secretions from the acinar cells and empty into Wirsung's duct, the major pancreatic duct that extends the entire length of the pancreas. Wirsung's duct empties the digestive enzymes into Vater's ampulla, located in the duodenum.

The pancreas also consists of clusters of cells that form spherical islands embedded within the lobules of acinar tissue known as the islets of Langerhans. These cells also are referred to as endocrine tissue because they have no ductal system and they release their products directly into the bloodstream. Four distinct cell types are present in the islets of Langerhans: A, B, D, and F cells. A cells secrete glucagon, B cells secrete insulin, D cells secrete somatostatin, and F cells secrete pancreatic polypeptide hormone. This endocrine tissue composes less than 1% of the pancreas.

**Function.** The pancreas has both an endocrine and an exocrine function. The islets of Langerhans, as just described, produce the endocrine products of insulin, glucagon, somatostatin, and pancreatic polypeptide hormone; these substances are released into surrounding capillaries, empty into the portal vein, and are distributed to target cells in the liver where these hormones enter the general circulation to reach other target tissue. (A detailed discussion of these hormones is beyond the scope of this discussion and can be found in other textbooks.) Table 9-3 summarizes the stimulant, the target tissue, and the action of these hormones.

Exocrine secretions (pancreatic juices), which are produced by the acinar cells, are odorless, colorless, watery, and alkaline (pH of 8.3). The primary components of pancreatic juice include water (97%) and bicarbonate. Electrolytes such as sodium and potassium in high concentrations and calcium and chloride in smaller concentrations also are present. Enzymes in the pancreatic secretions include trypsin, chymotrypsin, carboxypeptidase, amylase, lipase, cholesterol esterase, deoxyribonuclease, and ribonuclease. Trypsin is secreted in the form of trypsinogen, a precursor, and is activated to trypsin by enterokinase, an enzyme secreted by the cells in the duodenum. This precursor mechanism thus inhibits autodigestion of the pancreas, which can occur with acute pancreatitis. Pancreatic juices serve to digest foodstuff (by the enzymes) and to neutralize and dilute gastric hydrochloric acid (by the bicarbonate, electrolytes, and water). Average daily volume for pancreatic secretions is 700 to 1000 ml.

**Table 9-3**    Functions of pancreatic endocrine cells

| Cell | Hormone | Stimulant | Target tissue | Action (response) |
|------|---------|-----------|---------------|-------------------|
| A | Glucagon | ↓ Glucose<br>Exercise<br>↑ Amino acids<br>SNS stimulation | Hepatocyte<br>Myocyte | ↑ Glucose in bloodstream<br>↑ Gluconeogenesis<br>↑ Glycogenolysis<br>Mobilization fats<br>Mobilization proteins |
| B | Insulin | Glucose | Skeletal cells<br>Muscle cells<br>Cardiac cells | ↓ Blood glucose<br>↓ Fat mobilization<br>↑ Fat storage<br>↓ Protein mobilization<br>↑ Protein synthesis<br>↑ Glucogenesis |
| D | Somatostatin | Hyperglycemia | A cells<br>B cells | ↓ Blood glucose<br>↓ Glycogen secretion<br>↓ Insulin secretion |
| F | Pancreatic<br>polypeptide | Acute hypoglycemia | Gallbladder<br>Smooth<br>muscle | ↑ Gallbladder contraction<br>↓ Pancreatic enzyme |

From Thelan LA, Davie JF, Urden LD: *Textbook of critical care nursing: diagnosis and management*, St Louis, 1990, Mosby–Year Book.
*SNS*, Sympathetic nervous system.

Both hormonal and neural signals regulate pancreatic exocrine function. In response to stimulation by chyme in the intestine, the intestinal hormones secretin and cholecystokinin are released and transported to the pancreas via the portal system. In the presence of an acid chyme (pH below 4.5), secretin is released and acts on the pancreas to produce a high volume of fluid low in enzymes but rich in water and bicarbonate. The acid chyme that is delivered to the duodenum is thereby neutralized. Other effects of secretin production include increased bile secretion from the liver, decreased gastrin-induced gastric secretion and emptying, stimulation of insulin release, increased pancreatic flood flow, and potentiation of cholecystokinin.

The release of the intestinal hormone cholecystokinin is stimulated when the chyme present in the duodenum is rich in protein and fat. Cholecystokinin causes the pancreas to produce secretions that are rich in enzymes, low in volume, and high in bicarbonate and amylase. Additional effects of cholecystokinin include increased GI motility, increased pancreatic blood flow, slowed gastric emptying, inhibition of the lower esophageal sphincter, stimulation of sigmoid colon motility, relaxation of the hepatopancreatic ampulla, stimulation of gallbladder emptying, relaxation of the sphincter of Oddi, and release of insulin and glucagon.

Additional hormones are believed to influence the pancreas. Vasoactive intestinal peptide may mediate an increase in pancreatic fluid and bicarbonate secretion. Somatostatin, vasopressin, and calcitonin inhibit pancreatic exocrine function.

Neural influences on the pancreas are inhibitory stimulation by the sympathetic system and increased exocrine secretions and blood flow by the parasympathetic system. In addition, anticholinergic agents decrease enzyme production, whereas alcohol and histamines increase pancreatic secretions by stimulating gastric hydrochloric acid production.

**Blood Supply and Innervation.** Branches of the celiac, splenic, and superior mesenteric arteries form the pancreatic arteries and supply arterial blood to the pancreas. The splenic and superior mesenteric veins drain blood from the pancreas into the portal circulation.

Both sympathetic and parasympathetic fibers innervate the pancreas. The splanchnic nerves and celiac plexus (sympathetic nerves) contain the preganglionic fibers for pain and the postganglionic fibers for vascular control. Sympathetic fibers also innervate the acinar cells and stimulate secretion of enzymes. Parasympathetic stimulation by the vagus nerve controls both exocrine and endocrine pancreatic function and mediates the gastropancreatic reflex.

## Liver

**Structure.** The liver, the largest organ in the body, weighs 1200 to 1600 g (3 to 4 pounds); it is located in the right upper abdominal quadrant below the right diaphragmatic dome (Fig. 9-6). A thick capsule of connective tissue, Glisson's capsule, surrounds the liver; it is covered by serosa and contains blood vessels and lymphatics.

The liver is held in place by intraabdominal pressure and by the falciform ligament, which is formed from the peritoneum that covers the liver. This ligament attaches the liver to the anterior portion of the abdomen between the diaphragm and the umbilicus and also divides the liver into the right and left lobes.

Six times larger than the left lobe, the right lobe has three sections: right lobe proper, caudate lobe, and quadrate lobe. The left lobe has two sections.

The functional unit of the liver is the lobule; each lobe contains numerous lobules. Approximately 1 million lobules form the liver parenchyma. Each lobule comprises rows of hepatic cells held together with connective tissue. Between the rows of hepatic cells are capillaries or sinusoids that are branches of the portal vein and hepatic artery; central to each lobule is an intralobular vein that drains the lobule.

Although sinusoids are a type of capillary, they lack a definite cell wall and are lined with two types of cells: Kupffer's cells (phagocytic cells that belong to the reticuloendothelial system) and some nonphagocytic cells of modified epithelium. Kupffer's cells are significant in that they serve to phagocytose old or defective red blood cells and to detoxify harmful substances.

The liver also contains parenchymal cells or hepatocytes. These cells secrete bile and perform metabolic (not digestive) duties.

Of interest is the liver's ability to regenerate, which is thought to result from the volume of blood supplied to the liver and the proximity of the blood flow to the individual cells. Although factors such as age, hormone levels, and diet may affect the rate, regeneration is believed to occur within 3 weeks; normal function returns within 4 months. Generally, 70% of the liver can be destroyed without manifestation of symptoms.[5]

**Blood Supply.** The liver is unusual in that it receives blood from one artery and one vein. The portal vein supplies nutrient-rich blood from the intestines, pancreas, spleen, stomach, and mesentery. The hepatic artery divides and subdivides to supply oxygenated blood to lobules and cells; it empties into the hepatic vein and the inferior vena cava. Approximately one third of the total cardiac output (i.e., 800 to 1500 ml) is carried to the liver every minute through these two blood vessels.[13]

The portal vein carries the majority of the blood flow (75%) in the liver and branches into the sinusoids to supply each of the lobules. Sinusoids empty blood into the intralobular vein, which ultimately empties into the hepatic vein and the inferior vena cava.

Lymphatic vessels surround the hepatic veins and bile ducts. The lymph drains into these vessels from lymphatic spaces that are located between parenchymal cells. Carcinoma frequently metastasizes to the liver because of the considerable lymphatic and vascular supply.

**Function.** The liver is a complex organ that performs many metabolic and digestive functions. (A detailed discussion of the function of the liver can be found in any physiology textbook.) Briefly, the functions of the liver include bile formation, carbohydrate metabolism, protein metabolism, fat metabolism, steroid metabolism, vitamin storage, coagulation, mineral and water metabolism, and detoxification.

Bile production and secretion are continuous processes within the liver. Components of bile include water, bile salts, bilirubin, cholesterol, fatty acids, and lecithin. The predominant electrolytes present in bile are sodium chloride (145 mEq/L), chloride (100 mEq/L), bicarbonate (28 mEq/L), and potassium and calcium (5 mEq/L, respectively). Bile salts, the most abundant substance secreted into bile, are formed by the liver cells, with cholesterol serving as a precursor; cholesterol is either supplied by the diet or synthesized from fat metabolism.[5,8]

Bile salts function primarily (1) to emulsify fat globules into minute sizes to facilitate digestion and (2) to promote the absorption of lipids (cholesterol and fatty acids) across the intestinal mucosa. Fat absorption is important because when fats are not absorbed adequately, fat-soluble vitamins (A, D, E, and K) are not absorbed adequately. Bile salts also serve as a route to excrete bilirubin, cholesterol, and various hormones (sex, thyroid, and adrenal).[8]

Reabsorption of approximately 94% of the bile salts occurs in the terminal ileum; the reabsorbed salts are returned to the liver through the portal blood.[8] In the liver the bile salts are absorbed into the hepatic cells and then resecreted into the bile. The small amounts of bile salts lost are eliminated in the feces. This recirculation of bile salts, known as the enterohepatic circulation, is essential for maintaining normal daily flow of bile; otherwise the liver would not be able to synthesize enough of the salts to produce the normal amount of bile. The daily volume of bile production averages 600 to 1000 ml.

Bile also serves as a mechanism for excretion of bilirubin from the body. Bilirubin, the primary pigment in bile, is derived from the heme portion of hemoglobin during the degradation of red blood cells by Kupffer's cells. When bilirubin is released into the bloodstream, it combines with albumin to form a fat-soluble, unconjugated (indirect) bilirubin. When indirect bilirubin passes through the liver, the liver cells conjugate it to a water-soluble form (direct bilirubin), which is then excreted into the intestine. Here conversion of direct bilirubin to urobilinogen compounds occurs. Some of this urobilinogen is reabsorbed into the portal blood and recycled, whereas other forms of the urobilinogen compounds are excreted in the feces, thus giving feces their color.

The liver serves an important role in carbohydrate metabolism and storage by synthesizing glycogen (the stored form of glucose) from glucose, protein, fat, or lactic acid. Glycogen is then broken down as necessary and released by the liver to maintain normal blood glucose levels.

The liver has a vital role in protein synthesis and amino acid metabolism. Through a complex process amino acids can be formed from the metabolites of carbohydrates and fat. Plasma proteins important for maintaining normal serum osmotic pressure and blood clotting (such as prothrombin, factors V, VII, VIII, IX, and X, fibrogen, albumin, transferrin, and hepatoglobin) also are synthesized by the liver. Finally, the liver breaks down amino acids, thus producing ketoacids and ammonia. From these substances urea is formed, which is excreted in the urine.

Fat metabolism continues in the liver and involves conversion of triglycerides to glycerol and fatty acids, a process called *ketogenesis*. Synthesis of fat substances such as cholesterol, phospholipids, and lipoproteins also occurs in the liver.

Steroid metabolism is another function of the liver. Adrenocorticosteroids, glucocorticosteroids, testosterone, and aldosterone are metabolized and catabolized by the liver.

Vitamins such as $B_{12}$, $B_1$, riboflavin, $B_2$, nicotinic acid, pyridoxine, D, E, K, and A are stored in the liver. Bile and bile salts are required for vitamin D and K absorption to occur.

Coagulation is an extremely complex process that is influenced and regulated by the liver. Prothrombin, fibrinogen, and heparin are produced by the liver. Vitamin K, however, is necessary for the synthesis of prothrombin, and absorption of vitamin K across the intestinal mucosa requires the presence of bile salts. The liver also disposes of disintegrating red blood cells.

The liver functions to metabolize minerals and water. Ferritin, the storage form of iron, is stored primarily in the liver. Copper, calcium, magnesium, zinc, manganese, and cobalt also are stored in the liver.

Finally, the liver serves a unique function of detoxification of foreign and toxic substances. For example, certain medications are detoxified and excreted in the urine, whereas other medications (such as morphine and atropine) are stored to be released at a later time into the circulation. Kupffer's cells also serve to protect the body by phagocytosis of viruses, bacteria, dyes, and foreign proteins.

## Biliary System

**Structure.** The biliary system consists of the gallbladder and the biliary ductal system, which provide a passageway for bile from the liver to the intestine (Fig. 9-6). On a daily basis the liver produces an average of 600 to 1000 ml of fluid with a pH of 7.5. This liver bile, when produced, is golden or orange-yellow. When concentrated in the gallbladder, this fluid becomes tenacious and a dark golden brown; the pH decreases to below 7.

The duct system consists of two hepatic ducts that drain the liver and the cystic duct that drains the gallbladder. These converge to form the common bile duct. The common bile duct empties into the duodenum at Vater's ampulla. The sphincter of Oddi surrounds Vater's ampulla to control the flow of bile into the duodenum.

The gallbladder is a pear-shaped organ that lies on the underside of the liver (Fig. 9-6). It is approximately 7 to 10 cm long and 2.5 to 3.5 cm wide, with a capacity of 60 ml of bile.

**Blood Supply and Innervation.** The hepatic artery and cystic artery supply blood to the gallbladder. Venous drainage occurs via the cystic vein. Lymphatic drainage is abundant.

Innervation of the gallbladder is provided by the sympathetic (splanchnic) system and the parasympathetic (vagus) system. Sympathetic stimulation inhibits biliary smooth-muscle contraction; vagal stimulation causes contraction of the gallbladder and relaxation of Oddi's sphincter.

**Function.** The primary function of the gallbladder is to collect, concentrate, acidify, and store bile until it is needed for digestion. Normally the sphincter of Oddi is closed during fasting and between meals. During this time the continuous bile production by the liver increases pressure within this closed system so that as bile is passed into the hepatic ducts, it is forced into the cystic duct to be stored in the relaxed gallbladder (Fig. 9-6). Once in the gallbladder, concentration of the bile begins to occur.

Emptying of the gallbladder and the passage of bile into the duodenum therefore depend on the tone of Oddi's sphincter. This tone is influenced by the hormone cholecystokinin, which is released in response to the presence of fats in chyme. Anticholinergic agents decrease the tone of the gallbladder and Oddi's sphincter, whereas epinephrine and cholinergic drugs produce contraction of the gallbladder and stimulate of Oddi's sphincter. Sight, smell, and taste of food may stimulate the gallbladder; however, emotional states such as fear or excitement may decrease the flow of bile.

## SUMMARY

The normal anatomy and physiology of the GI tract establish the foundation for understanding alterations in function and anticipating normal function after surgical resection of any of its segments. The function of the GI tract is complex and interrelated; one part cannot be removed or altered without affecting another part of the tract. The nurse's understanding and anticipation of problems that can arise when the GI anatomy and physiology are altered are vital to providing good patient care.

# SELF-EVALUATION

## QUESTIONS

1. Which of the following organs is critical to life and health?
   a. Stomach
   b. Small bowel
   c. Ileocecal valve
   d. Large intestine
2. Identify the four layers of the intestinal wall, from inside to outside.
3. Describe the structure and function of the intramural plexus.
4. Which of the following is the most important function of the structures and secretions of the mouth?
   a. Mechanical breakdown of food particles
   b. Initiation of carbohydrate digestion
   c. Initiation of protein digestion
   d. Initiation of fat digestion
5. Match the daily volume of secretions to the appropriate organ:

   | | |
   |---|---|
   | a. Salivary glands | 1. 800 ml |
   | b. Stomach | 2. 1200 ml |
   | c. Small intestine | 3. 2000 ml |
   | d. Colon | 4. 3000 ml |
   | e. Pancreas | 5. None |
   | f. Biliary tree | 6. 1000 to 1500 ml |

6. Swallowing is initiated voluntarily but is completed on a reflex basis.
   a. True
   b. False
7. Explain the purpose of the pharyngoesophageal and the esophagogastric sphincters.
8. Explain why a transmural inflammatory process may cause a generalized inflammation of the peritoneum (peritonitis).
9. Explain the relationship between the mesentery and the peritoneum.
10. Identify two mechanisms that help to protect the gastric and duodenal mucosa from the ulcerating effects of gastric secretions.
11. Which of the following has a stimulant effect on gastric secretion?
    a. Duodenal distention
    b. Highly acidic duodenal contents
    c. Caffeine
    d. Fear
12. Briefly describe the five functions of the stomach.
13. Which of the following is known to *slow* the rate of gastric emptying?
    a. High-fat meal
    b. Liquid meal
    c. Carbohydrate meal
    d. Cholinergic medications (e.g., metoclopramide)

14. The absorptive surface of the small bowel is tremendously increased by which of the following?
    a. Villi
    b. Rugae
    c. Peyer's patches
    d. Taenia coli

15. The small intestine plays an important role in maintenance of fluid-electrolyte balance.
    a. True
    b. False

16. Blood flow for most of the small intestine is provided by the:
    a. Superior mesenteric artery
    b. Inferior mesenteric artery
    c. Celiac artery
    d. Portal artery

17. The major function of the duodenum is:
    a. Absorption of nutrients
    b. Neutralization of chyme
    c. Digestion of proteins
    d. Secretion of intrinsic factor

18. Most nutrients, vitamins, and minerals are absorbed in the:
    a. Ileum
    b. Duodenum
    c. Jejunum
    d. Cecum

19. Explain the impact of massive ileal resection on absorption of vitamin $B_{12}$.

20. Describe the structure and purpose of the ileocecal valve.

21. Explain the effects of the taeniae coli on the colon wall and implications for construction of loop colostomies.

22. The colonic mucosa contains villi and provides significant absorption of nutrients.
    a. True
    b. False

23. Which of the following is *not* a function of the anaerobic bacteria found in the colon?
    a. Synthesis of folic acid and some vitamins
    b. Breakdown of indigestible residue
    c. Production of intestinal gas
    d. Production of colonic mucus

24. Total colonic length in the adult averages:
    a. 5 to 6 feet
    b. 20 to 22 feet
    c. 2 to 4 feet
    d. 10 to 12 feet

25. Explain the significance of valves of Houston.

26. The rectum normally is empty.
    a. True
    b. False

**27.** Differentiation among gas, liquid, and solid is provided by sensory receptors located in the:
    **a.** Rectal wall
    **b.** Anal canal proximal to the dentate line
    **c.** Anal canal distal to the dentate line (anoderm)
    **d.** All of the above

**28.** Which of the following accurately describes the response of the anal sphincters to rectal distention?
    **a.** The internal sphincter contracts; the external sphincter relaxes.
    **b.** The internal sphincter relaxes; the external sphincter contracts.
    **c.** Both sphincters relax.
    **d.** Both sphincters contract.

**29.** "Mass movements" occur primarily in the left colon and are responsible for propelling the fecal bolus into the rectum.
    **a.** True
    **b.** False

**30.** Briefly describe the endocrine and exocrine functions of the pancreas.

**31.** The liver is capable of regeneration.
    **a.** True
    **b.** False

**32.** List the key functions of the liver.

**33.** The gallbladder's primary function is the collection, acidification, concentration, and storage of bile.
    **a.** True
    **b.** False

# SELF-EVALUATION
## ANSWERS

1. **b.** Small bowel
2. Four layers of intestinal wall:
      Mucosa
      Submucosa
      Muscularis
      Serosa, or adventitia
3. Meissner's plexus, located in the submucosal layer, and Auerbach's plexus, located in the muscularis, are jointly known as the intramural plexus. It is composed of nerve cell bodies and nerve fibers, or processes; the nerve fibers originate in receptor cells located in the bowel wall. These receptors are sensitive to local stimuli, such as stretch. The intramural plexus is the *primary* mediator of intestinal secretion and motility. Autonomic nerve fibers synapse on nerve cells in the intramural plexus and serve to modify its response, but autonomic stimulation is not critical to intestinal secretion or motility.
4. **a.** Mechanical breakdown of food particles
5. Volume of secretions:
      **a.** Salivary glands: 1000 to 1500 ml (*6*)
      **b.** Stomach: 2000 ml (*3*)
      **c.** Small intestine: 3000 ml (*4*)
      **d.** Colon: None (*5*)
      **e.** Pancreas: 1200 ml (*2*)
      **f.** Biliary tree: 800 ml (*1*)
6. **a.** True
7. The pharyngoesophageal sphincter prevents reflux of food and fluid from the esophagus into the mouth; the esophagogastric sphincter prevents reflux from the stomach into the esophagus.
8. The outer layer of the bowel wall, the serosa, is continuous with the visceral peritoneum, which covers abdominal organs. Inflammation of the serosa may spread to involve the peritoneal structures.
9. The mesentery is a double layer of peritoneum that encircles most of the small intestine and anchors it to the posterior abdominal wall. The mesentery is a vital support structure because it contains the blood vessels and nerves that nourish and innervate the bowel.
10. Two mechanisms:
      The surface membranes of the mucosal cells and the tight junctions between the mucosal cells
      Blanket of viscous and alkaline mucus that coats the mucosal surface
11. **c.** Caffeine
12. Five functions of the stomach:
      The stomach serves as a reservoir for ingested nutrients and provides controlled emptying into the duodenum.
      The stomach begins enzymatic digestion of proteins. The parietal cells produce HCl acid, which converts pepsinogen (secreted by the chief cells) into pepsin. Pepsin is a proteolytic enzyme.

The parietal cells secrete intrinsic factor, which is essential for absorption of vitamin $B_{12}$.

The stomach provides for limited absorption: some carbohydrates, alcohol, some medications.

The low pH of the stomach eliminates most of the ingested bacteria.

**13. a.** High-fat meal

**14. a.** Villi

**15. a.** True

**16. a.** Superior mesenteric artery

**17. b.** Neutralization of chyme

**18. c.** Jejunum

**19.** Absorptive sites for vitamin $B_{12}$ are located only in the terminal ileum. Significant ileal resection places the individual at risk for pernicious anemia and may necessitate life-long replacement of vitamin $B_{12}$.

**20.** The ileocecal valve is a one-way valve located at the junction between the ileum and the large intestine; it serves to regulate emptying into the large intestine and to prevent reflux of colon contents back into the small intestine.

**21.** The taeniae coli are three muscle bands that create sacculations in the colon wall known as haustrations. If a loop colostomy is opened parallel to the taeniae, the natural haustrations create two separate openings, one proximal and one distal; this separation provides almost complete diversion of the fecal stream.

**22. b.** False

**23. d.** Production of colonic mucus

**24. a.** 5 to 6 feet

**25.** The valves of Houston are three folds located in the rectum, two on the left and one on the right; they serve as landmarks and must be carefully negotiated during proctoscopic examination.

**26. a.** True

**27. c.** Anal canal distal to the dentate line (anoderm)

**28. b.** The internal sphincter relaxes; the external sphincter contracts.

**29. a.** True

**30.** *Endocrine:* Production of insulin, glucagon, somatostatin, and pancreatic polypeptide hormone

*Exocrine:* Secretion of pancreatic juices containing water, bicarbonate, and digestive enzymes. Acidic chyme stimulates production of fluid rich in bicarbonate and low in digestive enzymes. Chyme that contains significant amounts of protein and fat stimulates production of fluid rich in enzymes and bicarbonate.

**31. a.** True

**32.** Liver functions:

Bile formation
Carbohydrate, protein, and fat metabolism
Steroid metabolism
Vitamin storage
Coagulation
Mineral and water metabolism
Detoxification

**33. a.** True

## REFERENCES

1. Boarini J, Bryant R, Kennedy-Caldwell C: Anatomy and physiology of the digestive system. In Thelan L, Davie J, Urden L: *Textbook of critical care nursing: diagnosis and management*, St Louis, 1990, Mosby–Year Book.
2. Broadwell D: Gastrointestinal system. In Thompson JM et al, editors: *Mosby's manual of clinical nursing*, ed 2, St Louis, 1989, Mosby–Year Book.
3. Ganong WF: *Review of medical physiology*, ed 11, Los Altos, Calif, 1983, Lange Medical Publications.
4. Gantt L, Thompson C: Short gut syndrome in the infant, *Am J Nurs* 85:1263, 1985.
5. Given BA, Simmons SJ: *Gastroenterology in clinical nursing*, ed 4, St Louis, 1984, Mosby–Year Book.
6. Goldberg SM, Gordon PH, Nivatvongs S: *Essentials of anorectal surgery*, Philadelphia, 1980, JB Lippincott.
7. Greenberger, INJ: *Gastrointestinal disorders: a pathophysiologic approach*, ed 4, Chicago, 1986, Mosby–Year Book.
8. Guyton AC: *Textbook of medical physiology*, ed 6, Philadelphia, 1981, WB Saunders.
9. Kirsner JB, Shorter RG, editors: *Diseases of the colon, rectum, and anal canal*, Baltimore, 1988, Williams & Wilkins.
10. Murray N, Vanderhoof J: Short bowel syndrome in children and adults, *J Enterostom Ther* 14(4):168, 1987.
11. Rothenberger D: Anatomy and physiology related to continence and defecation. In Doughty D, editor: *Urinary and fecal incontinence: nursing management*, St Louis, 1991, Mosby–Year Book.
12. Seeley R, Stephens T, Tate P: *Anatomy and physiology*, ed 2, St Louis, 1991, Mosby–Year Book.
13. Thelan L, Davie J, Urden L: *Textbook of critical care nursing: diagnosis and management*, St Louis, 1990, Mosby–Year Book.

# 10 Pathophysiology and Diagnostic Studies of Gastrointestinal Tract Disorders

RUTH A. BRYANT
JOHN G. BULS

## OBJECTIVES

1. Describe the normal embryonic development that, when interrupted, results in Hirschsprung's disease, anorectal malformation, or malrotation.

2. Differentiate among the clinical presentation of:
   Hirschsprung's disease and meconium ileus
   Low anorectal malformation and high anorectal malformation
   Ulcerative colitis and Crohn's disease
   Diverticular disease and diverticulosis
   Necrotizing enterocolitis and malrotation

3. State the key diagnostic test for each of the following diseases:
   Hirschsprung's disease
   Anorectal malformation
   Colorectal cancer
   Familial adenomatous polyposis
   Necrotizing enterocolitis
   Volvulus
   Pseudomembranous colitis

4. Describe how the following diseases are identified:
   Extrahepatic biliary atresia
   Ulcerative colitis
   Crohn's disease
   Ischemic bowel disease

5. Distinguish among the following terms:
   Dynamic obstruction
   Adynamic obstruction
   Closed loop obstruction

6. State at least five risk factors for the development of colorectal adenocarcinoma.

7. Compare and contrast four gastrointestinal polyposis syndromes.

8. Compare and contrast the pathologic features of Crohn's disease and ulcerative colitis.

9. Describe at least four extraintestinal manifestations that may be present in the patient with ulcerative colitis and in the patient with familial adenomatous polyposis.

10. Define the categories in the modified Duke's colorectal cancer classification scheme.

11. Discriminate between signs and symptoms of a right colonic tumor and left colonic, or sigmoid, tumor.

12. Describe the current theory for the cause of necrotizing enterocolitis and one of the theories for the cause of inflammatory bowel disease.

13. Identify four classes of medications that may be used to manage ulcerative colitis and Crohn's disease; include their intended actions and side effects.

14. Describe the surgical treatment of extrahepatic biliary atresia and associated complications.

15. Compare the surgical treatment of the following disease processes:
    Hirschsprung's disease and necrotizing enterocolitis
    High and low anorectal malformations
    Ulcerative colitis and familial adenomatous polyposis
    Crohn's disease and ulcerative colitis
    Toxic megacolon and pseudomembranous colitis
    A 3-cm rectal carcinoma and an 8-cm rectal carcinoma

Several types of disorders occur that may require surgical creation of an intestinal stoma for either palliation or cure. These diseases vary from familiar processes such as adenocarcinoma in the adult to less familiar congenital diseases. In each case, surgical construction of the stoma is but one component of management. This chapter deals with the epidemiologic, pathologic, and clinical manifestations, diagnosis, and treatment of gastrointestinal (GI) disorders that may require intestinal diversion.

## CONGENITAL DISORDERS

The neonate with a congenital disorder of the lower GI tract (small intestine, colon, and rectum) often requires a diversion of the GI tract. For most infants these diversions are temporary, and the defect can be repaired as the infant grows. The majority of these congenital diseases are detected in the first few days of life and present life-threatening complications in the neonate. Hirschsprung's disease, anorectal malformations, and malrotation are the congenital anomalies discussed in this section.

### Hirschsprung's Disease

Hirschsprung's disease, originally described more than a century ago, occurs in approximately 1/5000 live births and is a major cause of intestinal obstruction in the neonate.[58] It affects all races but is less common in black persons. It appears to be autosomal recessive and sex linked; males are affected in greater number than females, approximately 4:1.[32,58]

**Pathophysiology.** Hirschsprung's disease, which is the absence of ganglion cells in the distal intestine, results in abnormal innervation of the bowel segment. Specifically, ganglion cells fail to develop in Auerbach's plexus (between the circular and longitudinal muscle), Henle's plexus (along the inner margin of the circular muscle), and Meissner's plexus (immediately beneath the muscularis mucosa). This aganglionosis of the intestinal wall always involves the internal anal sphincter and extends proximally from the anorectum for a variable distance. In about 80% of patients the lesion is limited to the rectum and sigmoid (referred to as *short-segment disease*). An additional 10% have more proximal involvement, with variable lengths of the colon affected (*long-segment disease*). The remaining 10% have total colonic aganglionosis (the absence of ganglion cells in the entire colon and for a variable extent of the small bowel).[4,47,49] Rarely is the entire GI tract affected.

Because normal peristalsis cannot occur in the aganglionic segment of bowel, a functional obstruction develops at the level of transition between normal and abnormal bowel. This obstruction produces a grossly dilated and hypertrophied proximal normal bowel, resulting in megacolon. A paradoxic appearance develops in that the abnormal aganglionic segment of bowel looks normal (i.e., collapsed and empty), whereas the normally innervated bowel actually appears abnormal (i.e., dilated and hypertrophied). The junction between the dilated, normally innervated proximal bowel and the distal aganglionic segment of bowel is cone-shaped and known as the *transition zone of narrowing* (TZN).

**Clinical Manifestations.** An increased awareness of this disease has now made it possible to establish the diagnosis of Hirschsprung's disease in the vast majority of neonates within the first week of life. Within the first 24 hours of birth, the healthy infant should spontaneously evacuate meconium. Therefore delayed passage or failure to pass meconium within the first 24 hours of life should alert the health care team to the possibility of the disease. The newborn also may manifest symptoms of intestinal obstruction such as bilious vomiting and abdominal distention. Hirschsprung's disease precipitates approximately 25% of the cases of neonatal intestinal obstruction.[32]

The diagnosis of Hirschsprung's disease in some patients is delayed. Although most are established within about 4 years after birth, in some the diagnosis is not established until adult life, although this delay is rare. The hallmark of Hirschsprung's disease in the older infant, child, or adult is chronic, intractible constipation that is unresponsive to medications or diet.[61] Bowel habits, however, are irregular. Although many days may pass between bowel movements, stool consistency can range from hard and pelletlike to pasty to voluminous, foul-smelling liquid. On digital examination the rectal vault is empty and the anal sphincter is tight.

A wide variety of anomalies (cardiovascular, limb, GI, and skeletal) have been reported to occur with Hirschsprung's disease. The two anomalies, however, that occur with greatest frequency are Down syndrome, which is reported in 5% to 10% of the infants, and urologic anomalies, which are noted in approximately 3% of the infants.[4,58] In addition, as many as 33% of the infants may have urologic complications that develop as a consequence of the fecal impaction compressing the urinary tract. These urologic complications include vesicoureteral reflux, hydronephrosis, and bladder dysfunction.[58]

**Diagnosis.** The definitive diagnosis of Hirschsprung's disease is established on histologic examination: histologically a rectal biopsy specimen is obtained to determine the presence or absence of ganglion cells in the bowel wall. In the child younger than 2 years of age, biopsy can be performed easily with a suction method, thereby avoiding the need for anesthesia or sedation. Because specimens obtained through suction generally are superficial (limited to the mucosa and submucosal tissue), the risk of perforation is minimal. In the child older than 2 years, rectal biopsy is best approached by means of a forceps so that a full-thickness specimen of the bowel wall can be obtained. Because the ganglion cells present in the TZN of the anal canal are scattered, specimens should be taken 2 to 3 cm above the dentate line to enhance accuracy.

Barium enema radiographs are helpful to diagnose Hirschsprung's disease in the older child. However, to avoid dilation of the narrowed aganglionic distal bowel, thereby rendering the TZN unrecognizable, the barium enema should be performed *without* cleansing the bowel and with use of a soft rubber catheter (not a balloon) to instill the barium. A normal result from examination does not rule out the disease, because a 20% false-negative rate is reported with contrast radiographs.[61] The classic radiographic appearance shows the distal bowel to be of a normal caliber for varying lengths, with the bowel most proximal to the TZN quite dilated, often containing large boluses of stool.

Anorectal manometry, a simple test that measures the anal sphincter pressure and demonstrates the anorectal reflex, may be conducted to *exclude* Hirschsprung's disease. When Hirschsprung's disease is limited to a short segment of bowel, anorectal manometry is more reliable than a barium enema examination. This test consists of positioning a probe (rectal balloon and transducer) in the anal canal at the level of the internal sphincter. As the rectal balloon is inflated, an anorectal response is elicited. Normally the anorectal response is relaxation of the internal sphincter, a response that excludes the diagnosis of Hirschsprung's disease. The failure of the internal sphincter to relax in response to rectal distention, however, cannot be used to confirm a diagnosis of Hirschsprung's disease.

**Management.** The treatment goals for Hirschsprung's disease are to provide prompt relief of the intestinal obstruction and, at a later date, to restore bowel function without interfering in bowel continence. These two goals are accomplished by using a staged surgical approach whereby the aganglionic bowel is first by-passed with an intestinal stoma. Most often this diversion is a loop right transverse colostomy. However, to ascertain that the colostomy is in fact located proximal to the aganglionic bowel, seromuscular biopsy specimens must be obtained intraoperatively at the TZN. If the TZN is not readily apparent, serial specimens must be obtained at progressively proximal intervals until normal ganglionic bowel is identified. The colostomy is closed after performing definitive surgery.

Definitive surgery (resection of the aganglionic segment) is delayed until the infant is 9 to 12 months of age or older. In the case of the older child or adult, definitive surgery is delayed for approximately 3 months after stoma construction. This waiting period is important because it provides time for the dilated and hypertrophied segment of bowel to return to a normal state, thus facilitating corrective surgery.

Options for definitive surgery include the Swenson, Duhamel, and Soave procedures.[58] The Swenson procedure (Fig. 10-1) first requires an abdominal approach to free the aganglionic segment and rectum down through the levator ani muscle until the perineal floor is reached. A small incision is made in the ganglionic bowel to serve as a marker identifying the TZN. From the perineal approach the colon is grasped and the rectum everted (intussuscepted) to exit through the anal opening. An incision is made through the anterior wall of the everted anal canal slightly above the dentate line. (To preserve sphincter control, anastomosis must be proximal to this line.) Through this anterior incision the proximal colon is extracted up to the marker that indicates normal bowel. Working at the anterior incision, the surgeon anastomoses normal proximal colon to the anterior portion of the

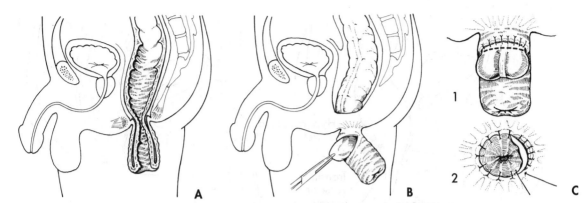

**Fig. 10-1** Swenson procedure for Hirschsprung's disease. **A,** Proximal bowel intussuscepted and exteriorized through anal opening. **B,** Proximal bowel pulled through anterior anal canal incision made slightly above dentate line, and anterior shared seromuscular layers anastomosed. **C,** Posterior half of aganglionic bowel resected completely, remainder of anastomosis completed, and ganglionic bowel returned to proper position in pelvis. (Modified from Spitz L: Hirschsprung's disease and anorectal anomalies. In Schwartz SI, Ellis H, editors: *Maingot's abdominal operations,* vol 2, ed 9, Norwalk, Conn, 1989, Appleton & Lange.)

**Fig. 10-2** Duhamel procedure for Hirschsprung's disease. Aganglionic colon has been resected, leaving distal rectum isolated from normal proximal colon. Normal proximal colon is brought down behind rectal wall. Common wall between the rectum and proximal bowel is severed, creating neorectum with aganglionic anterior wall and ganglionic posterior wall. (Modified from Spitz L: Hirschsprung's disease and anorectal anomalies. In Schwarts SI, Ellis H, editors: *Maingot's abdominal operations,* vol 2, ed 9, Norwalk, Conn, 1989, Appleton & Lange.)

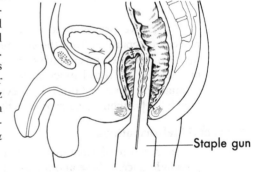

anal canal. Next the posterior half of the rectum is severed, thus leaving the aganglionic segment of bowel completely separated from normal bowel. Anastomosis of the normal proximal colon to the posterior anal canal can now be completed and the anal canal replaced in the pelvis. This procedure has been described as technically difficult because of the tedious dissection; the entire aganglionic segment of bowel is eliminated.

The Duhamel procedure (Fig. 10-2) is a rectrorectal pull-through technique by means of both an abdominal and a perineal approach but avoiding the tedious dissection required in the Swenson procedure. Basically the normal proximal colon is dissected, separating it from the diseased rectum. The normal proximal colon is brought down to the anus behind the diseased rectum. The common wall between the two segments is then eliminated, thus creating a new rectum. The anterior wall of the new rectum is aganglionic, whereas the posterior wall is ganglionic.

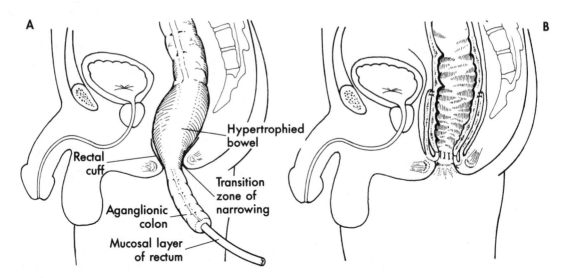

**Fig. 10-3** Soave procedure for Hirschsprung's disease. **A,** Dissected mucosal layers of rectum with attached aganglionic proximal bowel are pulled out through anal opening up to level of normal bowel or TZN. **B,** Normal proximal bowel anastomosed to seromuscular rectal cuff at dentate line. (Modified from Spitz L: Hirschsprung's disease and anorectal anomalies. In Schwartz SI, Ellis H, editors: *Maingot's abdominal operations,* vol 2, ed 9, Norwalk, Conn, 1989, Appleton & Lange.)

The Soave procedure (Fig. 10-3) is an endorectal pull-through technique in which mucosa is separated from the seromuscular layers of the rectum; the seromuscular layer of the rectum is then severed from the same layers of the proximal colon to create a rectal cuff of muscle. The rectal mucosal layer and attached proximal colon are then pulled down through the rectal cuff until the previously marked normal bowel is identified. Normal proximal bowel is then anastomosed to the dentate line and also tacked down to the rectal cuff.

### Anorectal Malformations

Anorectal malformations occur in approximately 1/5000 live births, with a slight male preponderance.[4] These anomalies encompass a wide variety of defects, often are associated with other major congenital disorders, and provide the most common cause of intestinal obstruction in the newborn.[59] An international classification scheme for anorectal malformations is listed in Table 10-1. Also referred to as *imperforate anus,* anorectal malformations are classified according to the position of the terminal bowel to the puborectalis muscle[56] (Fig. 10-4). Lesions that terminate above the pelvic floor musculature are considered high or supralevator anomalies and require extensive corrective surgery. Low anomalies lie below the pelvic musculature and can be repaired by a local perineal operative procedure. Intermediate anomalies are somewhere between these two extremes.

**Pathophysiology.** The embryologic changes that result in anorectal abnormalities are varied and complex. Although an in-depth discussion of embryology is beyond the scope of this text, a brief overview of fetal development is helpful in understanding the anatomy of these anorectal defects.

**Table 10-1**   Classification of anorectal anomalies

| Male | Female |
|---|---|
| A.  Low (translevator) | |
|     1.  *At normal anal site* | 1.  *At normal anal site* |
|         a.  Anal stenosis |     a.  Anal stenosis |
|         b.  Covered anus, complete |     b.  Covered anus, complete |
|     2.  *At perineal site* | 2.  *At perineal site* |
|         a.  Anocutaneous fistula (covered anus, incomplete) |     a.  Anocutaneous fistula (covered anus, incomplete) |
|         b.  Anterior perineal anus |     b.  Anterior perineal anus |
| | 3.  *At vulvar site* |
| |     a.  Anovulvar fistula |
| |     b.  Anovestibular fistula |
| |     c.  Vestibular anus |
| B.  Intermediate | |
|     1.  *Anal agenesis* | 1.  *Anal agenesis* |
|         a.  Without fistula |     a.  Without fistula |
|         b.  With rectobulbar fistula |     b.  With fistula |
| |         i.  Rectovestibula |
| |         ii.  Rectovaginal, low |
|     2.  *Anorectal stenosis* | 2.  *Anorectal stenosis* |
| C.  High (supralevator) | |
|     1.  *Anorectal agenesis* | 1.  *Anorectal agenesis* |
|         a.  Without fistula |     a.  Without fistula |
|         b.  With fistula |     b.  With fistula |
|         i.  Rectourethral |         i.  Rectovaginal, high |
|         ii.  Rectovesical |         ii.  Rectocloacal |
| |         iii.  Rectovesical |
|     2.  *Rectal atresia* | 2.  *Rectal atresia* |
| D.  Miscellaneous | |
|     Imperforate anal membrane | |
|     Cloacal exstrophy | |

From Berry CL, Keeling JW: Gastrointestinal system. In Berry CL, editor: *Paediatric pathology*, ed 2, New York, 1989, Springer-Verlag.

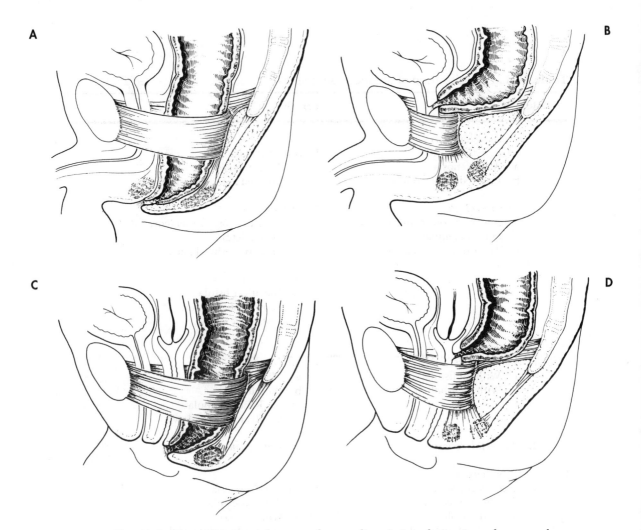

**Fig. 10-4**   Common types of anorectal anomalies. **A,** Low lesion in male: covered anus with or without anocutaneous fistula. **B,** High lesion in the male: anorectal agenesis with rectourethral fistula. **C,** Low lesion in female: ectopic anus with anovulvar or anovestibular fistula. **D,** High lesion in female: anorectal agenesis with rectovaginal fistula. (Modified from Spitz L: Hirschsprung's disease and anorectal anomalies. In Schwartz SI, Ellis H, editors: *Maingot's abdominal operations,* vol 2, ed 9, Norwalk, Conn, 1989, Appleton & Lange.)

In the embryo the cloaca serves as a common posterior cavity for the rudimentary structures that later formulate the GU tract and the intestinal tract (see Fig. 7-1). The cloaca is covered with a cloacal membrane. Between the fourth and sixth weeks of gestation, separation of the GU and GI tracts begins by the development of a urorectal septum. The developing urorectal septum follows a cephalid to caudal progression. As the urorectal septum develops, the cloacal membrane becomes invaginated into the perineum and atrophies once the urorectal septum formation is complete. At this point a common orifice is established for the urinary and genital tracts; likewise the anal orifice also is established. Finally, the urogenital tract begins to differentiate into male or female genital structures, and the anus migrates in a posterior fashion away from the developing urogenital tract.[32,35,58]

High or supralevator anorectal anomalies appear to be the result of a failure of the normal development of the urorectal septum in the embryo. In these defects the terminal bowel either ends in a blind pouch above the muscular floor of the pelvis or as a fistula into the bladder, vagina, cloaca, or the male urethra. Most often the anal opening is not present, such as with anorectal agenesis. Rarely the anal canal is present but does not connect with the terminal rectum (rectal atresia). Severe bowel obstruction commonly accompanies high anorectal anomalies.

Low or translevator anomalies are believed to result from irregularities in the normal migration of the anus and from irregularities in the development of genital folds. The rectum has developed normally and has descended properly through the pelvic musculature. However, the anal opening is abnormal. The anal opening may be properly placed but stenotic or it can be ectopic (e.g., opening at a perineal or a vulvar site). These defects are less serious than are high anomalies.

Intermediate anomalies consists of anal agenesis (rectum normal but anal opening is either absent or ectopic, so it communicates as a fistula low within the male urethra or female vagina) and anorectal stenosis. Because anorectal stenosis involves stenosis of a portion of the rectum in addition to the anus, it is important to distinguish this condition from anal stenosis.[35] Intermediate anorectal malformations typically are managed as if they were high anomalies to preserve structures important for continence.

The cause of these abnormalities is totally unknown, and to date no specific agent or agents can be incriminated. There appears to be no relationship to maternal age, parity, or family history.

Many different congenital anomalies accompany anorectal malformations. Anomalies in the lower portion of the urinary system are the most common and include vesicoureteral reflux, ectopic ureters, and vesicoureteral obstruction. Urogenital anomalies are present in almost 50% of the infants with high anorectal malformations and 20% of the infants with low anorectal malformations.[58] Cardiovascular anomalies also may be present and include ventricular septal defects and tetralogy of Fallot.

The acronym *VACTERL* reflects a syndrome of coexisting congenital anomalies, with anorectal malformations among the disorders.[60] *Vertebral defects occur predominantly in the sacral vertebrae, such as sacral agenesis and missing or deformed vertebrae. *Anorectal deformities include the numerous types of malformations already discussed. *Cardiovascular anomalies, as previously mentioned, may exist. *Tracheoesophageal defects refer predominantly to a tracheoesophageal fistula. *Esophageal atresia occurs in approximately 5% of the infants (with or without tracheoesophageal fistulas).[58] *Renal defects include renal dysplasia, hydronephrosis, and unilateral renal agenesis. *Limb defects may include webbed fingers or missing digits.

**Diagnosis.** Careful physical examination provides the data necessary to diagnose anorectal malformation in a majority of cases. Contrast studies such as fistulograms, however, may be performed to define the lesion more precisely.

Radiologic investigation can be quite informative regarding the level of the anorectal malformation in relation to the puborectalis muscle and is easily accomplished in the neonate. Because swallowed gas usually passes distally into the rectum within 6 to 12 hours after birth, a lateral radiograph of the pelvis of the inverted infant (i.e., an invertogram) can be taken and the position of intestinal gas in the terminal bowel ascertained. A radiopaque marker (barium paste) is applied to the anal site externally. With the infant in an upside down or prone position for 3 to 5 minutes, the meconium in the distal bowl is displaced by the gas. The distance from the distal bowel (as displayed by the gas shadow) to the skin of the perineum (as marked by the barium) can then be measured. A distance of less than 2 cm indicates a low malformation; distances of greater than 2 cm indicate supralevator malformation.

Errors do arise with the use of the invertogram to determine the level of the malformation.[49] The result may be misinterpreted as a high lesion (1) when the examination is conducted too early after birth so that the gas has not passed through the intestinal tract and (2) when the meconium is impacted into the distal bowel. Finally, because the infant's crying during the examination may depress the levator ani muscles, a high malformation may falsely appear to be a low lesion.

Magnetic resonance imaging and ultrasonography can be used to visualize the distal bowel in relation to the pelvic musculature and to avoid the aforementioned problems.[49] These two tests may have an advantage over the barium radiographs in that they also provide information about the status of the commonly affected GU system.

**Management.** One of the primary concerns at all times in the treatment of anorectal malformations is to preserve normal bowel control as much as possible. Therefore the precise anatomy of the lesion must be established on radiographic examination before surgical manipulation. Ultimately, surgical correction should create an anal opening and position the neoanus appropriately in the perineum so that maximum continence is possible.[58]

Low lesions should be managed with a local anoplasty without delay; high and intermediate lesions require a staged operation. If the level of the lesion remains in doubt after extensive diagnostic testing, initially the lesion should be managed as a high lesion to avoid muscle or nerve damage, thus preserving continence. A diverting colostomy is created once the level of imperforation is determined. Occasionally the rectovaginal fistula opening may be of adequate caliber to allow passage of stool; thus the need for a colostomy is delayed. Once the infant is older (6 to 12 months of age or older), definitive surgical correction is conducted. This delay is important to allow the pelvis to enlarge and the pelvic musculature (structures providing continence) to develop.[22] The colostomy is then closed during a third operation.

Surgical correction of the high anorectal deformity is accomplished with a pull-through procedure. Either the sacroabdominoperineral endorectal pull-through or the posterior sagittal anorectoplasty is used; the latter is more common. With the posterior sagittal anorectoplasty a perineal incision is made and the fistula identified so that after careful mobilization the fistula communication can be closed. The rectum is now further mobilized and repositioned anterior to the levator mechanism so that the rectum is surrounded by the striated muscle complex (thus external sphincter mechanism). The new anal opening is created. Anal dilations commonly are needed to maintain adequate patency. These are initiated 2 weeks after the anorectoplasty and continued for several months.[58] Reports on bowel control are varied. Incontinence or constipation has been reported and should be kept in mind, particularly during the bowel-training years.

## Malrotation

Malrotation is any abnormality in the rotation of the midgut and fixation of mesentery that occurs during fetal development. Severe complications, although rare, can result.

**Pathophysiology.** During fetal development the gut progresses through two stages. The first stage occurs when the midgut actually leaves the abdominal cavity and is extruded into the umbilical cord, creating a physiologic hernia. This temporary extrusion occurs because the gut develops at such a rate that it is too large to be contained within the abdominal cavity. The second stage occurs when the gut migrates in an orderly fashion to return to the abdominal cavity. In the process of returning, segments of the gut that become the colon and duodenojejunal loop rotate.

Deformities develop that can be categorized according to the stage within which they occurred.[59] Malrotations that occur during stage 1 result in an omphalocele (also termed an *exomphalos*). The umbilical hernia of extruded bowel that normally occurs in utero persists. Bowel contents are visible through a thin, transparent membrane that has an external surface of amnion and an internal surface of peritoneum.

An omphalocele may be further categorized as major or minor or as gastroschisis. A major omphalocele frequently is associated with congenital anomalies and an abdominal wall defect that is larger than 5 cm in diameter. A minor omphalocele rarely is associated with congenital anomalies, and the abdominal wall defect is less than 5 cm in diameter. Gastroschisis is the extrusion of variable amounts of bowel (stomach also may be present) through a defect to the right of the normally formed umbilicus. The bowel is characteristically foreshortened, thickened, and edematous, and loops of bowel are matted together. No covering membrane is evident. Congenital anomalies infrequently coexist.

Malrotation deformities that occur during stage II are varied.[58] Although in utero the bowel has returned to the abdominal cavity, rotation is either absent or abnormal; fixation of mesentery also is variable. Intestinal malformations that may develop include a failure of the duodenum to form a normal C loop, lowered position of the ligament of Treitz, inadequate fixation of the mesentery and intestine, and abnormal location of bowel segments (e.g., the ascending colon in the upper portion of the abdomen).[28] Consequently the severity of symptoms (such as ischemia and abdominal pain) is diverse, and the malrotation may go undiagnosed for many years.

The incidence of additional congenital malformations that may accompany malrotation is 10% to 20%.[59] These conditions include prune-belly syndrome, Hirschsprung's disease, biliary atresia, anorectal anomalies, and esophageal atresia.

**Clinical Manifestations.** In the neonate, malrotation may result in strangulating obstruction or recurrent subacute obstruction. Symptoms include abdominal distention and bilious vomiting. The older infant typically manifests a failure to thrive and early satiety.

**Management.** Treatment requires assessment of the extent of ischemia, resection of clearly necrotic bowel, and relief of symptoms. Malrotation often is accompanied by volvulus and, less commonly, intussusception, which requires repair.[4] Lysis of adhesive bands that may precipitate duodenal obstruction is warranted. The malrotation is not repaired by returning the intestine to a normal anatomic position. For example, both the ileum and jejunum may be located in the right lower quadrant of the abdomen and the right colon may be placed in the left upper quadrant.[28]

## EXTRAHEPATIC BILIARY ATRESIA

Extrahepatic biliary atresia is a rare disease with an incidence of 1/8000 live births, with a predominance in the female. Although the disease first was described more than 100 years ago, its cause remains unclear. Typical sources of potential harm such as irradiation, medications, and ischemic injury have no relationship to the onset of biliary atresia. Whether this disease exists at birth or develops after birth is unclear.[63]

**Pathophysiology.** Biliary atresia is characterized by the occlusion or complete destruction of part or all of the extrahepatic bile duct, thereby obstructing bile flow from the liver. On histologic examination the extrahepatic ducts, gallbladder, and periductal tissue show progressive inflammatory destruction that leads to fibrosis of the ducts and closure or atresia.[24] Without surgical correction the entire biliary system ultimately is obliterated, and death ensues from cirrhotic liver failure. The common bile duct, the common hepatic duct, or the right and left hepatic ducts may be involved.

**Clinical Manifestations.** The infant with biliary atresia has a normal birth weight and appears healthy and well nourished. Within the first 2 weeks of life jaundice and acholic stools are evident. The liver and spleen commonly are enlarged. Laboratory tests reveal conjugated hyperbilirubinemia; this abnormality, however, also is associated with other disorders in the neonate. With progression of the disease, biliary cirrhosis and periportal fibrosis develop.

**Diagnosis.** A number of diagnostic studies are employed primarily to distinguish biliary atresia from other causes of conjugated hyperbilirubinemia. These tests include liver biopsy, intubation of the duodenum for the presence of bile, ultrasonography, percutaneous cholangiography, and radionuclide hepatobiliary imaging.[24]

**Management.** Prompt, effective biliary drainage is the treatment goal for extrahepatic biliary atresia. The surgical procedure of choice to accomplish biliary drainage is the Kasai portoenterostomy.

The Kasai portoenterostomy (Fig. 10-5) requires the dissection and surgical removal of occluded or partially occluded extrahepatic duct remnants at the porta hepatis, which is a specific location on the underside of the liver where the right and left hepatic ducts exit (also referred to as the *hilar bifurcation of the portal vein*). The objective is to identify and expose hepatic bile ducts of adequate diameter so that biliary drainage is possible. A segment of jejunum is anastomosed to this area to allow bile to enter the GI tract.

A number of variations for achieving continuity of the GI tract have been developed in an attempt to reduce the incidence of postoperative ascending cholangitis.[63] Stoma construction from the jejunal conduit is common and can be performed as an end, a loop, or a double-barrel technique; some procedures eliminate the need for a cutaneous stoma.

Bowel continuity is restored by several methods. (1) The jejunal conduit can remain isolated from bowel continuity and be anastomosed cutaneously, thus creating an enterostomy. Usually a functional portion of distal bowel also is brought out to the skin (in a double-barrel fashion). Bile contents drain from the enterostomy and may be reinstilled through the functional bowel stoma. A modification of this is the double-barrel Mikulicz enterostomy, in which the common bowel walls of the jejunal segment and the distal bowel walls are severed and continuity automatically is achieved (Fig. 11-10) . It is anticipated that minimal bile will drain through the stoma. (2) The jejunal segment can be anastomosed to distal bowel so that bowel continuity is restored and a cutaneous stoma avoided. (3) The jejunal segment can be anastomosed to functional bowel and a cutaneous stoma created from

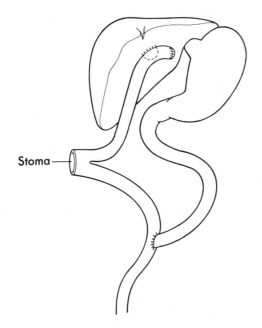

**Fig. 10-5** Kasai portoenterostomy surgical procedure for extrahepatic biliary atresia. (Modified from Zink M: Biliary atresia: nursing diagnoses and management, *J Enterostom Ther* 12[4]: 128, 1985.)

this section of bowel. In each of these techniques the jejunal segment serves as a conduit to allow bile to drain from the liver; although the configuration of anastomoses is variable, the principle is to drain bile from the liver, to deliver the bile to the gut, and to prevent cholangitis.[63]

Intrahepatic bile ducts remain patent during the first 2 to 3 months of life, after which time they begin to regress. Therefore the Kasai portoenterostomy is most effective if performed during the first 10 weeks of life.[24] Ascending cholangitis is a common complication of this procedure and does not seem to be altered by the separation of the jejunal conduit from fecal continuity.

Cutaneous bile drainage through the creation of an ostomy can be closed surgically from 3 months to 1 year after the original procedure. It also is recommended in patients with advanced liver disease and portal hypertension.[57]

Patients may have postoperative complications such as recurrent cholangitis, intrahepatic fibrosis, and portal hypertension. When cholangitis is suspected, intravenous administration of broad-spectrum antibiotics is essential to prevent deterioration of liver function.[24] Unfortunately, despite successful portoenterostomy, significant biliary cirrhosis with portal hypertension develops in as many as 73% to 90% of the affected children.[57] The only other surgical alternative for extrahepatic biliary atresia is liver transplantation.

## NEONATAL NECROTIZING ENTEROCOLITIS

Neonatal necrotizing enterocolitis (NEC), which occurs predominantly in the very small, sick infant, is a major cause of death in the preterm neonate, with a 30% to 50% mortality rate.[13] The incidence in preterm neonates weighing less than 750 g has been reported at 14% and 3% in neonates weighing between 1500 and 1750 g.[29] When NEC occurs in infants more than 1750 g, it typically is limited to those infants who have poly-cythemia, reduced cardiac output, or exchange transfusions.[13]

**Pathophysiology.** NEC is an acute necrosis of the intestine that always involves the distal terminal ileum. Variable lengths of contiguous small and large bowel also may be affected; occasionally the entire large and small bowel may be involved. Although patchy distribution of the necrotic lesions has been observed, it is uncommon. The depth of the necrotic lesions through the bowel wall varies.

The cause of NEC appears to be a combination of two events. First, the bowel mucosa is injured through some type of ischemic event. Next, the gut microflora invade the injured bowel mucosa.[4,13] Ischemic events that may injure the bowel mucosa include asphyxia at birth, arterial hypoxemia, and congenital heart disease (such as patent ductus arteriosus) because blood flow is shunted away from the gut. Finally, epithelial cells in the bowel mucosa also may be damaged by the osmolarity, the volume, or the composition of feeding solutions.[13]

On examination the affected bowel will appear plum colored and friable. Perforation of the affected bowel wall may occur.

**Clinical Manifestations.** NEC manifests by a constellation of suspicious but vague signs and symptoms. GI signs of NEC include ileus, abdominal distention, gastric retention of feedings, and episodes of gross or occult bloody diarrhea. If perforation has occurred, abdominal tenderness will result.

General symptoms in the infant also include apnea, lethargy, and temperature instability. Neutropenia is reported in one third of the infants with NEC; thrombocytopenia should be expected, although it may not develop for hours or days after clinical onset.[13] These general symptoms may exist for several days, progressively worsening and leading to deterioration in the infant's condition. Respiratory distress commonly develops, and the neonate often requires ventilatory support.

Confirmation of NEC can be obtained radiologically when an abdominal flat-plate roentgenogram demonstrates intestinal pneumatosis (i.e., gas trapped in the bowel submucosa) or free air in the peritoneal cavity (as a result of bowel perforation). Radiologic confirmation, however, often lags several days behind clinical suspicion of NEC.

**Management.** Medical management is promptly initiated when NEC is suspected. Feedings are halted, and a nasogastic tube is inserted to decompress the bowel. Supportive interventions are implemented as necessary to address the accompanying infectious, pulmonary, hematologic, and cardiovascular complications. Serial radiographs are obtained to monitor for evidence of intestinal pneumatosis or perforation. Once the acute episode resolves, parenteral fluids and parenteral nutritional support are continued for 10 to 14 days. Oral feedings are reintroduced slowly, and the infant is monitored closely for symptoms that indicate a recurrence of NEC.

Emergent surgical intervention is indicated when either perforation or gangrene is suspected. Symptoms may be as straightforward as demonstrated evidence of peritonitis or as vague as severe symptoms that persist more than 24 hours or progressive deterioration of the infant's condition. The operative procedure includes exploratory laparotomy, resection of necrotic bowel, and creation of a proximal intestinal stoma. Surgery also may be indicated at a later date to repair the intestinal strictures that develop in approximately 10% of the infants who survive the medical and surgical management of NEC.[13]

## OBSTRUCTIVE DISORDERS

Intestinal obstruction is a common surgical problem in the adult and pediatric patient, as well as in the neonate. It is broadly categorized into two types: adynamic and dynamic.

### Intestinal Obstruction

**Adynamic.** Adynamic obstruction is common and is the result of the absence of peristalsis in varying parts of the GI tract. The most familiar type of adynamic obstruction is the paralytic ileus. Many etiologic factors contribute to this problem, such as abdominal surgery, narcotic medications, retroperitoneal injuries or operations, spinal disease, injuries or operations, and metabolic derangements (e.g., hypokalemia). Adynamic obstruction most commonly is a temporary condition that resolves as soon as the initiating cause is removed.

Adynamic obstruction becomes more serious when it develops as a consequence of neurologic conditions. For example, the neuropathic changes that frequently accompany diabetes mellitus can affect both the autonomic and the peripheral nervous systems. Varying degrees of obstruction can then develop.

Ogilvie's syndrome is a relatively uncommon condition whereby the colon is functionally obstructed because of a lack of peristalsis. Massive dilation of the colon develops without organic cause. In extreme cases, Ogilvie's syndrome may result in a colonic perforation. The diagnosis is established by flat-plate radiographic studies of the abdomen that demonstrate the presence of distention. A meglumine diatrizoate (Gastrografin) enema radiograph confirms the absence of an obstruction; this procedure also tends to be therapeutic and to relieve the dilation.

**Dynamic.** Dynamic intestinal obstructions are precipitated by pathologic conditions and represent a medical-surgical emergency. The obstruction may be of the small intestine or the colon; obstructions of the small intestine are most common. The source of the obstruction can be within the lumen of the bowel, external to the bowel, or within the bowel wall.

Several diseases are associated with causing dynamic intestinal obstructions. In Western countries, intraabdominal adhesions from previous abdominal surgery is the most common cause of small intestine dynamic obstruction.[38] A strangulated hernia and Crohn's disease also contribute to the development of a dynamic obstruction in the small intestine.

The most common cause of a dynamic obstruction of the colon is malignancy, specifically, left-sided primary adenocarcinoma of the colon.[18] Recurrent or extensive pelvic malignancies such as ovarian cancer may cause a dynamic obstruction of the distal colon. Benign tumors of the colon rarely, if ever, reach a size to cause obstruction. If a benign tumor is present, intussusception must develop first before the lumen is compromised sufficiently to produce obstruction. Volvulus also results in an intestinal obstruction that can involve the entire colon or can be limited to the sigmoid colon. In the neonate, bowel obstruction can signal severe, life-threatening conditions such as Hirschsprung's disease, anorectal malformations, malrotation of the gut, and cystic fibrosis (specifically, a meconium ileus). Intussusception is the most common cause of bowel obstruction in children between 2 months and 5 years of age.[40]

**Diagnosis.** Obstruction of the colon usually develops with an acute onset of symptoms and little or no forewarning.[18] The diagnosis of intestinal obstruction is strongly suggested in the clinical setting of relatively sudden onset of abdominal cramps that accompany abdominal distention. The patient also has either difficulty in passing or an inability to pass stool or flatus.

Abdominal radiographs taken with the patient in both the erect and the supine posture often reveals an obstruction. Distended loops of small bowel that contain air fluid levels, accompanied by the absence of significant amounts of distention of the colon, are diagnostic of a dynamic (mechanical) small bowel obstruction. Similarly, massive distention of the colon with absence of gas distal to the point of obstruction is diagnostic of mechanical colonic obstruction.

Perforation is a serious complication of obstruction and may occur at the site of obstruction or proximal to the obstruction.[18] Proximal perforations commonly occur in the cecum and develop as a result of entrapment of fluid and gas in the segment of bowel between the intact ileocecal valve and the point of obstruction. This is a potential complication of any closed-loop obstruction (distal obstruction with intact ileocecal valve).

**Management.** Treatment of the intestinal obstruction requires immediate relief of the obstruction, generally with nasogastric suction. This approach serves the dual purpose of preventing possible bowel perforation in the face of megacolon and also provides relief from nausea and pain. In addition, the patient requires support of accompanying problems such as electrolyte imbalance, potential fluid imbalances, and hemodynamic instability. Surgical exploration and correction of the underlying cause are warranted for dynamic intestinal obstructions that affect the colon. A more conservative medical approach is typical in the management of dynamic obstructions of the small intestine, particularly when the causative agent is adhesions or Crohn's disease.

Specific treatment of obstructive disorders is dictated by the underlying cause for the obstruction, such as volvulus, intussusception, and meconium ileus, which are discussed next.

## Volvulus

**Pathophysiology.** Volvulus is the clockwise twisting of a section of the intestinal tract of the colon around the mesentery. Consequently, the vascular supply to the bowel is jeopardized, and a closed-loop obstruction often results. The severity of this complication is reflected in the high mortality rates that have been reported: up to 35%.[3]

Volvulus is a relatively unusual cause of intestinal obstruction in the United States; less than 10% of the cases of intestinal obstruction are due to a volvulus. In other parts of the world, however (such as Africa, the Middle East, and northern Europe), volvulus is a common cause of intestinal obstruction. This may reflect different dietary patterns, particularly with excessive intake of nondigestible vegetable fiber. In the United States the sigmoid colon is the most common site for a volvulus.

Sigmoid volvulus most often develops in patients who have a long redundant sigmoid colon attached to the retroperitoneum by a narrow mesosigmoid. Factors that produce a redundant bowel are variable. In the United States, bowel redundancies may develop in elderly residents of long-term care facilities, a condition caused by chronic constipation and resultant megacolon. In other parts of the world, a high-roughage diet and certain diseases (such as Chagas' disease) are implicated.

**Diagnosis.** Sigmoid volvulus should be suspected in any patient with colonic obstruction, particularly in an elderly resident of a long term-care facility. A typical diagnostic radiographic pattern shows a dilated segment of bowel that assumes a bent inner tube configuration arising from the left lower quadrant, with distention of the surrounding proximal bowel. If a contrast radiograph is obtained, it reveals the characteristic bird's-beak appearance that the site of torsion creates. A Gastrografin enema often confirms the diagnosis and more accurately localizes the point of obstruction.

Endoscopic evaluation shows a normal rectum, but as the site of torsion is approached, mucosal folds appear markedly swollen and assume a classic spiral configuration. Occasionally it is possible to pass the endoscope through this area into the twisted colon, resulting in a sudden gush of stool and gas and in detorsion. Although this entry usually is beyond the limit of the rigid proctoscope, the site of torsion may be reached with flexible instruments.

**Management.** Volvulus must be reduced and can be accomplished by means of sigmoidoscopy or by a surgical procedure. Because volvulus is associated with a high recurrence rate when reduced in a nonoperative fashion, surgical reduction may be recommended either emergently or electively after the first episode of volvulus.[3] An intestinal stoma (such as a loop transverse colostomy or loop ileostomy) may be indicated when the obstruction is severe or perforation has resulted.

## Intussusception

**Pathophysiology.** Intussusception refers to the invagination of one part of the intestine into itself. The intussusception is composed of two parts: the intussusceptum (the invaginating portion of the intestine) and the intussuscipiens (the part of intestine that contains the intussusceptum). Peristalsis advances the intussusceptum farther into the intussuscipiens.

Although intussusception may occur at any age, 60% to 85% of the cases are encountered in the first 2 years of life. Classically, intussusception affects well-nourished, otherwise healthy, white male infants 6 to 9 months of age in whom severe episodes of abdominal colic develop.[4] In these instances the intussusception is idiopathic, although there appears to be some association with gastroenteritis and respiratory tract infection.

Intussusception occasionally develops in the neonatal period, when almost invariably it is caused by an identifiable "leading point" (or pathologic condition at the apex of the intussusception). Most commonly this point is intestinal duplication, Meckel's diverticulum, a polyp, or an intestinal tumor.

Intussusception in the adult is a rare but an important cause of intestinal obstruction. In all cases there is an identifiable cause found at the leading edge. The cause can vary from a benign condition such as a Meckel's diverticulum or an intestinal polyp to a malignant tumor, particularly in the ileocecal valve or distal sigmoid.

**Clinical Manifestations.** The clinical manifestations of intussusception become clear once the twofold effects of this disease are understood. First, incomplete intestinal obstruction is created when the lumen of the intussusceptum is compressed by the surrounding intussuscipiens. This phenomenon results in the colic that is classic in this condition. Second, the vascular supply of the intussusception is obstructed at the site of the invagination because of the acute angulation of the vessels. This process creates immediate congestion of the venous and lymphatic flow and edema in the surrounding tissue. Musocal cells become engorged with blood and mucus and subsequently exude into the lumen of the bowel. Rectal passage of this exudate mixed with stool is characterized as "red currant jelly," a classic manifestation. If the venous congestion increases, the arterial inflow may be compromised significantly enough to produce intestinal necrosis and gangrene.

**Diagnosis and Management.** Diagnosis of intussusception is established by clinical symptoms, physical examination, and radiographic examination. On physical examination a sausage-shaped mass is palpable either through the abdomen or through a digital rectal examination. Symptoms of acute intestinal obstruction may develop in the adult; occasionally the intussusception may prolapse out through the anus.

A contrast enema radiographic examination often is necessary to confirm the diagnosis of intussusception and demonstrates obstruction to the flow of contrast medium at the head of the intussusception. The "meniscus" sign or a "coiled-spring" sign often appears as a result of the diffusion of barium between the two opposing layers of the intussusception. Surgical resection of the intussusception is indicated and most often does not require a diversion.

## Meconium Ileus

Meconium ileus is accountable for approximately 15% of the cases of neonatal small-bowel obstruction.[4] It can occur with Hirschsprung's disease and is the earliest manifestation in 10% of infants with fibrocystic disease of the pancreas.[50] Meconium ileus in the infant with fibrocystic disease of the pancreas develops because of the pancreatic enzyme deficiency and hyposecretion of water and electrolytes from the pancreas, biliary system, and small intestine.[32]

**Pathophysiology.** Meconium ileus results in enormous distention of the proximal ileum, with sticky, tenacious, dark-green to black meconium. The wall of this segment of bowel becomes hypertrophied in an attempt to propel the thick stool. The ileum distal to this area becomes contracted, narrowed, and filled with pelletlike stool; the colon is collapsed and empty. The meconium stool in the proximal ileum is tenacious enough to induce intestinal obstruction. In as many as 50% of the infants, perforation, gangrene, volvulus, atresia, or meconium peritonitis may develop.[59]

**Clinical Manifestations.** A failure to pass meconium or difficulty in passing meconium should suggest this condition. Symptoms of intestinal obstruction also may manifest in the infant.

**Management.** Treatment of meconium ileus is largely conservative and medical. Hyperosmolar enemas (such as Gastrografin) delivered by use of fluoroscopy primarily to diagnose the problem also have been shown to be therapeutic. By drawing fluid into the intestinal lumen and emulsifying the stool, the hyperosmolar enema disimpacts the stool.[58] When successful, results should be observed promptly. If unsuccessful, the procedure should not be repeated. Acetylcysteine (Mucomyst), a wetting agent, also may resolve the meconium obstruction and can be delivered by nasogastric intubation.[50]

When these medical measures are ineffective or complications are suspected (volvulus or perforation), surgical intervention to evacuate the meconium mass is warranted. This may be effectively accomplished by dissecting the dilated bowel and reanastomosing the bowel ends. In some cases a temporary ileostomy such as a double-barreled Mickulicz or the Bishop-Koop ileostomy is necessary. These two procedures provide access to the meconium plug, relief of the obstruction, and continuity with the distal bowel. The stomas created by these two procedures usually are quite flush with the skin but are expected to serve as a safety valve, producing only minimal stool (mostly mucus) once the distal bowel is disimpacted. If necessary, acetylcysteine or Gastrografin can be instilled into the meconium plug and distal bowel to clear any contents.[56]

## COLON AND RECTAL MALIGNANCIES

Colorectal cancer has become a major health care problem and is a common cause of death in the Western countries. Excluding skin cancers, colon, lung, and breast are the three leading sites for new cancer cases annually in the United States. More than 120,000 new cases of colorectal cancer are diagnosed per year, and the 5-year survival is less than 50%.[20,54]

Colon and rectal malignancies are either primary (arising from the bowel) or metastatic (spreading from adjacent or distant sites). Adenocarcinomas are the most common primary malignancy and are the focus of discussion in this section. Epidermoid or squamous malignancies (which arise from the squamous and columnar cells in the transition zone of the anal canal) also are primary malignancies but occur less frequently than do adenocarcinomas. Metastatic colon and rectal malignancies can develop from lymphoma, leiomyosarcoma, malignant melanoma, and cancer of the breast, ovary, prostate, and lung.

### Adenocarcinoma

The prevalence of adenocarcinoma of the colon and rectum is highest in developed countries; the United States has one of the highest rates in the world. Colon cancer occurs almost equally in both sexes, whereas rectal cancer has a slight male predominance. Although the reported frequency of adenocarcinoma in different segments of the large bowel varies, in general the frequency, in descending order, is rectum, sigmoid, cecum, ascending colon, transverse colon, descending colon, splenic flexure, and hepatic flexure.[5] This frequency distribution of colorectal cancer is changing; a proximal migration, and thus more right-sided cancers, has been observed.

**Etiology.** The cause of colorectal cancer is unknown, of course, but may be the interaction of several factors.[5] Much epidemiologic study focuses on the influence of diet, specifically, a low intake of fiber and a high intake of animal fat and red meat.[39] It is theorized that fiber reduces the exposure of potential carcinogens to the bowel mucosa (1) by reducing intestinal transit time and (2) by diluting the carcinogens in a bulky stool. In addition, higher fat and animal protein intake may contribute to the establishment of bacterial flora, with enzymatic activity that results in the formation of carcinogenic metabolites.[19] International comparisons show a high correlation between the incidence of colorectal cancer and these dietary factors.[7,48]

Other etiologic factors for colorectal cancer have been studied.[17] Previous cholecystectomy has been implicated, although evidence is inconclusive. Alcohol consumption, particularly beer, has been associated with a higher incidence of rectal cancer in several countries. It is speculated that by interacting with the diet, beer may influence either fecal flora or the fecal steroid concentration. Finally, low serum cholesterol levels may increase the risk of colorectal cancer, although the data for this relationship are insufficient.[16,62]

**Risk Factors.** Several factors have been identified to be associated with an increased risk for the development of colorectal cancer. Although colon cancer can occur at any age, it is most common between the ages of 50 and 80 years. Risk increases slightly at 40 years of age and increases sharply at age 50 years. The risk doubles with each decade thereafter up to the age range of 75 to 80 years.[34]

Patients with a previous colorectal cancer that has been *cured* are at an increased risk (5% to 10%) for the development of a new malignancy in the colon.[62] These lesions are referred to as *metachronous* lesions and are distinct from those colorectal tumors that are not cured and have spread to new sites within the bowel.

There is growing support for the theory that a large percentage (if not all) colorectal cancers develop from benign adenomatous polyps, the so-called polyp-cancer sequence.[16,20] A polyp is a mass of tissue protruding from the intestinal tract. Adenoma is a generic term for three types of benign epithelial polyps: tubular, tubulovillous, and villous.[34] The tubular adenoma is most commonly pedunculated and the most common large-bowel tumor. Villous adenomas, which form a soft, flat tumor that arises from a large mucosal surface, typically populate the rectum and rectosigmoid. Tubulovillous adenomas, an intermediate type of polyp, are smaller and more compact than the villous tumor, and often become pedunculated. A malignancy is more likely to occur in larger polyps, in tubular adenomas, and in polyps with a villous changes.

The polyp-cancer sequence, however, may be an oversimplification. Whereas much research has been conducted[43] supporting the belief that benign polyps have the potential to degenerate into a malignancy, much of the evidence implicating polyps is circumstantial. Although the removal of polyps certainly may decrease the incidence of colorectal cancer, to date no conclusive evidence implicates each polyp that arises in the colon as premalignant.

Genetic predisposition is found in patients with hereditary syndromes such as familial adenomatous polyposis, the cancer family syndrome, and hereditary site-specific colon cancer.[36,37] Familial adenomatous polyposis (FAP), also referred to as *Gardner's syndrome*, is characterized by multiple adenomatous polyps of the colon; less frequently, polyps may develop in the stomach and small intestine. Colon cancer inevitably develops in all affected individuals. Prophylactic excision of the colon in affected family members should be undertaken before malignancy develops.

The cancer family syndrome has been recognized only recently.[36,37] The following criteria characterize this syndrome: (1) an increased number of all types of adenocarcinomas, especially colon and endometrial carcinomas, develop; (2) cancer develops in affected persons at a younger age than does cancer of the same site in the general population; (3) multiple primary malignant neoplasms develop in affected persons; and (4) the genetic transmission is autosomal dominant.

Hereditary, site-specific colon cancer is similar to the cancer family syndrome, except that the site is limited specifically to the colon. Patients with this type of tendency have a higher frequency of cancer in the proximal colon than does the general population or do patients with familial adenomatous polyposis.[37,46]

Ulcerative colitis has long been associated with an increased incidence of colorectal cancer. Although the data that suggest the degree of risk posed are controversial, it is agreed that risk is influenced by two variables: duration of active disease and extent of inflammatory changes within the colon. When the ulcerative colitis is universal (the entire colon and rectum are involved), the incidence of malignancy after the disease has been present for 10 to 15 years is between 3% and 12%.[25] Disease limited to the left side of the colon and present for 20 years presents a risk of up to 30%. The risk of cancer in patients who have extensive disease or total colonic involvement is noticeably increased in 8 to 10 years after onset of symptoms. Malignancy develops in patients with ulcerative colitis at a significantly younger age (37 years) than in the average patient with colorectal cancer (58 years of age).[33]

Less information is available on the risk of colorectal cancer in patients with Crohn's disease of the colon. Although their risk is higher than that of the general population, it is not considered significant enough to warrant prophylactic screening or colon resection.

**Pathophysiology.** On macroscopic examination, colorectal malignancy may assume a variety of shapes. The focus of malignancy can occur in an otherwise benign polyp. Most commonly the shape of adenocarcinoma is ulcerative; it varies in size and shape and may be extensive enough to involve the circumference of the bowel (anular). The edges of the ulceration are everted, and the floor is irregular, hard, and friable. If other areas of tissue are involved, this lesion may become fixed.

Less commonly, the tumor may assume a large exophytic mass that protrudes into the lumen of the bowel. This is quite common on the right side of the colon, where the tumor may become large without invading the bowel wall or surrounding tissues.[18]

Biologic behavior of colorectal cancer is somewhat variable. At one time it was believed that a sequence of events occurred that enabled the tumor to spread initially in the local area. Penetration through the bowel wall followed, and only then would the local lymph nodes become involved. Finally, distant lymph nodes become involved. Ultimately, blood-borne metastases to remote areas of the body occurred.

It now appears more likely that this sequence of events happens in a sporadic, haphazard manner largely determined by biologic factors involving host-tumor relationships that are poorly understood. Distant and lymphatic spread of colorectal tumors appears to occur early rather than late and often is predetermined, inasmuch as the survival rate for treated colorectal cancer has not changed during this last century.[16]

**Staging.** A method of classifying colon and rectal cancer was first described by Duke in 1932 and has undergone modifications over the years.[62] A modified Dukes' classification system is listed in the box below. The tumor-node-metastasis (TNM) classification, described in the box on p. 320, also may be used.

---

**STAGING SYSTEM FOR COLORECTAL CANCER: MODIFIED DUKES' CLASSIFICATION SYSTEM (GITSG*)**

| | |
|---|---|
| **A**<br>Tumor limited to mucosa (carcinoma in situ) | **C₁**<br>One to four tumor-involved lymph nodes |
| **B₁**<br>Tumor penetrates muscularis mucosa | **C₂**<br>Five or more tumor-involved lymph nodes |
| **B₂**<br>Tumor penetrates through muscularis propria (serosa where present) | **D**<br>Distant metastases |

*Gastrointestinal Tumor Study Group.

---

## TNM* STAGING SYSTEM FOR COLORECTAL CANCER

**TX**
Depth not specified

**$T_0$**
No demonstrable tumor

**$T_{1s}$**
Carcinoma in situ (no invasion of lamina
  propria)

**$T_1$**
Tumor confined to mucosa and
  submucosa

**$T_2$**
Tumor invading muscularis propria but
  not extending through muscularis
  propria

**$T_3$**
Tumor through entire thickness of bowel
  wall; through entire muscularis propria,
  and through serosa when present; may
  or may not invade adjacent structures

**$N_X$**
Nodes not assessed

**$N_0$**
No nodal metastasis identified

**$N_1$**
Regional node metastasis identified

**$M_X$**
Distant metastasis not assessed

**$M_0$**
Distant metastasis not identified

**$M_1$**
Distant metastasis reported

---

*Tumor, Nodes, Metastasis.*

**Clinical Manifestations.** Colorectal cancer can be symptomless and diagnosed on routine health examinations and screening. The initial symptoms may be intermittent, subtle, and easily dismissed by the patient. Unfortunately, symptoms portend late-stage disease. The symptoms associated with colorectal cancer relate to its ability to obstruct, ulcerate, bleed, invade surrounding tissue, perforate, and cause pain. The extent to which these conditions develop will be influenced by the type of tumor growth (e.g., exophytic or ulcerative) and its location in the GI tract.

The most common complaint is rectal bleeding, with either bloody or tarry stools. Bowel habits change, with a tendency for either obstructive symptoms or irritative symptoms. Obstructive symptoms of the left colon include constipation, paradoxic diarrhea, and cramping pain. Obstructive tumors in the cecum or right colon may precipitate such obstructive symptoms as abdominal distention, nausea, and vomiting. Rectal cancers generally produce tenesmus, narrowed caliber of stool, bleeding, and urgency that may result in incontinence.

**Diagnosis.** In the presence of any of the aforementioned symptoms, particularly rectal bleeding or a family history of colon cancer or previous bowel disease such as ulcerative colitis or polyps, the patient requires a full colorectal evaluation. In most cases this examination is performed by use of fiberoptic colonoscopy with biopsy. Rigid proctoscopy with an air-contrast barium enema can be substituted for the fiberoptic colonoscopy. Attention should be given to examination of the flexures because lesions may be missed as a result of inadequate visualization with currently available techniques.

Laboratory tests do not serve a diagnostic function with colorectal cancer. Initially carcinoembryonic antigen (CEA) was described to be a tumor-specific test for colon cancer that would provide a diagnosis in symptom-free patients. This description has turned out to be erroneous because of the high number of false-positive and false-negative results. CEA is elevated in patients who smoke or have conditions such as inflammatory bowel disease, renal disease, and alcoholic cirrhosis. CEA, however, may be useful in postoperative follow-up. After colectomy for adenocarcinoma is performed, a previously elevated CEA declines; a gradual postoperative rise may signal a recurrence.

Fecal occult blood tests are not diagnostic tools; however, their role in screening for colorectal cancer is worthy of discussion. Such tests are "based on the assumption that smaller, earlier, and (consequently) more favorable lesions might bleed enough to leave detectable residues of blood in the feces."[16] Because colonic tumors characteristically bleed intermittently and rectal lesions tend to bleed less than right-sided lesions, it is important to obtain a series of fecal occult blood tests and to conduct follow-up tests in high-risk populations by means of proctoscopy or flexible sigmoidoscopy.

Although Hemoccult is a familiar test for occult blood in the stool, it is associated with high false-positive and false-negative results. The HemoQuant test, which is a similarly simple test for occult blood in stools, has greater sensitivity and specificity.[1]

**Management.** Surgical resection is the treatment of choice for primary adenocarcinoma of the colon and rectum. The surgical approach is determined by the anatomic site of the lesion (with consideration of the three major blood vessels that supply the colon and rectum) and the presence or absence of adjacent organ involvement.

The operative procedure of choice for cancer of the cecum and ascending colon is a right hemicolectomy; for cancer in the transverse colon the procedure of choice is an ileocolic anastomosis to the descending colon, and for cancer located in the descending colon the operative procedure of choice is a left radical hemicolectomy. Tumors in the sigmoid colon may be limited to the sigmoid or may require resection of the left colon, depending on the position of the lesion in the sigmoid.

Resection for cancer of the rectum depends on the level of the lesion within the rectum. Generally, tumors in the upper third of the rectum can be resected with a low anterior resection, referred to as an *LAR*. Abdominoperineal resection is the widely accepted and most appropriate procedure for cancers located in the distal 6 cm of the rectum. The surgical approach for cancer located in the midrectum (7 to 11 cm from the anal verge) is more controversial. With the development of the end-to-end circular anastomotic stapler, an extended low anterior resection with coloanal anastomosis is now technically feasible while still obtaining safe margins.[61] This procedure is sphincter-saving as compared with the time-honored abdominoperineal resection and consequent sigmoid colostomy. Although concerns are expressed about reported high recurrence rates at the suture line after low anterior resection, survival rates of near 50% are comparable to abdominoperineal resection.[5]

## GASTROINTESTINAL POLYPOSIS SYNDROMES

GI polyposis syndromes are characterized by the presence of multiple benign polyps in the GI tract. Universally the principal organ affected is the colon; in many of the syndromes, however, polyps also develop in the stomach and small intestine. These syndromes are categorized according to the histologic character of the polyp, that is, as an adenoma or a hamartoma (nonneoplastic, tumorlike projections). The most familiar polyposis syndrome is FAP and is described in more detail later in this section. Because proctocolectomy (with an ileoanal reservoir, continent ileostomy, or conventional ileostomy) is the treatment of choice for FAP, the nurse who cares for patients with ostomies should be familiar with this syndrome and its distinction from other polyposis syndromes.

### Peutz-Jeghers Syndrome

Peutz-Jeghers syndrome (PJS) is characterized by hamartomatous polyps in the stomach, small intestine, and colon. The predominant concentration is in the jejunum and ileum. PJS also is typified by mucocutaneous pigmentation (melanin spots) that are particularly noticeable around the mouth. Abdominal pain as a result of small-bowel intussusception, obstruction by a large polyp, or bleeding are the primary symptoms.[9] Treatment of PJS is largely conservative; associated GI carcinomas are rare.

### Juvenile Polyposis Syndromes

Juvenile polyposis syndromes (JPS) consist of hamartomatous polyps typically in the rectum; polyps also may be present in the colon and, less commonly, in the stomach and small intestine. JPS have been described in both children and adults. Rectal bleeding and malnutrition are common symptoms. JPS have been suggested to comprise actually four separate but similar syndromes.[53]

### Turcot Syndrome

Turcot syndrome is characterized by adematous polyps in the colon and the coexistence of a malignant tumor of the central nervous system (such as a glioblastoma or medulloblastoma). The colonic polyps most often are tubular and premalignant. Turcot syndrome, which is genetically transmitted, has been detected in persons between the ages of 10 and 25 years.[53]

### Familial Adenomatous Polyposis

Familial adenomatous polyposis is an inherited condition; the condition is transmitted through a non–sex-linked, autosomal dominant mendelian gene. Recently the abnormality was found to exist on chromosome 5, resulting in generalized cellular growth disorder. This disorder dictates the development of benign and malignant lesions in different body organs.[26]

The disease develops in approximately 50% of the offspring of the affected parent. Although rare, occurring at a frequency of 1/24,000 births,[53] FAP is the most common of polyposis syndromes. It has been reported in white, Oriental, Arab, American Indian, and African and American black persons.

**Pathophysiology.** FAP is characterized by adenomas that occur earlier, grow more abundantly and faster, and become malignant at a younger age than in the normal population.[26] Typically the adenomas in FAP are tubular and either sessile or pedunculated.

Numerous small (less than 0.5 cm) polyps are present; a diagnosis can be made when at least 100 adenomatous polyps populate the colon and rectum. The polyps may be isolated or situated in groups separated by normal-appearing mucosa. Often the polyps are so dense that they are said to carpet the colon. It is now recognized that the distribution of polyps in FAP, also called *familial polyposis coli,* is not limited to the colon and rectum; polyps also may develop throughout the stomach and small intestine.

FAP is one of the most unfailingly premalignant conditions known. If left untreated, cancer invariably develops somewhere in the colon about 15 years after the appearance of polyps. Colon malignancies have been detected at an average age of 39 years, approximately 20 years earlier than among the general population without polyposis.[53]

**Clinical Manifestations.** Classically, multiple polyps appear in the colon early in the teenage years. FAP is diagnosed at a mean age of 24 years when a family history of FAP is known and between 20 and 40 years of age in the absence of family history. Although a family history is typical, sporadic cases appear after several generations. FAP is diagnosed when these persons seek routine screening because of a family history of polyposis, during routine proctoscopic examinations, or after the development of GI symptoms.

FAP can be symptomless even in the presence of a colon lined with polyps. The most common symptoms that occur early and, in fact, motivate the patient to seek medical consultation are changes in bowel habits (mild to moderate diarrhea) and rectal bleeding. Patients also may have abdominal pain, weakness, and weight loss.

Within the syndrome of FAP a portion of the patients manifest a variety of extracolonic conditions (benign and malignant), commonly referred to as *Gardner's syndrome.* In addition to the polyps in the colon, rectum, small intestine, duodenum, and stomach, these patients have associated cutaneous and subcutaneous soft tissue tumors (such as desmoid tumors of the abdominal wall or bowel mesentery and epidermoid or sebaceous cysts on the face, neck, and trunk), skeletal changes (such as osteomas in the mandible, maxilla, or long bone), and miscellaneous tumors (such as periampullary carcinoma and thyroid carcinomas). Stomach polyps have been observed in as many as 50% of persons with FAP.[26] These polyps are nonadenomatous and do not seem to have malignant potential. Polyps in the duodenum also are common and affect as many as 90% of those with FAP.[9] Duodenal polyps are all adenomatous. After colon cancer, cancer of the duodenum is the next most common cause of death in cases of FAP.[26]

Patients with FAP often exhibit congenital hypertrophy of the retinal pigmentation epithelium. This condition is not a disease; rather it seems to be more of a birthmark for the disease because it has been observed in young children and infants before other manifestations are present.[26]

**Diagnosis.** Ideally FAP should be diagnosed during routine screening of otherwise symptomless patients who have relatives known to have the disease. Screening should commence at a young age (10 to 13 years of age) because, although polyps most typically do not appear until the teenage years, patients have been described with *malignancy* before the age of 15 years. Adenomas form by the age of 20 years in 80% of the persons who inherit the disease.[26] Confirmation of FAP is made with fiberoptic proctosigmoidoscopic or colonoscopic examination. Air-contrast barium enema examination also demonstrates polyps; however, fiberoptic endoscopic examination often is preferable.

Laboratory tests do not serve to confirm the diagnosis of FAP. Certain tests, however, do indicate complications the patient may have before the disease is diagnosed. For example, iron deficiency anemia may develop as a result of bleeding or abnormal serum electrolyte levels in the presence of severe diarrhea.

**Management.** Prophylactic surgical resection of the colon and rectum is the agreed upon treatment for FAP before malignant changes occur. The exact timing of this resection and the extent of resection (or type of procedure) to be performed, however, are controversial. Generally resection is advised at the time of diagnosis.

Curative resection consists of those operations that remove the colon and the rectum, thus eliminating the risk of colorectal cancer. Total proctocolectomy and ileostomy (Brooke or continent) has long been accepted as the standard surgical procedure for FAP. Sphincter-saving procedures that avoid the need for a permanent stoma, such as the restorative proctocolectomy with ileoanal reservoir, also are surgical options for the patient with FAP. These surgical procedures are discussed in more detail in Chapters 4 and 11.

Total colectomy with ileorectal anastomosis is an alternative procedure that leaves a length of rectum that can be easily examined by means of endoscopy. With this procedure, rectal polyps must be periodically fulgurated; proctoscopic examination and fulguration of polyps are recommended every 6 months. Obviously it is essential that candidates for this procedure be informed preoperatively of the necessity of proctoscopic examination at 6-month intervals. When patient compliance with follow-up examinations is a concern, the appropriateness of the ileorectal anastomosis must be reconsidered. This procedure sometimes is preferred in symptomless children when routine and regular follow-up examinations are feasible.

## INFLAMMATORY BOWEL DISEASE

Diarrhea caused by inflammatory changes of the large intestine has been a problem plaguing human beings for millennia. In most cases diarrhea is due to infectious agents. It was not until the late 1800s that an entity of noninfectious diarrhea was established. Although inflammatory bowel disease can be interpreted to include all disease processes that create an inflammation within the bowel, the term as used here refers specifically to Crohn's disease and ulcerative colitis. Because epidemiology and etiology are similar for these two diseases, these issues are discussed together. An in-depth discussion of each particular disease then follows.

### Epidemiology

Crohn's disease is most common in the northern temperate zones of Europe and North America. Ulcerative colitis, which is common in Europe and North America, also has been reported in Australia, South Africa, Japan, and South America.[15] Both diseases affect people of western heritage, especially those from northern Europe or from the northern part of eastern Europe, with a preponderance of white versus nonwhite, Jewish versus non-Jewish, and urban versus rural populations. Israeli Jews, however, have a low incidence of both diseases.[2] No obvious variation in the incidence of ulcerative colitis or Crohn's disease in relation to social class is known.

Although a genetic mechanism of transmission of inflammatory bowel disease has not been identified, multiple occurrences of ulcerative colitis or Crohn's disease in the same family have been reported.[30] The sex distribution appears to be equal. Both diseases occur at all ages, but peak incidence of ulcerative colitis is in teenagers and young adults (15 to 25 years of age). Crohn's disease is rare in childhood and peaks between the ages of 20 and 35 years and 55 and 70 years.[2,41]

The average annual incidence of ulcerative colitis is approximately 4 to 7 per 100,000 persons. The incidence of Crohn's disease is slightly less and estimated from 1 to 7 per 100,000. Prevalence (number of patients affected at any one point in time) is estimated to be 40 to 100 per 100,000 persons for ulcerative colitis and between 10 and 100 per 100,000 persons for Crohn's disease.[41] The incidence of Crohn's disease, however, appears to be on the increase, whereas that of ulcerative colitis remains stable.[30]

Epidemiologic data for Crohn's disease and ulcerative colitis are difficult to obtain and interpret for a number of reasons. First, Crohn's disease is diagnosed essentially by description. To further confuse the data, the diagnostic distinction between Crohn's disease and ulcerative colitis is difficult to make in about 10% to 15% of the colitis cases.[2] Such cases contain features of both diseases and therefore are termed *indeterminate colitis*. Acute ileitis that affects the distal ileum adds even more confusion to the data because these cases have been classified as Crohn's disease in some studies; yet acute ileitis often is caused by infections such as *Yersinia enterocolitica* and other microorganisms and nematodes. In fact, chronic disease develops in only a small number of patients with acute ileitis.

## Etiology

Ulcerative colitis and Crohn's disease typically are referred to as idiopathic because the origin of these two diseases continues to be elusive. The focus of research has been on genetic, infectious, immunologic, and dietary causes.

A genetic association with human leukocyte antigen (HLA)–B27 has been described. Patients with ulcerative colitis who have this antigen were found to be more likely to have ankylosing spondylitis. As yet, however, no genetic marker for ulcerative colitis has been found.[30]

Much emphasis has been placed on infection as being either a primary or a secondary factor in the cause or perpetuation, or both, of inflammatory bowel disease. Certainly ulcerative colitis and Crohn's disease are not considered contagious. However, the role of infection in the disease process is intriguing because of the obvious inflammatory process taking place in the lumen and outside the bowel wall and because of the relatively recent recognition of new bacterial causes of intestinal inflammation (such as *Campylobacter* organisms). Although considerable indirect evidence implicates infection, to date no conclusive evidence supports viral, chlamydial, or bacterial agents as causative.[31]

A variety of possible deficiencies in immunologic processes have been investigated. The GI tract contains its own immune system, which includes Peyer's patches, gut-specific lymphocytes, mast cells, Paneth's cells, and secretory immunoglobulin A (IgA). Working in coordination with the systemic immune system, the GI tract contributes to maintaining the body's immunologic status. Deficiencies in particular components of both the systemic and gut-specific immune system are under investigation. These include diminished lymphocyte responsiveness, inhibited peripheral leukocyte migration, toxicity of either circulating or gut lymphocytes for colonic epithelial cells, increased suppressor T-cell activity, alterations in helper and suppressor T-cell ratios, and malfunction of the lymphocytes, neutrophils, macrophages, and immunoglobulins within the intestinal bowel wall.[30] Although poorly understood or defined, the role of the immune system in the pathogenesis of ulcerative colitis holds much promise and currently is the focus of research efforts.[31]

Dietary factors (such as milk, chemical food additives, and deficient dietary fiber) historically have been implicated as causing inflammatory bowel disease. No evidence exists to substantiate these factors as contributory.[31]

Stress, maladaptation, and emotional difficulties do not cause ulcerative colitis or

Crohn's disease. Similarly, personality traits in no way contribute to these diseases. Although such psychogenic factors frequently were cited in early research, it has become clear that the presence of emotional stress or psychologic status with inflammatory bowel disease more reasonably represents the *impact* of a recurrent and unpredictable disease. Although many patients with inflammatory bowel disease are found to be anxious, inquiring, and introspective, this should not be interpreted as precipitating the disease.

## Chronic Ulcerative Colitis

The term *ulcerative colitis* is used to describe a disease of unknown cause characterized by inflammatory changes of the mucosa of the rectum and colon. Ironically ulcers may or may not be present; when present they usually are microscopic. The patient generally has varying degrees of toxemia because of the many local and systemic complications. Actually, the term *idiopathic proctocolitis* more accurately describes this disease; however, because of common usage, ulcerative colitis has gained widespread acceptance.

**Pathophysiology.** Pathologic features that accompany ulcerative colitis depend on the severity and duration of the disease. Ulcerative colitis commences confluently from the dentate line of the anal canal and ceases sharply at the ileocecal junction. The disease extends for variable distances in a proximal progression from the anal canal; the most severe disease is found distally in the sigmoid and rectum. Transition from normal to abnormal mucosa can be abrupt or gradual over several centimeters.

The mucosa, which is diffusely red, friable, and edematous, bleeds on contact. Submucosal vessels are obscured by the edema, thus creating a characteristic roughened or granular appearance. Blood and mucus ooze from the mucosa and pool in the lumen of the bowel. The presence of pus and ulcers, which vary in size, shape, and distribution, usually indicates severe acute disease. Ulcers concomitant with normal mucosa should raise the suspicion of another disease such as Crohn's disease or acute infectious colitis.

Chronic inflammation results in scarring of the submucosa and the muscular layers of the bowel, thus creating a shortening of the colon and a loss of haustra, which is readily demonstrated on barium enema radiologic examination. The external appearance of the colon may exhibit some changes, although these appear insignificant in comparison with the dramatic changes in the mucosal appearance.

Classic manifestations of microscopic changes of the mucosa and surrounding tissue have been described. The earliest lesion seen is that related to the crypts of the mucosa. Small crypt abscesses, along with nonspecific inflammatory cell infiltrates of the lamina propria, are present. As the disease persists and worsens, the mucosal surface becomes flat and the mucosal folds are lost. Inflammatory changes quite characteristically do not involve the deeper layers of the bowel or the serosa.

Polypoid changes of the mucosa in the form of pseudopolyps are common. These pseudopolyps actually consist of edematous mucosal tissue that is located between areas of denuded mucosa and protrudes into the lumen of the bowel. Occasionally granulation tissue with severe inflammation may take on the appearance of a polyp. Pseudopolyps are nonadenomatous and do not represent a malignant threat. Adenomatous polyps of the colon can coexist with ulcerative colitis and thus may be difficult to distinguish.

**Clinical Manifestations.** Symptoms of ulcerative colitis are a combination of diarrhea, rectal bleeding, crampy abdominal pain, weight loss, and anemia; they are the same for

## CLINICAL SEVERITY RATING FOR ULCERATIVE COLITIS

**SEVERE**
Diarrhea with six or more stools per day
Macroscopic blood in stool
Mean evening temperature >99.5° F
*or*
≥100° F temperature on at least 2 of 4 days
Tachycardia (mean pulse rate >90/min)
Anemia (hemoglobin concentration ≤ 75%
   of normal)
ESR >30 mm/hr

**MILD**
Diarrhea with four or fewer stools per day
Only small amounts of macroscopic blood
   in stools
No fever
No tachycardia
Anemia present but not severe
ESR <30 mm/hr

**MODERATE**
Symptoms between extremes of severe
   and mild

*ESR,* Erythrocyte sedimentation rate.

adults and children. Clinical severity of each attack of ulcerative colitis can be categorized as severe, moderate, or mild, as described in the box above.

Rectal bleeding is both the most common as well as the initial symptom associated with ulcerative colitis. In most situations blood loss is the result of inflammatory mucosal changes and the oozing of blood into the lumen. Profuse bleeding from ulcerations occurs in more severe cases, and anemia may result from bloody diarrhea.

Diarrhea, a common problem with all degrees of ulcerative colitis, is described as both bloody and mucoid. The frequency of diarrhea can vary widely and is a function of several factors. Stool volume is increased by the mucosal exudation of mucus, pus, and blood combined with deficiency in the ability of the mucosa to reabsorb sodium and water. Colonic and particularly rectal capacity is reduced because of muscle shortening, spasm, and scarring. Transit time is decreased by abnormal motility caused by prostaglandin release from the bowel mucosa.

Abdominal pain, which is associated with the desire to defecate, is created by the scarred, shortened taeniae coli. The pain, described as crampy, typically is located over the left lower quadrant of the abdomen. Bowel evacuation relieves the abdominal pain. As the disease becomes more severe, abdominal pain commonly abates because the significant damage to the bowel wall and muscles interrupts the transport motility of the colon and the gastrocolic reflex.

Weight loss depends on the severity of the disease. With mild disease the patient generally feels well; as disease progresses, nutritional intake and impaired mucosal absorption compromise the patient's nutritional status.

Elevated temperature may occur with ulcerative colitis but generally is associated with severe and extensive disease. An elevated temperature concomitant with malabsorption should suggest sepsis.

**Diagnosis.** In all situations it is imperative to distinguish the symptoms of ulcerative colitis from other diseases such as Crohn's disease and an infection. Table 10-2 lists the clinical features of ulcerative colitis that distinguish it from Crohn's disease.

**Table 10-2**    Comparison of clinical and pathologic features of ulcerative colitis and Crohn's disease

|  | Ulcerative colitis | Crohn's disease |
|---|---|---|
| **CLINICAL FEATURES** | | |
| Gender | Equal | Equal |
| Diarrhea | Very common | Common |
| Rectal bleeding | Very common | Uncommon |
| Abdominal pain | Common | Common |
| Fever | Uncommon (but does occur) | Common |
| Abdominal mass | Rare | Common |
| Perianal disease | Rare | Common |
| Toxic megacolon | More common than in Crohn's disease | Rare |
| **PATHOLOGIC FEATURES** | | |
| **Macroscopic** | | |
| Distribution | Continuous from rectum | Skip lesions |
| Thickened mesentery | Rare | Common |
| Serositis | Absent | Common |
| Bowel wall | Normal size | Thickened |
| Small bowel involvement | Terminal ileum only as backwash | May occur |
| Fistula | Rare | May occur |
| Strictures | Rare | Common |
| Pseudopolyps | Frequent | May occur |
| Cobblestoning of mucosa | Rare | Common |
| Ulcers | Shallow | Rake (deep, longitudinal) |
| **Microscopic** | | |
| Granulomas | Never | Common |
| Depth of inflammation | Mucosa and submucosa | Transmural |
| Crypt abscesses | Common | Uncommon |
| Fibrosis | Rare | Common |

Visualization of the mucosa of the colon and rectum and biopsy are essential in the diagnostic process. A complete endoscopic or roentgenographic colon examination is not necessary in the acute phase. The diagnosis is established by a combination of visualization of the changes in the rectum and the sigmoid, of biopsy, and of exclusion of other possible diseases. Serial proctosigmoidoscopy examinations generally are sufficient to evaluate the activity of the disease and response to therapy. Complete colonoscopy or barium enema is necessary to provide cancer surveillance and to evaluate the extent of disease in patients with long-standing disease. One of these procedures also is required to establish the extent of disease before surgery or to exclude other diseases.

**Complications.** The numerous complications that may accompany ulcerative colitis can be categorized as local, general, and extraintestinal.

Local complications are limited to the colon and consist of stricture and cancer. Stricture formation is rare in ulcerative colitis. (It occurs more commonly in Crohn's disease.) Therefore, when a stricture is observed in a patient with ulcerative colitis, a carcinoma must be suspected as the cause. When strictures do occur, they are smooth and fusiform, with tapered margins. Strictures are more common with extensive long-standing disease.

Colon cancer is well known to be a potential complication of disease that is long-standing and involves the total colon. Carcinoma in the patient with ulcerative colitis usually is difficult to diagnose, particularly in the presence of pseudopolyps, and tends to be multicentric in origin. The cancer usually arises about 20 years earlier than do adenocarcinomas in the nonpolyposis general population, and survival rates are considered to be poorer.[33]

General complications associated with ulcerative colitis include massive hemorrhage and toxic megacolon. Although general oozing of blood from colonic mucosa is typical of ulcerative colitis, massive hemorrhaging is infrequent and tends to occur without significant disease activity. Emergency colectomy usually is needed to resolve the hemorrhaging.

Toxic megacolon is a life-threatening complication and represents a severe attack of colitis, with total or segmental dilation of the colon (typically the transverse colon). Toxicity may be reflected by the presence of several of the following symptoms: temperature elevation, tachycardia, leukocytosis, hypoalbuminemia, and anemia. In addition, patients may have mental changes, hypotension, dehydration, abdominal tenderness, and electrolyte disturbance. Often, previously severe diarrhea suddenly improves. Extreme dilation of the transverse colon (measuring 5 cm or more) can be ascertained by observation, percussion, and flat-plate radiograph.

Treatment of toxic megacolon requires immediate decompression of the bowel, with GI intubation and administration of corticosteroids. Intravenous antibiotics and nutritional support may be instituted. Barium enema and colonoscopic examinations are contraindicated when toxic megacolon is suspected. The bowel is monitored closely for response to treatment and signs of impending perforation; emergency surgery is indicated in the threat of perforation. A subtotal colectomy and ileostomy most commonly are performed in such circumstances.

Children with ulcerative colitis often have additional complications such as growth retardation, delayed puberty, and profound malnutrition. These symptoms are the combined effects of corticosteroid therapy and an inability to meet the metabolic demands of growth and development. At times these problems are significant enough to warrant surgical resection.[44]

Extraintestinal complications, including pathologic processes that involve the joints, skin, liver, and eyes, have been reported with ulcerative colitis.[14] Joint complications primarily include arthritis (especially peripheral arthritis, spondylitis, or coincidental rheumatoid arthritis). Although difficult to evaluate clearly, peripheral arthritis and rheumatoid arthritis appear to regress after total proctocolectomy.

Skin complications, which include lesions such as pyoderma gangrenosum, are discussed in Chapter 3. Liver dysfunction includes cholestasis, fatty infiltration, pericholangitis, and sclerosing cholangitis. The inflammatory changes typical of pericholangitis affect the bile ducts and the connective tissues around the hepatic artery and portal vein. Colectomy does not appear to significantly affect the progression or lack of progression of this disease. The significance of observed sclerosing cholangitis is uncertain because of its relatively recent observation since the advent of bile duct imaging techniques such as endoscopic retrograde cholangiopancreatography.[14]

Ocular lesions such as uveitis have been noted, although they are not considered common extraintestinal complications of ulcerative colitis. Uveitis, which tends to occur more frequently in women, resolves within 6 to 8 weeks, regardless of therapy, and is unlikely to recur after colectomy.[14]

**Management.** Medical management is the primary treatment for ulcerative colitis. Medications that are used include antidiarrheal agents, sulfasalazine, and corticosteroids. The exact mechanism of the action of sulfasalazine is not completely understood. Sulfasalazine is a combination of sulfapyridine and 5-aminosalicylic acid (5-ASA). The medication undergoes little digestion in the stomach and small intestine.[11] Colonic bacteria break the bond binding the two ingredients, which releases 5-ASA. This ingredient remains in the colon, contacting the mucosal surface, and is excreted in the stool. The active ingredient of sulfasalazine, 5-ASA, appears to act topically on colonic mucosa to inhibit the inflammatory process.[52] Therapeutic response may not be observed for 3 to 4 weeks after sulfasalazine is initiated and often is continued for 1 to 2 or more years. Side effects develop, which appear to be precipitated by the sulfapyridine, not 5-ASA.

New forms of oral and rectal preparations of 5-ASA and 4-ASA have been promising in controlling symptoms, particularly the rectal preparations for disease limited to the distal sigmoid and rectum.[21] Rectal preparations of 5-ASA, which allow direct application of the active ingredient of sulfasalazine to the mucosa by means of a retention enema, are indicated when the disease is limited to less than 60 cm of distal colon. It is believed that oral sulfasalazine provides only limited effectiveness because it is not in contact with the mucosa long enough and because it becomes encased in stool. Rectal preparations do not replace the need for oral sulfasalazine; patients who are taking oral sulfasalazine should continue to do so when rectal 5-ASA is initiated. Although oral sulfasalazine may not deliver enough of the medication to the distal colon to obtain beneficial effects, it appears to be sufficient to control symptoms in the right colon.[21]

Oral preparations of 5-ASA (coated) are being investigated as a method to administer the medication by means of a time-released capsule or according to the pH of the contents of the patient's GI tract.

Corticosteroids are used to reduce inflammation during acute disease and severe episodes. Doses are initially high (in the range of 40 to 80 mg daily) for severe episodes or acute disease and then tapered according to disease activity and therapeutic response. Sulfasalazine often is used in conjunction with corticosteroids. Long-term use of steroids has not been shown to prevent relapse or to maintain remission.[27] Rectal corticosteroids also are used to control or treat distal disease; however, rectal 5-ASA quickly is gaining preference because it can be administered over a long period of time without the adverse effect of corticosteroids.

Definitive surgical intervention (curative resection of the colon and rectum) is obtained by means of (1) total proctocolectomy with ileostomy or continent ileostomy, (2) restorative proctocolectomy and construction of an ileoanal reservoir, or (3) ileoanal anastomosis.[44] The type of procedure selected is largely a function of the patient's preference and age, the severity of the disease, and, of course, the surgeon's preference.

## Crohn's Disease

Granulomatous intestinal disease that shows no evidence of tuberculosis or actinomycosis has been described sporadically for several centuries. It was not until Burrill Crohn and colleagues at Mount Sinai Hospital in New York presented a collected series in 1932 that what is now known as *Crohn's disease* was described.

Many different terms have been used for this disease, which reflects the lack of complete adequacy of any of the terms. Although *granulomatous enteritis* or *colitis* can be an appropriate description, granulomas do not appear in almost one third of the cases. *Regional* or *segmental enteritis* or *colitis* also can be misleading because total involvement, particularly of the colon, is by no means rare. *Transmural colitis* is a term used to differentiate the process from idiopathic proctocolitis; however, in severe cases of ulcerative colitis all layers of the bowel may be involved. Consequently Crohn's disease is the universally preferred term for this pathologic process.

It is now realized that Crohn's disease is a chronic, progressive, granulomatous, inflammatory disease that can affect any part of the alimentary tract from the mouth to the anus. The underlying cause is totally unknown; thus, descriptions of the disease continue to be based on anatomic, clinical, radiologic, and pathologic criteria (Table 10-2).

**Pathophysiology.** Crohn's disease is predominantly a full-thickness (transmural) disease of the bowel wall. Yet submucosal, muscular, or serosal disease may dominate in different sites. The extent of the inflammatory process varies in character from hyperemia, serosal edema, and curious spiraling of superficial serosal vessels in acute disease to purplish discoloration and marked fibrosis in chronic disease. Diseased areas often are separated by normal unaffected areas, producing "skip" lesions. The number of pathologic changes in Crohn's disease can be approached most clearly through a discussion of distribution, mucosal abnormalities, bowel wall abnormalities, and radiographic appearance.

*Distribution.* The anatomic distribution of Crohn's disease is not continuous; disease can be present at various sporadic sites throughout the alimentary tract. In the classic pattern the last few centimeters of terminal ileum are affected. Terminal ileal involvement is extremely common; however, exclusive involvement is not typical. The colon alone may be affected, but most often the ileum and colon are simultaneously involved. Although the anal canal typically is involved, which can occur in isolation, most often it is associated with Crohn's colitis (disease located in the colon). Mouth lesions are rare and seem to occur more frequently when Crohn's disease affects the colon rather than the ileum alone. Esophageal, stomach, and duodenal involvement also are relatively rare but tend to occur in conjunction with small bowel disease.

*Mucosal abnormalities.* The mucosal change characteristic of Crohn's disease is the presence of ulcerations. Both aphthoid ulcers (canker sores) and deep, longitudinal rake ulcers can be observed. Aphthoid ulcers are small, discrete, superficial ulcers with a white sloughing base and bright red hyperemic edge. Normal, uninvolved mucosa often surrounds ulcers. The mucosa typically assumes a cobblestone appearance because of the ulcers' criss-cross pattern and the protrusion of surrounding edematous mucosa into the bowel lumen. Large, irregular, haphazardly arranged serpiginous ulcers also are typical of Crohn's disease that involves the colon and in fact may extend into the perianal skin.

Ulcers may be limited to the submucosa but classically are deep. Penetration through the full thickness of the bowel wall creates such complications as abscesses, fistulas, and adhesions. The absorptive function of the mucosa is grossly reduced by the presence of ulcers, which contain mainly lymphocytes and which exude pus.

*Bowel wall abnormalities.* Bowel wall changes invariably include a thickened bowel wall, rigidity, and loss of peristalsis. These changes occur because of localized edema, submucosal lymphatic dilation, and fibrosis. Mural thickening also leads to impingement of the lumen or stenosis.

External to the bowel wall, edema and fatty inflammation may extend into the root of the mesentery near the involved bowel. In long-standing cases, fibrosis develops, making the mesentery thick, short, and rigid. Lymph nodes adjacent to the affected segment are visibly enlarged and firm and may be matted together. When transected, lymph nodes typically have a fleshy appearance, often with necrosis.

***Radiologic appearance.*** On radiographic examination the appearance of the bowel and mucosal surface in Crohn's disease can be both varied and informative. It is, however, difficult to identify distinct radiologic patterns that correspond to acute, subacute, or chronic stages of the disease.

Small-bowel disease is demonstrated by a small-bowel follow-through radiograph. Mucosal folds appear thickened, rigid, and partially fused. The contour of the lumen appears irregular. Although superficial ulcers may not be detectable, deeper ulcers appear as spicules or "rose thorns." Streaks of barium outline and expose these ulcers. Filling defects reveal inflammatory pseudopolyps and skip areas.

The thickened intestinal wall and narrowed lumen are demonstrated on radiographic examination by wide separation of the neighboring loops of intestine. Pseudodiverticula, which are highly characteristic of the disease, are created by the protrusion of normal intestine between thickened folds and skip lesions.

Fibrosis, muscle spasms, and loss of mesenteric flexibility produce a picture of a rigid, narrowed lumen without mucosal pattern. With long-standing fibrosis the more severe degrees of segmental constriction (of varying lengths) assume a characteristic pipe-stem appearance that often is called the "string sign" because the narrowed disease segment appears as a thin linear shadow. Proximal dilation of normal bowel may develop and commonly suggests chronic intestinal obstruction.

Localized perforation may be visible as extravasation of barium outside the lumen of the bowel. The perforation may form a localized abscess or a fistula to a surrounding viscus or another part of the intestine.

Finally, deformity of the cecum or ascending colon is common when Crohn's disease is located in the distal ileum. Because the thickened segment of ileum may impinge on the medial wall of the cecum, a characteristic concavity is produced. Direct extension of the disease subsequently produces narrowing and mucosal irregularity of the cecum.

**Clinical Manifestations.** The severity and extent of clinical manifestations are influenced by many factors, including the underlying inflammatory process occurring within the bowel. Fever, abdominal pain, and diarrhea are common. Abdominal pain is described as colicky and may be diffuse or located over a diseased area. Rectal bleeding is uncommon, although occult blood may be detected in the stool. Additional manifestations include malaise, anorexia, nausea, vomiting, weight loss, and malnutrition.

Physical examination may reveal an abdominal mass in the right lower quadrant of the abdomen and perianal disease (such as fistulas or fissures). Children may have slowed growth patterns before the onset of intestinal symptoms.[55]

**Complications.** Several complications may accompany Crohn's disease. These include free perforation, strictures, abscess, fistula, perianal disease (such as fistula, abscess, and skin lesions), malnutrition, massive hemorrhage, and toxic megacolon.

**Diagnosis.** Establishment of the correct diagnosis of Crohn's disease after initial investigation occurs only in a small number of patients because the mucosal changes revealed by radiographic examination and colonoscopy are nonspecific. In most cases a firm diagnosis is not established until a series of events have occurred over time. During the early stages of the disease, lack of a firm diagnosis does not pose a problem because treatment is directed at relief of the symptoms.

Given these constraints, the diagnosis of Crohn's disease generally is made by corroborating a constellation of findings: clinical manifestations, examination of the bowel (with endoscopy or radiographic studies, or both), exclusion of other possibilities (such as ulcerative and infectious colitis), and histologic features. Patterns of histologic observations are more significant in the diagnosis than is one specific histologic feature.

Briefly, granulomas are the hallmark of the disease. Composed of epithelial cells with or without giant cells, granulomas are seen in any of the bowel wall layers; lymph nodes near the involved segment also may contain granulomas. The absence of granulomas, however, cannot exclude Crohn's disease because granulomas are not present in all cases. Mucosal fissures (linear ulcers) are lined with a layer of necrotic cells, underlying macrophages, and inflammatory cells. Edema, dilated lymphatic vessels, and collagen deposits also are revealed.

**Management.** Crohn's disease is treated primarily with medical therapies. Because no known cure exists for this disease, the treatment goal is to reduce bowel inflammation, correct nutritional deficiencies, and provide symptomatic relief of intestinal and extraintestinal manifestations. As with ulcerative colitis, the medications typically used to achieve these objectives include sulfasalazine, corticosteroids, and antidiarrheal agents, as already discussed.

Immunosuppressive agents have been substituted for corticosteroid therapy to reduce inflammation. Such medications (azathioprine, 6-mercaptopurine) are controversial; however, they may be indicated to eliminate the undesirable effects of corticosteroid therapy (such as growth retardation). Close observation is mandatory because bone marrow depression, leukopenia, arthralgias, infection, and hypersensitivity are frequent adverse effects. These agents are commonly intended for long-term use (several months to years).

Metronidazole (Flagyl), which is used in Crohn's disease, appears to be slightly more effective than sulfasalazine.[42] Indications for use include allergic, intolerant, or unresponsive reactions to sulfasalazine. In some studies metronidazole has been found to be effective in healing indolent perianal disease.[12] Reactions to metronidazole include metallic taste, urticaria, dark urine, reversible neutropenia, headache, vertigo, and peripheral neuropathy. The mechanism of metronidazole is unknown, but it may be related to the suppression of cell-mediated immunity.[42]

Nutritional support is provided through dietary modifications, vitamins, oral supplements, or parenteral nutrition as needed. Dietary modifications are not routinely prescribed; rather the patient should identify those foods that are well tolerated and those that tend to aggravate symptoms.

Certain dietary modifications may be beneficial in the presence of specific complications. When the bowel is stenotic, roughage should be eliminated to reduce the risk of partial or complete obstruction. A low-residue diet may reduce the diarrhea associated with severe attacks. Lactose intolerance should be confirmed with a lactose tolerance test before milk products are eliminated from the diet because these products are commonly good sources of nutrients. Finally, extensive resection or disease in the small bowel may result in malabsorption syndromes and diarrhea that can be reduced with a low-fat diet.

In general, surgery usually is delayed in Crohn's disease until complications develop. Indications include progressive obstructive symptoms, fistula formation, perforation, hemorrhage, and a failure to respond to medical therapy. Failed medical therapy includes persistent symptoms, complications of corticosteroid therapy, side effects of sulfasalazine, and, in children, impaired growth and failure to thrive.

Total proctocolectomy with end ileostomy is the preferred procedure for Crohn's disease that is confined to the colon and rectum. Resection with restoration of continuity (such as right hemicolectomy, ileocolic resection, or subtotal colectomy with ileorectal anastomosis) is also used to resect diseased bowel.

## DIVERTICULAR DISEASE

Diverticular disease has been recognized for several centuries, but clarification of the various aspects of this disease occurred only in the twentieth century. It is now postulated that two forms of diverticular disease exist. One form is the presence of multiple diverticula scattered throughout the entire colon but without accompanying muscular abnormality of the colon. *Diverticulosis* is the proper term for this condition. Bleeding is the usual complication, although complications of this diffuse diverticulosis are uncommon. The other form of diverticular disease, *diverticular disease*, is the presence of diverticula, predominantly confined to the sigmoid colon, in conjunction with muscular abnormalities of the colon. Complications such as perforation and obstruction occur with this form of the disease. Diverticulitis, then, refers to an acute inflammation of the diverticular disease.

**Epidemiology.** The prevalence of diverticular disease and diverticulosis is difficult to define. Although millions are estimated to have diverticulosis, symptoms of diverticular disease develop in only 1/5 persons.[23] Autopsy studies suggest a 5% incidence at 50 years of age; this number increases dramatically to a 50% incidence at 80 years of age.[45] Diverticular disease seems to affect both sexes equally.

Contributory factors to diverticular disease are Western life-style, dietary changes (particularly the low-fiber diet), and geographic, genetic, and ethnic factors. Diverticular disease is uncommon in Japan, Africa, Asia, and many parts of South America. This demographic observation has led to the recognition of the role of dietary habits (low fiber and highly refined carbohydrates) in the pathogenesis of the disease.

**Pathophysiology.** It is important to clarify terminology before a discussion of the process of diverticular disease. The presence of one outpouching is a *diverticulum;* the plural form of the word diverticulum is *diverticula* (not diverticuli).

A colonic diverticulum is a herniation of the mucosa and submucosa through the circular muscle of the colon, which forms a sac. There is no bowel musculature in the diverticula. In as many as 90% of the cases diverticula are confined to the sigmoid and left colon.[45] A right-sided distribution (limited to the cecum and proximal right colon) has been observed in the Hawaiian population.

The anatomic distribution of diverticula is quite uniform. Diverticula are related to the taeniae coli and to the entry points of small blood vessels (considered to be a weak spot in the colonic wall). Classically the diverticula appear in two rows between the mesenteric and the antimesenteric taeniae (Fig. 10-6). The circular muscle between the two antimesenteric

**Fig. 10-6**   Diverticulum is evident between mesenteric and antimesenteric taeniae.

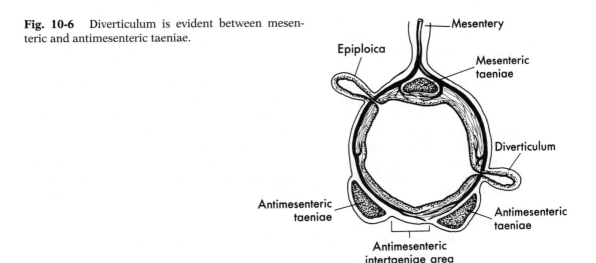

taeniae always is free of diverticula. Each individual diverticulum may vary in size from 1 mm to several centimeters. When diverticula are large, a distinction must be made between the standard acquired pulsion diverticula and the congenital large diverticulum. The latter usually involves all layers of the bowel wall and probably represents a type of reduplication of the intestine.

Small blood vessels are found to lie close to the neck of each diverticulum. They also may be found in relation to the fundus of the diverticulum, with small blood vessels radiating over the surface. The diverticula close to the mesenteric taenia may be completely obscured by the mesentery and the fatty epiploic appendices, making them difficult to observe.

In most cases muscular abnormalities, as well as the diverticula, are present. Thickened muscular crescents with shortening of the longitudinal taeniae are common. It is not known for certain whether diverticulosis or muscular thickening is the initial change; usually both manifestations coexist in patients with diverticular disease. Muscle abnormalities, however, are believed to play an important role in the pathogenesis of this disease.

Studies have shown a significant increase in intralumenal pressure in the colon of the patients with established diverticular disease. Excessive segmentation of the colon, particularly the sigmoid, has been suggested to result in isolated areas of high pressure. In fact, this pressure is high enough to induce herniation of the mucosa through the weak spot in the colonic wall caused by the entry and exit of small blood vessels. This pressure accounts for the constant distribution of diverticula in relation to the taeniae coli of the bowel wall. It is rare to observe diverticula on the antimesenteric border of the colon, which is not a site for vascular entry and exit.

Dietary habits typical of Western societies are believed to contribute to the muscle abnormality and excessive segmentation of the colon.[8] Such diets typically contain highly refined and fiber-deficient foods. The result is believed to be a stool that requires excessive segmentation to promote advancement and that prolongs its intestinal transit. A high-fiber diet tends to produce a frequent, bulky stool.

When diverticular disease exists with no muscular abnormality (such as with diverticulosis), a collagen tissue abnormality may cause the disease. This causative factor may better explain the type of diverticulosis that develops in the older person (because such collagen abnormalities may develop as one ages) and in the ascending colon (where intraluminal pressures are low).

Many of the previously accepted concepts of nomenclature, pathogenesis, pathophysiology, and management of diverticular disease are changing as more understanding and experience are acquired. Historically *diverticulosis* was the term used to denote symptomless diverticula of the colon. Pain was assumed to result from inflammation of the diverticula and consequently was termed *diverticulitis*. This concept, however, is not always sustained with histologic evidence of inflammation. It is now clear that the pain associated with acute diverticular disease is not necessarily due to inflammation; rather it is more likely due to sustained muscle spasm and secondary ischemia. Many patients receiving surgical procedures for diverticulitis, in fact, have no evidence of inflammation. It is therefore preferable to consider the terms *asymptomatic diverticular disease* and *symptomatic diverticular disease* to distinguish more accurately the presence or absence of symptoms in conjunction with diverticula.

When an inflammatory process occurs, it is believed to be an inflammation of the bowel wall that extends to adjacent peritoneum, pericolic fat, and mesenteric fat. This extension develops because the diverticulum is thin walled. An acute inflammatory reaction can result in a large, tender, palpable mass that adheres to other organs or segments of bowel. This adherence actually may serve to isolate a perforation or prompt fistulization.[43]

**Clinical Manifestations.** The majority of patients with diverticulosis remain symptom-free throughout life. The presence of diverticula usually is detected inadvertently when the patient is having examinations for other problems. A prediverticular state associated with repeated attacks of pain in the left lower quadrant of the abdomen often precedes the appearance of diverticula and is characterized by muscle thickening and shortening of the colon. These symptoms often are indistinguishable from those of irritable bowel syndrome. Some diverticula can regress; clinical signs of diverticulitis develop only in 10% to 25%.[45]

Inflammation of diverticula,—that is, diverticulitis—occurs more often in the older-aged person, commonly affects the sigmoid colon, and rarely involves the rectum. Less commonly the descending or ascending colon is affected. Diverticulitis is characterized by an increase in the severity of abdominal pain. This pain typically is located in the left lower abdominal quadrant, is persistent, and may extend to the lower portion of the back. Diarrhea or constipation often precede the attack, and nausea and vomiting may accompany the pain. Fever and leukocytosis may occur concomitant with abdominal tenderness over the involved bowel segment.

**Complications.** Several complications may accompany diverticulitis. In the acute phase perforation occurs with varying degrees of surrounding peritonitis that can be localized. These variations have led to a classification of acute diverticulitis grades 1 to 4, depending on the amount of local inflammation and the presence of pus with or without peritonitis. This classification is used to compare therapies in the acute phase.

Chronic inflammatory change either may be localized to a short area or may involve a long segment of colon. A chronic inflammatory phlegmon results; usually associated with an intermesenteric abscess, it often extends to other viscera as a secondary process.

Fistula formation caused either by acute or by chronic diverticular inflammation results from perforation and abscess formation. Colovesical, colocutaneous, or cologenital fistulas may develop, depending on the anatomy and gender of the patient. In most cases the fistula is small and usually emanates from a single perforated diverticulum.

Profuse lower GI hemorrhage usually occurs in the absence of acute or chronic diverticular inflammation. Bleeding may be profuse and life threatening. In the majority of cases, bleeding ceases spontaneously without need for any direct intervention. In a small number of patients, bleeding must be controlled either by radiographic or surgical interventions. Bleeding angiodysplasias have been found in a large number of patients whose original diagnosis was bleeding from diverticular disease.

Acute large-bowel obstruction can result from chronic diverticular disease. In all cases a coexisting carcinoma of the colon must be considered and excluded. Complete large-bowel obstruction rarely develops in patients with acute diverticular inflammation, although some degree of partial bowel obstruction is common.

**Diagnosis.** An investigation of diverticular disease begins with either contrast radiograph or endoscopic visualization. Contrast barium enema studies have the advantage of demonstrating the presence of diverticular, as well as the extracolonic, complications that may accompany the disease. The drawbacks of endoscopic evaluation are its occasional failure to reveal diverticula and difficulty in completing the procedure because of the presence of distortion, angulation, narrowing, and fixation of the bowel. Computed tomography (CT) scan evaluation is useful for the evaluation and occasional therapy of pericolic abscesses. Laboratory tests are not useful to diagnose the presence of diverticula but do reveal leukocytosis or anemia.

**Management.** The presence of asymptomatic colonic diverticula requires no specific treatment. Prophylactic measures such as increased dietary fiber, however, should be encouraged to prevent symptomatic disease.

Symptomatic diverticulosis is managed according to severity of symptoms. Bowel rest (such as clear liquids in mild attacks) and antibiotics are instituted. More severe attacks, particularly those that suggest concurrent complications, require hospitalization. Oral intake of food and fluids is not permitted; nasogastric intubation may be indicated to relieve nausea and vomiting. Opiate analgesics (such as morphine) are contraindicated because of their hypertonic effect on the bowel. Demerol, however, has less hypertonic effect.[8,45] Parenteral antibiotics are warranted.

When acute episodes resolve, the patient should be instructed in the importance of adding fiber either through the diet or with supplements. Medications such as cathartics, enemas, and antidiarrheal agents for symptomatic relief of constipation or diarrhea are to be avoided.

Surgical intervention is indicated in the presence of complications or in an attempt to relieve unrelenting acute attacks. Elective operations are preferred when possible because of the associated lower morbidity and mortality. Surgical procedures achieve resection of the affected segment with a primary anastomosis or temporary diverting intestinal stoma, depending on the extent of diverticular disease, coexisting disease, and the presence of complications.

# RADIATION ENTERITIS

Radiation therapy commonly is used for the treatment of pelvic malignancies, particularly gynecologic tumors and prostate and bladder carcinomas. Intestinal damage from irradiation may result, particularly that of the small bowel, because of the fixation of the bowel to the pelvis after previous pelvic surgery.

Radiosensitivity varies within the GI tract. The small intestine is the most radiosensitive of the intraabdominal organs. Doses of radiation greater than 45 Gy to the small bowel and 55 Gy to the rectum may cause bowel damage.[6]

**Pathophysiology.** Radiation that affects the intestine causes obliterative endarteritis of the smaller arteries, with ischemia and fibrosis in the submucosa and mesentery. This is a permanent change and produces avascularity. Consequently inflammation develops and may persist and progress over many years.

Early effects of irradiation, in the form of mucosal damage, become apparent within a few days. The degree of damage depends in part on total dosage but always on fractionation of the dose. These changes usually are minor and transitory, healing within 2 to 4 weeks.

Late changes are the result of ongoing obliterative endarteritis. This condition results in chronic inflammation, with the bowel wall becoming more pale and thick. Fibrosis may cause narrowing and, in fact, may be mistaken for Crohn's disease. Stricture formation, ulceration, and even perforation, with fistula formation from the involved segment, may develop.

**Management.** Radiation damage has been estimated to become devastating and life threatening in as many as 10% of the patients receiving irradiation.[6] Treatment of radiation complications depends on type of complications and patient prognosis. Surgical resection or bypass of the diseased segment may be warranted when the disease is severe or limited to a specific segment of bowel. Radiation affects the connective tissue to a degree that wound healing is impaired, complicating attempts at surgical removal of the affected bowel. Surgical intervention, however, for repair or control of severe disease should not be automatically excluded. Good results have been reported with the use of techniques for continent urinary diversion, for example, after previous pelvic irradiation.[38]

## PSEUDOMEMBRANOUS COLITIS

Pseudomembranous colitis is a condition that affects mainly the colon and rectum and is characterized by the formation of elevated yellowish-white mucosal plaques. Pseudomembranous colitis is believed to result from the two toxins produced by *Clostridium difficile* that cause diarrhea and enterocolitis. Originally pseudomembranous colitis was associated with the use of antibiotics, particularly clindamycin. With the identification of *C. difficile*, it has become clear that pseudomembranous colitis actually is a severe form of a variety of antibiotic-associated conditions.

**Clinical Manifestations.** Diarrhea occurs most commonly during antibiotic therapy, although it develops in some patients 4 to 6 weeks after cessation of therapy. Fever, leukocytosis, and abdominal cramps also are present. Stools, which are watery and offensive, do not contain gross evidence of mucus or blood. Complications are severe and include protracted diarrhea, electrolyte imbalance, hypoalbuminemia, and toxic megacolon.

**Diagnosis.** Diagnosis is established by tissue culture assay for *C. difficile* toxin or by stool culture (although results take longer to obtain by the latter method). The histologic appearance of plaques also is characteristic.

**Management.** Once diagnosis is established, treatment requires identification of the precipitating antibiotic and discontinuation of its administration. Antiperistaltic medications should not be used for the diarrhea because of the potential for toxic megacolon. Inasmuch as this disease may be spread from patients who are excreting the organism, precautionary measures should be instituted. Antimicrobial agents may be indicated in severe cases to eradicate the toxin-producing organism. Oral vancomycin, metronidazole, tetracycline, and bacitracin may be used.[10] After adequate therapy the disease may relapse in a small percentage of patients. Surgical resection is not warranted for pseudomembranous enterocolitis.

## INFECTIOUS ENTERITIS

Many organisms have been implicated in the precipitation of infectious diarrhea: bacterial, viral, parasitic, and fungal. The box below lists some of the more common causes of infectious enteritis. In all cases a severe toxic colitis or enteritis can develop. Symptoms mimic inflammatory bowel disease, which must be considered in the differential diagnosis. Most often, symptoms are short-lived and self-resolving. Investigation requires stool culture to identify the offending organism. A careful travel history often is helpful in the diagnosis. Appropriate antibiotic therapy is instituted after a diagnosis is established.

---

### COMMON CAUSES OF INFECTIOUS ENTERITIS

**BACTERIAL**
*Shigella*
*Salmonella*
Gonococcal
Syphilitic
Tuberculosis
Pathogenic *Escherichia coli*
Staphylococcal enterocolitis
*Yersinia enterocolitica*
*Campylobacter*
Pseudomembranous enterocolitis

**PARASITIC**
Amebiasis
Schistosomiasis
Balantidiasis
Cryptosporidiosis

**VIRAL**
Lymphogranuloma venereum
Cytomegalovirus
Behçet's syndrome
Herpesvirus proctitis

**FUNGAL**
Histoplasmosis
Blastomycosis

## ISCHEMIC DISORDERS

Colonic ischemia may be the result of catastrophic vascular accidents, usually resulting in varying degrees of colonic infarction and serious consequences. Recently, however, it has been recognized that noncatastrophic forms of colonic ischemia also exist. In fact, these forms account for one of the more common disorders of the large intestine seen in elderly persons. It is suggested that the second peak incidence (late 50s to 70s) observed with ulcerative colitis and Crohn's disease actually may be an ischemic event.[30]

A spectrum of clinical problems and pathologic findings exists, ranging from completely reversible damage to colonic gangrene with perforation and peritonitis. Ischemic injury to the colon can be classified according to the severity of injury: (1) reversible ischemic colitis, (2) transient ischemic colitis, (3) chronic ischemic colitis, (4) ischemic colonic stricture, and (5) colonic gangrene. The initial presentation may be identical in all cases and is not predictive of the course of the disease.

Reversible ischemic colitis can be mild or severe. Mild reversible ischemic colitis produces submucosal and intramural hemorrhages and edema. These conditions usually are transitory and resolve as a result of reabsorption within 1 to 2 weeks. In more severe cases ischemia of the overlying mucosa results in sloughing, with ulceration and inflammation; resolution occurs over a period of 4 to 8 weeks.

Irreversible lesions occur in those patients in whom the clinical course does not resolve rapidly. This result may be the extreme of transmural gangrene or lesser degrees of damage, which can cause severe ulceration with local sepsis. If untreated, lesser degrees of ischemia may heal over a long period but inevitably result in a stricture. Although these localized strictures may resolve over a period of 12 to 24 months, in the majority of cases a resection is warranted either because of nonhealing of the original lesion or because of obstructive problems precipitated by the stricture.

Ischemic colitis usually is diagnosed after an ischemic episode occurs and blood flow to the affected segment has returned to normal. The colon damage resulting from such an ischemic insult persists, however, and produces mild to moderate problems, usually causing diarrhea, often bloody. Although severe complications can develop, most episodes are noncatastrophic, with transient symptoms and pathologic changes.

Early diagnosis is imperative in colonic ischemia to ensure appropriate management and to identify patients in whom irreversible changes are occurring. A combination of radiographic, colonoscopic, and clinical findings is necessary to establish the diagnosis of ischemic colitis. Barium enema examination reveals "thumb printing," or pseudotumors, that is, changes generated by submucosal hemorrhage and edema. These signs are invariably segmental but are found only relatively early in the evolution of the disease because they disappear within days as the edema and hemorrhages resolve. Persistence of "thumb printing" after 1 week suggests a diagnosis other than ischemic colitis.

Visual inspection of the affected colonic mucosa by colonoscopy reveals the same changes. Submucosal hemorrhage, which may be accompanied by superficial mucosal ulceration and sloughing, is particularly evident. Biopsy specimens reveal submucosal hemorrhage characteristic of the disease.

## TRAUMA

Abdominal and pelvic trauma are common problems encountered in Western cultures. Blunt trauma caused by traffic or industrial accidents can result in multiple intraabdominal injuries, including damage to the colon and rectum. These injuries are the result of shearing force and often cause extensive damage, including mesenteric disruption and devascularization of large segments of intestine.

Penetrating trauma from stab wounds or gunshot injuries usually result in lesser degrees of injury and often are localized. Gunshot injuries can be further complicated by differing muzzle velocity. Low-velocity injuries such as those caused by small handguns often result in minimal localized trauma. High-velocity injuries from powerful rifles, however, can result in extensive surrounding tissue damage. Because of the small size of the entry wound, this damage often is not readily apparent.

In all cases of blunt abdominal trauma or in suspected cases of blunt abdominal trauma, radiographic examination and peritoneal lavage help delineate the problem. In many instances exploratory laparotomy is necessary to definitively exclude or diagnose the problem.

Treatment is based largely on both the degree of injury and associated problems. Isolated colon injuries with trauma rarely occur without the involvement of other organs.

## SUMMARY

Numerous pathologic conditions develop throughout the life span that warrant an intestinal diversion of some type. These diversions may be temporary or permanent, curative or palliative. In each situation intestinal diversion is but one component of the treatment, and complex, often long-term medical therapies accompany diagnosis and management of the disease. It is imperative that the nurse be familiar with these diseases so that the care provided can be truly in concert with the patient's total needs and health care goals.

# SELF-EVALUATION

## QUESTIONS

1. Hirschsprung's disease is characterized by the:
   a. Presence of a proximal migration of ganglionic cells
   b. Presence of a distal migration of ganglionic cells
   c. Absence of the proximal migration of ganglionic cells
   d. Absence of the distal migration of ganglionic cells

2. The neonate with symptoms of intestinal obstruction, failure to pass meconium, dilated hypertrophied proximal ileum, and narrowed distal ileum filled with pelletlike stool is likely to have which of the following diseases?
   a. Hirschsprung's disease
   b. Malrotation
   c. Meconium ileus
   d. Necrotizing enterocolitis

3. Anorectal malformations are classified as high, low, or intermediate by determining the position of the terminal bowel to which structure?
   a. Dentate line
   b. Puborectalis muscle
   c. Pubic symphysis
   d. Transition zone of narrowing

4. Describe the difference among diverticulitis, diverticulosis, and diverticular disease.

5. Compare and contrast five pathologic features and five clinical manifestations of Crohn's disease and ulcerative colitis.

6. Biopsies are used to confirm the diagnosis of the following diseases *except:*
   a. Anorectal malformation
   b. Colorectal cancer
   c. Familial adenomatous polyposis
   d. Hirschsprung's disease

7. Which of the following statements is true of extrahepatic biliary atresia?
   a. Ascending cholangitis is a common complication of corrective surgery.
   b. For best results the Kasai portoenterostomy should be performed between 10 and 15 weeks of life.
   c. Biliary atresia is a congenital disorder.
   d. The neonate with biliary atresia typically is premature and underweight.

8. Episodes of gross or occult bloody stools in the neonate is a suspect symptom for which of the following diseases?
   a. Hirschsprung's disease
   b. Malrotation
   c. Necrotizing enterocolitis
   d. Ulcerative colitis

9. Define each of the following terms: dynamic obstruction, adynamic obstruction, and closed-loop obstruction.

10. State the disease that is typically associated with the following diagnostic features:
    Granulomas
    Pneumotosis intestinalis
    Air-fluid levels demonstrated by a flat-plate radiograph
    Transition zone of narrowing (TZN)
    Bird's-beak appearance demonstrated on contrast radiograph of colon
11. A colorectal tumor that is contained within the bowel wall and does not involve lymph nodes is a Dukes' stage:
    a. A
    b. B
    c. C
    d. D
12. Which of the following gastrointestinal polyposis syndromes is characterized by hamartomatous polyps and melanin spots around the mouth?
    a. Familial adenomatous polyposis
    b. Juvenile polyposis syndromes
    c. Peutz-Jeghers syndrome
    d. Turcot syndrome
13. Desmoid tumors, osteomas, and duodenal polyps may be extraintestinal manifestations of which disease?
    a. Ulcerative colitis
    b. Familial adenomatous polyposis
    c. Crohn's disease
    d. Turcot syndrome
14. Briefly describe five risk factors for the development of colorectal cancer.
15. The surgical procedure that is *not* a curative operation for ulcerative colitis or familial adenomatous polyposis is:
    a. A low anterior resection
    b. A total proctocolectomy with continent ileostomy
    c. An ileoanal reservoir
    d. A panproctocolectomy with ileostomy
16. The Soave and Swenson procedures are corrective surgical techniques for:
    a. High anorectal malformations
    b. Hirschsprung's disease
    c. Meconium ileus
    d. Intussusception
17. Which of the following statements about the use of medications for medical management of inflammatory bowel disease is true?
    a. The active ingredient in sulfasalazine is sulfapyridine.
    b. Long-term use of oral corticosteroids helps prevent relapses of the disease.
    c. Rectal 5-ASA cannot be used over a long period because of adverse effects.
    d. Metronidazole is used more commonly in Crohn's disease than in ulcerative colitis.
18. Radiation effects on the bowel are transitory and resolve within 2 to 4 weeks.
    a. True
    b. False

# SELF-EVALUATION

## ANSWERS

1. **d.** Absence of the distal migration of ganglionic cells
2. **c.** Meconium ileus
3. **b.** Puborectalis muscle
4. *Diverticular disease* describes the presence of diverticula in the colon and the concurrent muscular abnormalities of the colon (shortening of the longitudinal taeniae and thickened muscular crescents). Abdominal pain may result from muscle spasms, or an inflammatory process *(diverticulitis)* may cause symptoms such as temperature, pain, leukocytosis, and nausea. Complications such as perforation and obstruction may occur with this disease. *Diverticulosis* is the presence of diverticula scattered throughout the colon, without muscle abnormality of the colon. Diverticula are present in many persons who are unaware of them because they are symptomless. Complications rarely accompany diverticulosis.
5. Comparison and contrast of Crohn's disease and ulcerative colitis:
   *Pathologic features*
   Ulcerative colitis
   Continuous from rectum; limited to colon
   Bowel wall, serosa, and mesentery normal
   Terminal ileum rarely involved
   Fistula and strictures rare
   Involves mucosal and submucosal layers only
   Pseudopolyps common
   Crypt abscesses common
   Ulcers rare; shallow if present
   Crohn's disease
   Most commonly involves ileum
   Sporadic involvement of intestine (skip lesions)
   May involve all of GI tract
   Transmural involvement of bowel layers
   Fistulas and strictures may develop
   Mucosa assumes a cobblestone appearance
   Rake ulcers common and deep
   *Clinical manifestations*
   Ulcerative colitis
   Rectal bleeding very common
   Fever uncommon
   Abdominal mass rarely palpated
   Perianal disease rare
   Toxin megacolon may develop
   Diarrhea and abdominal pain common

Crohn's disease
Rectal bleeding uncommon
Fever common
Abdominal mass often palpated over area of active disease
Perianal disease may develop
Toxic megacolon rarely develops
Diarrhea and abdominal pain common

**6. a.** Anorectal malformation

**7. a.** Ascending cholangitis is a common complication of corrective surgery.

**8. c.** Necrotizing enterocolitis

**9.** Definitions

*Dynamic obstruction:* Dynamic obstruction is a surgical emergency. The source of the occlusion can be from within the lumen of the bowel, from external compression of the bowel, or from within the bowel layers. Adhesions are the most common cause of small intestinal dynamic obstructions whereas colon cancer is the most common cause of large bowel dynamic obstructions.

*Adynamic obstruction:* This type of obstruction, which results from an absence of peristalsis such as in paralytic ileus, is a temporary condition that resolves once the initiating cause is corrected.

*Closed-loop obstruction:* A closed-loop obstruction is created by an obstruction in the colon and a patent ileocecal valve. Because this valve normally is closed to prevent reflux into the ileum, it also serves to trap colonic material (gas and feces) between the site of obstruction and the ileocecal valve. Distention of the bowel can then develop, with the potential for perforation.

**10.** Features and diseases

Granulomas: Crohn's disease
Pneumotosis intestinalis: Necrotizing enterocolitis
Air-fluid levels demonstrated by a flat-plate radiograph: Bowel obstruction
Transition zone of narrowing: Hirschsprung's disease
Bird's-beak appearance demonstrated on contrast radiograph of colon: Volvulus

**11. b.** B

**12. c.** Peutz-Jeghers syndrome

**13. b.** Familial adenomatous polyposis

**14.** Risk factors

Diet: Low fiber, high animal fat, alcohol consumption
Age: 50 to 80 years of age
History of previously cured colorectal malignancy
Presence of benign adenomatous polyps
Genetic predisposition (familial polyposis, cancer family syndrome, and hereditary site-specific colon cancer)
History of ulcerative colitis

**15. a.** A low anterior resection

**16. b.** Hirschsprung's disease

**17. d.** Metronidazole is used more commonly in Crohn's disease than in ulcerative colitis.

**18. b.** False

## REFERENCES

1. Alquist DA et al: Fecal occult blood levels in health and disease: a study using HemoQuant, *N Engl J Med* 312:1422, 1985.
2. Baba S et al: Symposium: inflammatory bowel disease–spectrum, *Dis Colon Rectum* 33:232, 1990.
3. Bak MP, Boley SJ: Sigmoid volvulus in elderly patients, *Am J Surg* 151:71, 1986.
4. Berry CL, Keeling JW: Gastrointestinal system. In Berry CL, editor: *Paediatric pathology*, ed 2, New York, 1989, Springer-Verlag.
5. Boarini J: Gastrointestinal cancer: colon, rectum, and anus. In Gorenwald SL et al, editors: *Cancer nursing: principles and practice*, ed 2, Boston, 1990, Jones & Bartlett.
6. Bralow SP, Marks G.: Radiation injury to the gut. In Berk JE, editor: *Bockus gastroenterology*, ed 4. Vol 4: *Intestine, part two*, Philadelphia, 1985, WB Saunders.
7. Bresalier RS, Kim YS: Diet and colon cancer: putting the puzzle together, *N Engl J Med* 313:1413, 1985 (editorial).
8. Bryant RA: Diverticular disease, *J Enterostom Ther* 13:114, 1986.
9. Burt RW, Samowitz WS: The adenomatous polyp and the hereditary polyposis syndromes, *Gastroenterol Clin North Am* 171:657, 1988.
10. Chang T: Antibiotic-associated injury to the gut. In Berk JE, editor: *Bockus gastroenterology*, ed 4. Vol 4: *Intestine, part two*, Philadelphia, 1985, WB Saunders.
11. Das KM: Sulfasalazine therapy in inflammatory bowel disease, *Gastroenterol Clin North Am* 18:1, 1989.
12. Duffy LF et al: Peripheral neuropathy in Crohn's disease patients treated with metronidazole, *Gastroenterology* 88:681, 1985.
13. Egan EA, Agarwal S: Neonatal necrotizing enterocolitis. In Lebenthal E, editor: *Textbook of gastroenterology and nutrition in infancy*, New York, 1989, Raven Press.
14. Farmer RG: Ulcerative colitis: complications. In Berk JE, editor: *Bockus gastroenterology*, ed 4. Vol 4: *Intestine, part two*, Philadelphia, 1985, WB Saunders.
15. Farmer RG: Ulcerative colitis: history and epidemiology. In Berk JE, editor: *Bockus gastroenterology*, ed 4. Vol 4: *Intestine, part two*, Philadelphia, 1985, WB Saunders.
16. Finne CO III: Cancer of the colon: ruminations on the past and future, *J Enterostom Ther* 13:196, 1986.
17. Finne CO III: Advances in colorectal cancer, *J Enterostom Ther* 18:82, 1991.
18. Fitchett CW, Hoffman GC: Obstructing malignant lesions of the colon, *Surg Clin North Am* 66:807, 1986.
19. Foltz AT: Nutritional factors in the prevention of gastrointestinal cancer, *Semin Oncol Nurs* 4:239, 1988.
20. Fry RD, Fleshman JW, Kodner IJ: Cancer of the colon and rectum, *Clin Symp* 41(5):2, 1989.
21. Ginsberg AL: Topical salicylate therapy (4-ASA and 5-ASA enemas), *Gastroenterol Clin North Am* 18(1):35, 1989.
22. Goldberg SM, Nivatvongs S: Anorectal diseases. In Berk JE, editor: *Bockus gastroenterology*, ed 4. Vol 4: *Intestine, part two*, Philadelphia, 1985, WB Saunders.
23. Haubrich WS: Diverticula and diverticular disease of the colon. In Berk JE, editor: *Bockus gastroenterology*, ed 4. Vol 4: *Intestine, part two*, Philadelphia, 1985, WB Saunders.
24. Howard ER: Extrahepatic biliary atresia. In Schwartz SI, Ellis H, editors: *Maingot's abdominal operations*, ed 9, vol 2, Norwalk, Conn, 1989, Appleton & Lange.
25. Isbell G, Levin B: Ulcerative colitis and colon cancer, *Gastroenterol Clin North Am* 17:773, 1988.
26. Jagelman DG: Extra-colonic manifestations of familial adenomatous polyposis, *Oncology* 5(2):23, 1991.
27. Jewell DP: Corticosteroids for the management of ulcerative colitis and Crohn's disease, *Gastroenterol Clin North Am* 18:21, 1989.
28. Jewett TC Jr, Karp P: Congenital lesions of the gastrointestinal tract. In Lebenthal E, editor: *Textbook of gastroenterology and nutrition in infancy*, New York, 1989, Raven Press.
29. Kanto WP Jr. et al: Perinatal events and necrotizing enterocolitis in premature infants, *Am J Dis Child* 141:167, 1987.

30. Kirsner JB: Chronic inflammatory bowel disease: overview of etiology and pathogenesis. In Berk JE, editor: *Bockus gastroenterology,* ed 4. Vol 4: *Intestine, part two,* Philadelphia, 1985, WB Saunders.

31. Kirsner JB: Inflammatory bowel disease: its present and its future, *Am J Gastroenterol* 84:1358, 1989.

32. Klosterman AR: Congenital anomalies of the gastrointestinal tract. In Broadwell DC, Jackson BS: *Principles of ostomy care,* St Louis, 1982, Mosby-Year Book.

33. Korelitz BI: Inflammatory bowel disease and cancer. In Berk JE, editor: *Bockus gastroenterology,* ed 4. Vol 4: *Intestine, part two,* Philadelphia, 1985, WB Saunders.

34. Leaper DJ: Tumours of the colon. In Schwartz SI, Ellis H, editors: *Maingot's abdominal operations,* ed 9, vol 2, Norwalk, Conn, 1989, Appleton & Lange.

35. Louw JH, Cywes S: Embryology and anomalies of the intestine. In Berk JE, editor: *Bockus gastroenterology,* ed 4. Vol 4: *Intestine, part two,* Philadelphia, 1985, WB Saunders.

36. Lynch HT et al: Familial heterogeneity of colon cancer risk, *Cancer* 57:2212, 1986.

37. Lynch HT et al: Hereditary nonpolyposis colorectal cancer-Lynch syndromes I and II, *Gastroenterol Clin North Am* 17:679, 1988.

38. Mannel RS, Braly PS, Buller RE: Indiana pouch continent urinary reservoir in patients with previous pelvic irradiation, *Obstet Gynecol* 75:891, 1990.

39. Margovich MJ et al: Dietary factors and colorectal cancer, *Gastroenterol Clin North Am* 17:727, 1988.

40. McLane AM, McShane: Bowel elimination: alteration. In Thompson JM et al, editors: *Mosby's manual of clinical nursing,* ed 2, St Louis, 1989, Mosby–Year Book.

41. Mendeloff AI: Epidemiologic aspects of inflammatory bowel disease. In Berk JE, editor: *Bockus gastroenterology,* ed 4. Vol 4: *Intestine, part two,* Philadelphia, 1985, WB Saunders.

42. Meyers S, Janowitz HD: Crohn's disease: medical management. In Berk JE, editor: *Bockus gastroenterology,* ed 4. Vol 4: *Intestine, part two,* Philadelphia, 1985, WB Saunders.

43. Muto R, Bussey HJR, Morson BC: The evolution of cancer of the colon and rectum, *Cancer* 36:2251, 1975.

44. Orkin BA et al: The surgical management of children with ulcerative colitis: the old vs the new, *Dis Colon Rectum* 33:947, 1990.

45. Parks TG: Diverticular disease of the colon. In Schwartz SI, Ellis H, editors: *Maingot's abdominal operations,* ed 9, vol 2, Norwalk, Conn, 1989, Appleton & Lange.

46. Pietroiusti A et al: Report of a family with hereditary site-specific colon cancer, *Cancer* 57:2438, 1986.

47. Raffensperger JG: Hirschsprung's disease. In Berk JE, editor: *Bockus gastroenterology,* ed 4. Vol 4: *Intestine, part two,* Philadelphia, 1985, WB Saunders.

48. Reddy BS and Cohen LA: *Diet, nutrition and cancer: a critical evaluation,* vol 1, Boca Raton, Fla, 1986, CRC Press.

49. Riddlesberger MM Jr: Congenital abnormalities of the gastrointestinal system. In Lebenthal E, editor: *Textbook of gastroenterology and nutrition in infancy,* ed 2, New York, 1989, Raven Press.

50. Roback SA, Boarini J: Common conditions requiring gastrointestinal stomas in infants, *J Enterostom Ther* 15:162–166, 1988.

51. Robinson MG: New oral salicylates in the therapy of chronic idiopathic inflammatory bowel disease, *Gastroenterol Clin North Am* 18:43, 1989.

52. Sack DM, Peppercorn MH: Drug therapy of inflammatory bowel disease, *Pharmacotherapy* 3:158, 1983.

53. Schwabe AD, Lewin KJ: Benign tumors of the colon: polyposis syndromes. In Berk JE, editor: *Bockus gastroenterology,* ed 4. Vol 4: *Intestine, part two,* Philadelphia, 1985, WB Saunders.

54. Silverman AL et al: Clinical features, evaluation and detection of colorectal cancer, *Gastroenterol Clin North Am* 17:713, 1988.

55. Slater G, Aufses AH Jr: Granulomatous colitis and ulcerative colitis. In Schwartz SI, Ellis H, editors: *Maingot's abdominal operations,* ed 9, vol 2, Norwalk, Conn, 1989, Appleton & Lange.

56. Smith ED: The bath water needs changing, but don't throw away the baby: an overview of anorectal anomalies, *J Pediatr Surg* 22:335, 1987.

57. Smith S et al: Stoma-related variceal bleeding: an under-recognized complication of biliary atresia, *J Pediatr Surg* 23:243, 1988.
58. Spitz L: Hirschsprung's disease and anorectal anomalies. In Schwartz SI, Ellis H, editors: *Maingot's abdominal operations,* ed 9, vol 2, Norwalk, Conn, 1989, Appleton & Lange.
59. Spitz L: Neonatal internal obstruction and intussusception in childhood. In Schwartz SI, Ellis H, editors: *Maingot's abdominal operations,* ed 9, vol 1, Norwalk, Conn, 1989, Appleton & Lange.
60. Wesson D: The intestines. Part 1, congenital anomalies. In Walker WA et al, editors: *Pediatric gastrointestinal disease: pathophysiology, diagnosis, management,* vol 1, Philadelphia, 1991, BC Decker.
61. Wheatley MJ et al: Hirschsprung's disease in adolescents and adults, *Dis Colon Rectum* 33:622, 1990.
62. Winawer SJ, Enker WE, Lightdale CJ: Malignant tumors of the colon and rectum. In Berk JE, editor: *Bockus gastroenterology,* ed 4. Vol 4: *Intestine, part two,* Philadelphia, 1985, WB Saunders.
63. Zink M: Biliary atresia: nursing diagnoses and management, *J Enterostom Ther* 12:128, 1985.

# 11 Gastrointestinal Surgical Procedures

WILLIAM C. McGARITY

## OBJECTIVES

1. Define the following terms: end stoma; double-barrel stoma; loop stoma.

2. Identify indications for permanent ileostomy and for temporary ileostomy.

3. Briefly describe the surgical procedure for construction of an end stoma (ileostomy or colostomy) and a loop stoma (ileostomy or colostomy).

4. Identify causative factors for each of the following complications:
   a. Mucocutaneous separation
   b. Stomal necrosis
   c. Peristomal skin breakdown
   d. Prolapse
   e. Retraction
   f. Stenosis
   g. Fistula formation
   h. Parastomal hernia
   i. Intestinal obstruction

5. Explain why food blockage may occur in the patient with an ileostomy.

6. Identify indications for temporary colostomy and for permanent colostomy.

7. Explain why an ileostomy may be preferable to a cecostomy for the patient who requires decompression of the right colon.

8. Identify two indications for a double-barrel colostomy.

9. Explain why it is more difficult to obtain a tension-free anastomosis of stoma to skin in the obese patient.

I wish to thank Jessie Moore for her assistance in the preparation of this chapter.

**Table 11-1** Gastrointestinal surgical procedures

| Surgical procedure | Synonymous terms | Description | Fecal diversion | Indications | Nursing concerns |
|---|---|---|---|---|---|
| Abdominoperinal resection | APR, Miles procedure | Wide resection of the rectum, surrounding tissues, and lymph nodes is accomplished by an abdominal and perineal approach | Permanent sigmoid or descending colostomy | Rectal cancer | Patient has both an abdominal and a perineal wound; sexual dysfunction common |
| Low anterior resection | LAR | Wide resection of upper portion of rectum includes at least a 2-cm distal margin from tumor to anal verge; procedure includes a hypogastric lymph node dissection in addition to the mesenteric dissection; splenic flexure may be mobilized | Occasionally a temporary colostomy to protect anastomosis | Rectal cancer (middle to upper one third of rectum) | Long-term cure rates are not known; bowel habits may be altered slightly |
| Hartmann's pouch | | End stoma is created from proximal bowel; distal bowel is closed and left in pelvis | Temporary or permanent colostomy, depending on disease | Trauma, incontinence, diverticulitis, rectal cancer (palliative), obstruction, Hirschsprung's disease | Patient may have mucus discharge from rectal segment |

| Procedure | Description | Stoma | Indications | Comments |
|---|---|---|---|---|
| Subtotal colectomy<br>Segmental resection | Diseased portion of the colon is removed: may be a one-, two-, or three-staged procedure: *one-stage procedure:* diseased colon is removed, and bowel is reanastomosed; no stoma is created; *two-stage procedure:* diseased colon is removed, and temporary stoma is created; later (usually 6 to 8 weeks), stoma is taken down; *three-stage procedure:* stoma is created to resolve immediate problem (e.g., obstruction); next, diseased colon is removed; finally stoma is taken down | Possibly a temporary colostomy | Diverticulitis, colon cancer, perforation, trauma, Crohn's disease, intestinal ischemia, obstruction, intestinal fistulas, chronic ulcerative colitis (not curative), familial adenomatous polyposis (not curative) | Bowel habits may be altered slightly |
| Ileorectal anastomosis | Colon is removed, and ileum is anastomosed to rectum (total colectomy) | Temporary ileostomy may be performed to protect anastomosis | Crohn's disease, chronic ulcerative colitis (not curative), familial polyposis (not curative); atonic colon | Patient has frequent, loose stools and urgency; number of stools decreases over time as bowel adapts; perianal skin care is important |

Modified from Thelan LA, Davie JK, Urden LD: *Textbook of critical care nursing: diagnosis and management,* St Louis, 1990, Mosby–Year Book.

*Continued*

**Table 11-1** Gastrointestinal surgical procedures—cont'd

| Surgical procedure | Synonymous terms | Description | Fecal diversion | Indications | Nursing concerns |
|---|---|---|---|---|---|
| Ileoanal anastomosis | | Colon and rectum are removed, and ileum is sutured to the anal canal | Temporary ileostomy if performed in two stages | Chronic ulcerative colitis, familial polyposis, atonic colon | Patient has frequent, loose stools and urgency; number of stools decreases over time as bowel adapts; perianal skin care is important |
| Total proctocolectomy with Brooke ileostomy | Panproctocolectomy | Colon, rectum, and anus are removed; narrow resection of rectum to preserve nerve function | Permanent Brooke ileostomy | Chronic ulcerative colitis, familial polyposis, Crohn's disease | Patient has both an abdominal and a perineal wound; bladder and sexual dysfunction possible |
| Total proctocolectomy with continent ileostomy | Kock pouch | Colon, rectum and anus are removed; approximately 45 cm of the distal ileum is used to construct internal reservoir and nipple valve; Brooke ileostomy may be converted to a Kock pouch | Permanent continent ileostomy | Chronic ulcerative colitis, familial adenomatous polyposis | Postoperatively stoma is catheterized continuously to avoid over-distention of pouch and tension on the many suture lines; approximately 14 to 21 days after surgery catheter is removed, and patient must intubate stoma to empty the reservoir; pouchitis; reoperation rate high |

| Ileoanal reservoir | Restorative proctocolectomy, IAR, J pouch, S pouch, Park's pouch, endorectal ileal pouch–anal anastomosis | Procedure is usually performed in two stages: *stage 1*: abdominal excision of colon and part of rectum; mucosectomy of rectal stump to dentate line; construction of terminal ileal reservoir; ileostomy; *stage 2*: ileostomy takedown | Temporary ileostomy (usually 6 to 8 weeks) | Chronic ulcerative colitis, familial polyposis | "High" ileostomy results in large-volume output and potential fluid and electrolyte depletion; after stage 2, bowel function is variable; patient may have frequent, liquid stools, transient incontinence, and perianal skin irritation; conditions improve with pouch adaptation; pouchitis; long-term results (e.g., nutrition and cancer) are unknown |

The possibility of having a permanent colostomy or ileostomy threatens a patient's integrity, both physically and mentally. Because many patients will live with the stoma for the remainder of their lives, the construction of an ideal stoma is vitally important to minimize complications and to prevent pouching difficulties.

Several important factors must be considered in recommending stoma surgery. The patient must be prepared both physically and psychologically; the surgeon must execute the technical procedure with skill; continuous postoperative support and care must be provided for the patient; and the patient must be assisted to deal with the changes in body image and life-style. Table 11-1 describes the various surgical procedures and their advantages, disadvantages, and nursing implications.

Historically, ostomy care was frequently neglected. Too often the surgeon regarded the construction of a stoma as a final therapeutic step rather than as one phase in the continued care of the patient. Construction of an optimal stoma is now recognized as an important component of the surgical procedure, and long-term rehabilitative management is accepted as the standard for follow-up care.

## STOMA TYPES

### Sites

Almost any portion of the small or large intestine can be exteriorized to form a stoma. The fecal diversions most commonly created, however, are the ileostomy and the colostomy. Most ileostomies are performed by use of the distal small bowel, usually the terminal ileum. Colostomies most commonly are performed in the cecum, transverse colon, left colon, and sigmoid colon.

The typical abdominal location for a particular stoma is determined by the anatomic location of the bowel segment. For example, ileostomies and cecostomies commonly are located in the right lower abdominal quadrant, whereas descending and sigmoid colostomies usually are located in the left lower quadrant. Transverse colostomies may be located in either the right upper quadrant or the left upper quadrant. Although the typical location for a stoma is determined by the anatomic location of the segment to be exteriorized, actual site selection must be based on assessment of the patient's abdominal contours (as discussed in Chapter 1). If the usual site does not provide an appropriate pouching surface, an alternate site must be selected; in this case the surgeon must be notified regarding alternate site location and rationale.

### Surgical Construction

Stomas commonly are constructed in one of three ways: end, loop, or double barrel.

**End Stoma.** An end stoma is constructed by dividing the bowel and bringing out the proximal end as a single stoma (Fig. 11-1). Most commonly the distal portion of the gastrointestinal tract is surgically removed. In some cases, however, the distal segment is oversewn and left in the abdominal cavity with its mesentery intact. The distal end may also be oversewn and secured to the anterior peritoneum near the stoma site as shown in Fig. 11-2. An end colostomy or an end ileostomy is then constructed. When the distal bowel is oversewn rather than removed, the procedure is known as a Hartmann's pouch (Fig. 11-3). If

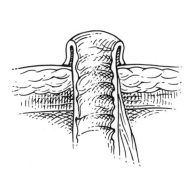

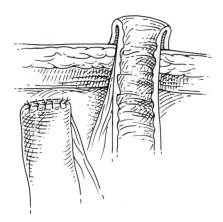

**Fig. 11-1**    Cross-sectional view of end stoma.

**Fig. 11-2**    Cross-sectional view of end stoma with distal bowel oversewn and secured to anterior peritoneum at stoma site.

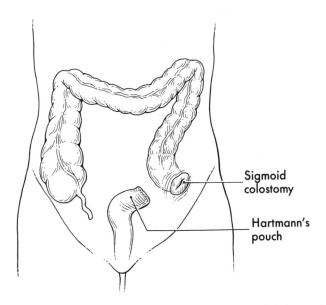

**Fig. 11-3**    Sigmoid colostomy. Distal bowel is oversewn and left in place to create Hartmann's pouch.

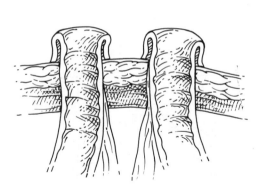

**Fig. 11-4** Cross-sectional view of double-barrel stoma.

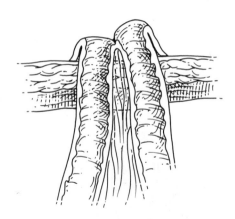

**Fig. 11-5** Cross-sectional view of loop stoma.

the distal bowel is removed, the stoma is permanent; if the distal bowel remains intact and oversewn, the potential exists for the bowel to be reanastomosed and the stoma to be closed (referred to as "takedown").

**Double-Barrel Stoma.** A double-barrel stoma is constructed when the bowel is divided and both the proximal and distal ends are brought to the surface as two separate stomas. One is a proximal, functioning stoma; the other is a distal, nonfunctioning stoma. Usually a bridge of skin is closed between the two stomas. The distal stoma generally is referred to as a mucous fistula (Fig. 11-4). A double-barrel stoma usually is temporary.

**Loop Stoma.** A loop stoma is constructed by bringing a loop of bowel to the abdominal surface and then opening the anterior wall of the bowel to provide fecal diversion (Fig. 11-5). The loop of bowel may be opened either transversely or longitudinally. This results in one stoma with a proximal and distal opening and an intact posterior wall that separates the two openings. A loop stoma usually is temporary.

## ILEOSTOMY

### Indications

Permanent ileostomies are less common today than they were a few years ago. Today an ileoanal reservoir rather than a permanent ileostomy is constructed in most patients who have familial adenomatous polyposis or ulcerative colitis. Strict criteria should be followed in selecting patients for the ileoanal procedure. Occasionally, if the ileoanal reservoir procedure cannot be performed, a Kock pouch, or internal continent ileostomy, is constructed[6,7,8] (see Chapter 4).

A permanent ileostomy is constructed when the entire colon, rectum, and anus are removed; this procedure is known as total proctocolectomy or panproctocolectomy (Fig. 11-6). The most common indication for this procedure is Crohn's colitis. This procedure may

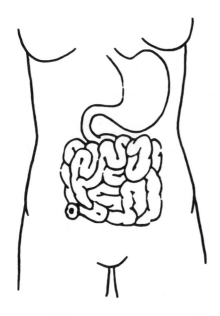

**Fig. 11-6** Abdominal view of ileostomy with colon, rectum, and anus removed, as with total proctocolectomy. However, ileostomy can be constructed and rectum, colon, and anus left intact.

also be performed in patients with familial adenomatous polyposis or chronic ulcerative colitis; however, these patients often are candidates for a continent procedure such as the ileoanal reservoir. An uncommon indication for permanent ileostomy is chronic constipation caused by loss of colonic motility or by failure of pelvic floor relaxation.

Temporary ileostomies sometimes are constructed in conjunction with other surgical procedures. For instance, a loop ileostomy may be constructed proximal to an ileoanal reservoir; this proximal diversion protects the newly constructed reservoir and anastomosis.[4,6,7,8] Usually the ileostomy is closed after the reservoir and anastomosis have healed, normally in 2 to 3 months. A temporary ileostomy may also be constructed to provide proximal diversion in the patient with obstruction of the ascending colon or to provide bowel rest for the patient with Crohn's colitis. In the infant temporary ileostomy may be indicated for necrotizing enterocolitis or total colon Hirschsprung's disease (aganglionosis).

## Types

**End Ileostomy.** An end ileostomy, frequently referred to as a *Brooke ileostomy*, was named after Bryan Brooke of London, who in 1952 described the technique used today.[2] Until that time the end of the small bowel was simply brought out through the abdominal wall, with 4 to 6 cm protruding, and allowed to mature on its own. Partial obstruction of the stoma as a result of serositis and edema usually developed in patients having this procedure, and resulted in cramping abdominal pain, watery diarrhea, and fluid-electrolyte imbalance. Brooke's technique was to evert the distal end of the ileum, exposing the mucosa, and to suture the stoma to the dermal layer of the skin.[1] This technique, known as *maturing* the stoma, has eliminated ileostomy dysfunction.

Most end ileostomies are brought out through an incision in the right lower abdominal quadrant (Fig. 11-6). The site of the stoma should be marked preoperatively with the

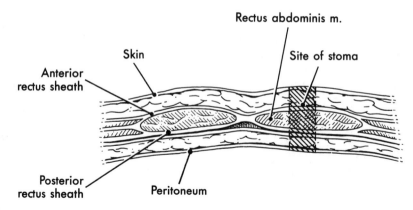

**Fig. 11-7**    Lateral view of abdominal wall illustrating proper location of stoma through rectus abdominis muscle.

patient in lying, sitting, and standing positions. The site should be on a flat surface of the abdominal wall. It should not be on a fold, near an old scar, or near a bony prominence. The stoma should be brought through the rectus fascia and muscle (Fig. 11-7). The stoma is usually positioned between the anterosuperior iliac spine and the umbilicus or just below the level of the umbilicus and through the rectus muscle, as discussed in Chapter 1.[4]

The laporotomy incision ideally is made just to the left of the midline and beveled in to the midline so that after surgery the incision is clear of the pouching surface.

A circular disk of skin, the size of a quarter, is excised from the abdominal wall at the previously marked stoma site. A vertical incision is then made through the subcutaneous tissue layer, and the fat is dissected to create an opening for the stoma. Some surgeons prefer to excise the subcutaneous tissue; however, excision reduces tissue support for the stoma and can contribute to retraction of the peristomal tissue and skin. A circular incision, similar to that made in the skin, is made through the anterior rectus sheath. (In some centers a cruciate incision, as opposed to a circular incision, is made into the fascia; either approach is acceptable, but the cruciate incision is more likely to extend and cause tearing of the fascia.) The fibers of the rectus muscle are separated, and the posterior rectus sheath and peritoneum are opened.[4] Two fingers are pushed through the hole to ensure the correct diameter of the opening through the abdominal wall; the exit wound must be large enough to prevent compression of the bowel but not overly large, since this causes predisposition to parastomal hernia formation.[4] The ileum is then passed through the opening in the abdominal wall, with the mesentery oriented in the cephalad position and with at least 6 cm of ileum extending beyond the skin surface[4] (Fig. 11-8). It is important to avoid tension on the bowel or mesentery because tension can result in retraction or ischemia of the stoma. (If the patient is obese, it can be difficult to mobilize the bowel sufficiently[7] to obtain a tension-free anastomosis because of fat deposits in the mesentery, which render the bowel less mobile, and because of the thickness of the abdominal wall.) The ileum is sutured to the parietal peritoneum to prevent prolapse and retraction of the stoma. To complete closure of the mesenteric hiatus, the mesentery is sutured to the parietal peritoneum from the exit wound in the abdominal wall to the duodenum, incorporating the falciform ligament above.

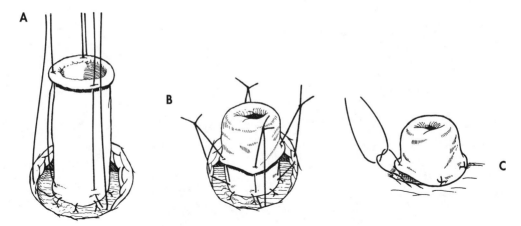

**Fig. 11-8**  Construction of Brooke stoma. **A,** Bowel advanced through abdominal wall; mesentery trimmed from bowel, and bowel secured to anterior rectus sheath. **B,** Sutures are placed through cut edge of bowel, seromuscular layer of bowel at skin level, and subcutaneous tissue to facilitate eversion of bowel, thus maturing stoma. **C,** Matured stoma is secured at skin level.

The distal end of the ileum is amputated to provide the everted stoma at least 2 cm of length. It is important for this loop of bowel to have a good blood supply. The end of the ileum is then everted and sutured to the dermis of the skin (Fig. 11-8). The ideal height of a matured stoma is about 2 cm. Such protrusion ensures that the stoma drains effectively into the pouching system, which helps prevent skin problems. It is important to avoid excessive stomal protrusion, which causes predisposition to complications such as stomal laceration. Fig. 2-1 shows three stomas: one with no protrusion, one with adequate protrusion, and one with excessive protrusion.

In summary, the technique for construction of an end stoma should include the following:

1. Stoma placement in a favorable site
2. Location of the exit wound within the rectus muscle to prevent parastomal hernia
3. Sufficient mobilization of the bowel to provide a tension-free anastomosis
4. Immediate maturation of the stoma by suturing it to the dermal layer of the skin

Immediately after completion of the operative procedure, a pouching system is applied over the stoma. The ileostomy should begin functioning in 2 to 3 days.

The end ileostomy is usually created in conjunction with total proctocolectomy (removal of the entire colon, rectum, and anus), which is most commonly indicated for the patient with inflammatory bowel disease (chronic ulcerative colitis or Crohn's disease) or familial adenomatous polyposis. When resecting the rectum in cases of benign disease, the surgeon uses a narrow rectal dissection to preserve the autonomic nerves that are vital for sexual function.

**Loop Ileostomy.** A loop ileostomy is usually temporary and is positioned at the same site as the end ileostomy. The exit wound through the abdominal wall is constructed in the

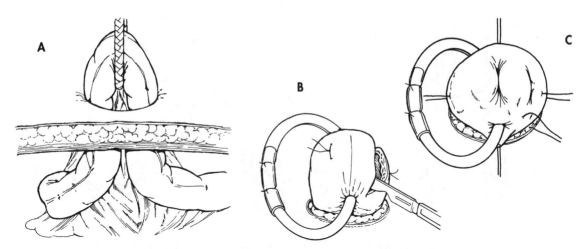

**Fig. 11-9** Loop ileostomy construction. **A,** Loop of bowel exteriorized. **B,** Support device placed to maintain position of bowel on abdominal surface. Distal bowel of ileum is incised, mesentery to mesentery. Stitch placed to designate proximal bowel. **C,** Loop ileostomy matured with protruding functional limb.

same manner as the end ileostomy, as previously described. A loop of ileum is brought through the opening without tension (Fig. 11-9). It should protrude 3 to 4 cm above the surface of the skin. The loop is held in this position with a No. 20F red rubber catheter or another support device, which is inserted through the mesentery of the loop of ileum.[10] Distal to the midline the loop is opened, and both ends are matured with a technique similar to that for maturing an end ileostomy (Fig. 11-9). This process provides the functioning proximal end with a longer stoma that fits easily into a pouching system. Spillover into the distal bowel is rarely a problem. After a few weeks the distal stoma recedes.

If complete diversion is needed, the distal limb can be stapled closed or the distal limb can be severed from the proximal bowel, closed, and left in the peritoneal cavity, as described for the Hartmann's pouch procedure (Fig. 11-3).

A pouching system is applied immediately after the surgical procedure. The support device is removed approximately 1 week after surgery.[4]

A loop ileostomy is most commonly constructed to provide temporary diversion after the ileoanal reservoir procedure. A loop ileostomy may also be performed to provide proximal diversion for the patient with an obstructing lesion in the ascending colon.

**Double-Barrel Ileostomy.** A double-barrel ileostomy is rarely constructed. The surgeon may perform this procedure, however, when complete diversion of the fecal stream is required or when the surgical procedure involves resection of a necrotic segment and both ends of the remaining bowel must be monitored for viability. For example, the double-barrel ileostomy is commonly performed after segmental resection in the infant with necrotizing enterocolitis.

A variation of the double-barrel ileostomy is the Mikulicz ileostomy, which is sometimes performed in the infant with meconium ileus. In this case the following goals are associated with the surgical procedure: (1) to provide proximal diversion until the obstructing meconi-

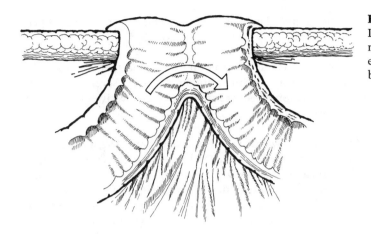

**Fig. 11-10** Mikulicz procedure. Loop of bowel is created, and common wall (spur) is crushed, thus establishing continuity of distal bowel.

um is removed, (2) to provide access to the distal bowel so that mucolytic agents that will dissolve the meconium plug can be instilled, and (3) to permit stool to pass through the distal bowel once the obstruction is removed. The Mikulicz procedure involves formation of a side-by-side double-barrel ileostomy; the two limbs of bowel are sutured together with a side-to-side anastomosis, and the double-lumen stoma is then converted to a single-lumen stoma by means of a crushing clamp, which destroys the wall separating the two limbs of bowel (Fig. 11-10). Additional procedures sometimes performed for management of meconium ileus include the Bishop-Koop procedure and the Santulli procedure; both procedures address the aforementioned goals. The Bishop-Koop procedure involves division of the ileum proximal to the obstructing meconium; the distal limb of the ileum is brought to the abdominal wall as an end stoma, and the end of the proximal limb is anastomosed to the side of the distal limb. This technique is known as an *end-to-side* anastomosis. The Santulli procedure also involves division of the ileum proximal to the obstructing meconium; in this procedure the proximal limb of the ileum is brought to the abdominal wall as an end stoma, and the end of the distal limb is anastomosed to the side of the proximal limb (a *side-to-end* anastomosis). The ileostomy is closed after the meconium ileus has been resolved.

## Complications

A number of complications may occur following construction of an ileostomy. Complications that can occur with any stoma are discussed later in this chapter; complications that more commonly occur after ileostomy are described here.

**Mucocutaneous Separation.** Mucocutaneous separation can result from inadequate suturing of the end of the ileum to the skin or from infection, tension, delayed healing (e.g., the patient on a regimen of corticosteroids), or necrosis. Usually healing occurs with conservative management, as described in Chapter 2. If excessive scarring occurs, stenosis of the stoma may develop later and may require surgical revision.

**Edema of Ileal Stoma.** Mild edema may occur soon after surgery but usually subsides after a few days. Severe edema may develop if the exit wound is too small, resulting in compression of the blood supply to the stoma. Later, edema may result from an improperly sized pouch, trauma, or recurrent inflammatory disease of the bowel.

**Obstruction.** Obstruction may be the result either of an exit wound that is too small or of a twist in the bowel as it was brought through the abdominal wall. Severe edema also may cause an obstruction. If the obstruction does not respond to conservative management, the problem should be surgically corrected.

**Peristomal Skin Breakdown.** Breakdown of the peristomal skin is the most common ileostomy complication. Mechanical, chemical, allergic, and infectious causes contribute to peristomal skin breakdown. Mechanical damage may be caused by pressure from the pouch (belt tabs, for example), frequent pouch changes, or the stripping effect of adhesives on the skin. Chemical damage can result from stool, glues, solvents, or soap residue in prolonged contact with the skin. Allergic peristomal skin reactions can be triggered by any product used in pouching. Peristomal skin infections can be either bacterial or fungal. Management of peristomal skin breakdown requires thorough assessment to determine the etiologic factors; treatment must then address the causative factors as well as the breakdown, as discussed in Chapters 2 and 3.

**Food Blockage.** Food blockage is a complication unique to patients with ileostomies. It is a mechanical obstruction caused by high residue and poorly chewed food that lodges in the distal small bowel, usually just proximal to the stoma. The symptoms of a food blockage are abdominal cramping; liquid, foul-smelling output; high pitched, tinkling bowel sounds; and stomal edema. These symptoms may progress to the absence of stomal output, as well as a silent atonic bowel, with abdominal distention, nausea, and vomiting.

Patients should be taught preventive measures: limited intake of high-fiber foods, thorough chewing of food, and adequate fluid intake. Patients also must be taught the signs of partial or complete obstruction and appropriate home-relief measures such as a warm bath and peristomal massage. Failure to respond to these measures mandates physician notification. A digital examination by the physician or ET nurse usually confirms the blockage, which may be relieved by repeated saline lavage (see Chapter 2).

**Intestinal Obstruction.** Intestinal obstruction is usually due to adhesions or herniation of the loop of bowel around the ileostomy stoma. Occasionally the obstruction responds to conservative treatment. If the obstruction does not respond to conservative management, laporotomy is required to correct the cause of the obstruction.

**Stomal Bleeding and Polypoid Granulomas.** Bleeding of the stoma may be caused by trauma or by recurrent inflammatory bowel disease. Although granulomas usually result from the trauma caused by an ill-fitting pouch, they also may be due to recurrent inflammatory bowel disease.

## COLOSTOMY

### Indications

A colostomy may be constructed on either a temporary or a permanent basis. A temporary colostomy may be required for infants with a congenital disorder such as

Hirschsprung's disease or atresia of the rectum. Trauma is a frequent indication for temporary colostomy. Other indications for a temporary colostomy include complications that result from diverticular disease, obstruction of the colon, perforation of the colon, and volvulus of the colon. A temporary proximal colostomy also may be performed to "protect" a low anterior anastomosis while the anastomosis heals.[4] (A low anterior anastomosis may be performed after resection of a midrectal carcinoma; the subsequent colorectal anastomosis is performed through an anterior abdominal incision and must be constructed *low* in the pelvis. A protective colostomy may be indicated on a temporary basis because of the technical difficulties involved in obtaining a secure anastomosis.)

A permanent colostomy most frequently is indicated for the patient who requires an abdominoperineal resection (APR) of the rectum for the treatment of low rectal carcinoma.[2,4]

## Sites

**Cecum.** Cecostomies rarely are performed today. They are inadequate for decompression of the colon, and they present a difficult nursing problem. If decompression of the right colon is necessary, a Brooke or a loop ileostomy functions much more effectively and is easier to manage than is a cecostomy.

The two types of cecostomies are tube and skin flush. A tube cecostomy sometimes is used for temporary decompression of the colon. Closure does not require another surgical procedure. The tube is simply removed, and provided there is no distal obstruction, the fecal fistula will close (Fig. 11-11). A skin-flush cecostomy is performed by suturing the cecum to the skin, but a surgical procedure is required for closure.

**Transverse Colon.** A colostomy created from the transverse colon is usually temporary and is usually constructed as a loop. Occasionally, if the remaining distal colon has been removed, it is necessary to construct an end transverse colostomy. Complicated diverticular disease, Hirschsprung's disease, and sigmoid colon obstruction may be managed by means of a transverse colostomy.

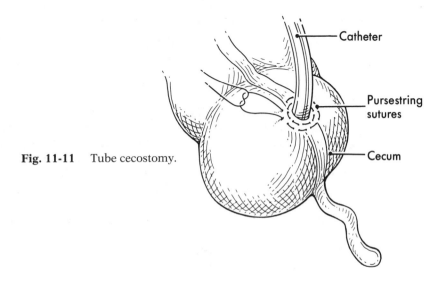

**Fig. 11-11**   Tube cecostomy.

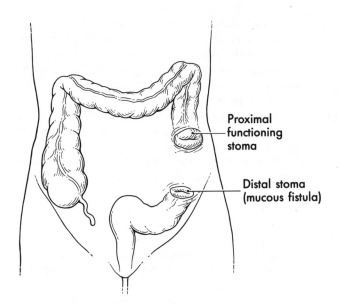

Proximal
functioning
stoma

Distal stoma
(mucous fistula)

**Fig. 11-12** Abdominal view of descending colostomy with distal bowel in place and exiting to skin as mucous fistula.

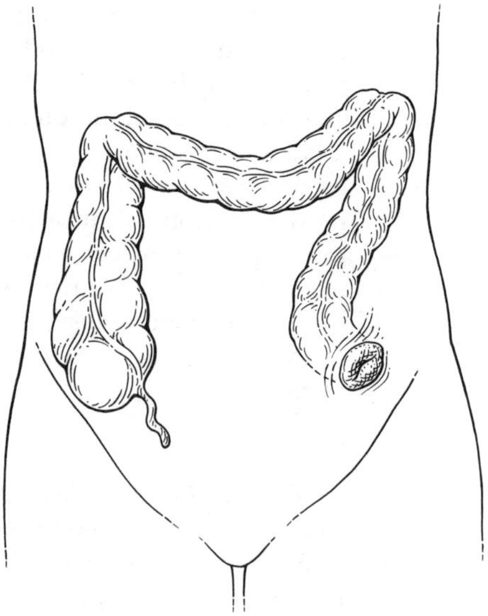

**Fig. 11-13** Abdominal view of sigmoid colostomy with rectum and anus removed, as with abdominal perineal resection.

**Descending or Sigmoid Colon.** For conditions such as severe radiation proctitis or a newly repaired rectovaginal fistula, a temporary sigmoid colostomy may be used to bypass the rectum. An end sigmoid colostomy and Hartmann's pouch may be constructed in cases of perforation of the sigmoid colon (Fig. 11-3). Sometimes the distal segment is brought out as a mucous fistula (Fig. 11-12). A permanent end sigmoid colostomy is required when the rectum is removed, such as with the APR (surgical removal of the rectum and anus by means of a combined abdominal and perineal approach) (Fig. 11-13). This procedure is most commonly performed for management of low rectal carcinoma but may also be required for management of benign disease such as Crohn's disease that affects the rectum and perianal tissues. The APR, also known as the *Miles* procedure, was first described in 1908 by an English surgeon, W. Ernest Miles.[2,3]

Removal of the rectum produces a perineal wound, as well as an abdominal incision. In the past the perineal wound usually was packed and left to heal by secondary intention. Current management usually involves primary closure of the perineal wound, except in the case of hemorrhage, when packing may be required for hemostasis. Penrose drains or wound sumps connected to low intermittent suction commonly are used to provide drainage of the operative site during the early postoperative period.[3]

Complications of rectal resection include bladder dysfunction, sexual dysfunction, and complications of wound healing. Bladder and sexual dysfunction usually are caused by damage to the pelvic nerves and most commonly are seen after wide rectal dissection for carcinoma.[2,5]

Both APR and total proctocolectomy involve removal of the rectum, with a resulting perineal wound. The procedures differ, however, in that total proctocolectomy involves

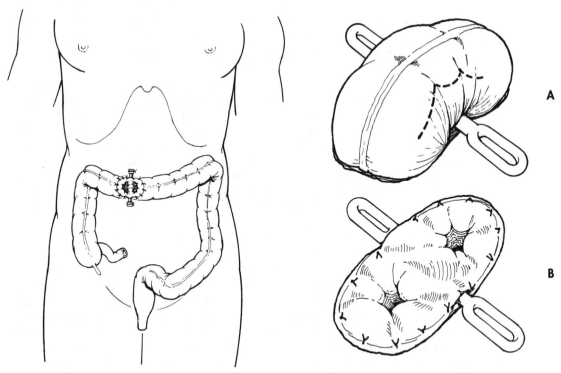

**Fig. 11-14** Abdominal view of loop colostomy in transverse colon.

**Fig. 11-15** Loop colostomy construction is much the same as construction of loop ileostomy. **A,** Stoma is created with longitudinal incision through sacculations in colon. **B,** Loop colostomy matured.

removal of the entire colon, rectum, and anus, whereas APR involves removal only of the rectum and anus. Total proctocolectomy is more commonly performed in cases of benign disease, whereas APR is usually performed for management of cancer of the low rectum; thus APR usually involves a wide excision of the rectum (to remove lymph nodes) and more commonly results in bladder and sexual dysfunction caused by nerve damage.[2,5]

## Types

**Loop Colostomy.** The most common type of colostomy is a loop colostomy. Loop colostomies usually are constructed in the transverse colon, although other segments of the colon also can be brought out as a loop (Fig. 11-14). A loop colostomy is usually temporary; it is commonly constructed when diversion is needed and a minimal surgical procedure is desired (e.g., in the presence of colon obstruction or diverticular abscess formation). If the loop colostomy is a planned procedure, the site should be marked before surgery.

If the transverse colon is used, the loop colostomy should be brought through the rectus muscle and rectus fascia. A transverse incision is made through the skin, the anterior and posterior rectus fasciae, and the rectus muscle. A loop of the transverse colon is brought through the incision, without tension, to provide 2 to 3 cm of colon above the level of the skin. The loop must then be supported on the abdominal wall until primary healing to the abdominal wall occurs; failure to support the loop until healing occurs may result in retraction of the loop to an intraabdominal position (Fig. 11-15).

A number of approaches are used to stabilize the loop on the abdominal wall. A variety of external support devices have been described; these devices are placed beneath the loop through the mesentery. In the past, support devices commonly used included glass or plastic rods; however, these devices are bulky, which makes colostomy management more difficult. Currently recommended devices include the flat bridge and the red rubber catheter; these devices are much less bulky and thus facilitate colostomy care. Surgeons who prefer the red rubber catheter cite the deformability of the catheter as an advantage; both the catheter and the stoma can be inserted into a pouching system.[10] A modification of the external support is the use of a "whistle-tip" catheter, which is placed through a subcutaneous tunnel under the loop, with the ends of the catheter exteriorized and sutured into place at a distance from the stoma. This approach also facilitates postoperative management, since the pouching surface is free of a support device.

Alternatives to the use of external support devices include the use of a fascial or fascial-skin bridge and construction of a loop-end stoma. A fascial or fascial-skin bridge involves conservation of a narrow tissue flap when the skin, subcutaneous tissue, and fascia are incised to create an opening for the loop of bowel; this tissue flap is then positioned underneath the loop of bowel and across the tissue defect and is sutured into place.[9] The loop-end stoma is a variation of surgical construction that eliminates the need for a support device, either internal or external. The loop of bowel is divided with a gastrointestinal stapling device; the proximal limb of the bowel and the antimesenteric corner of the distal limb of the bowel are then brought through the abdominal wall, opened, and matured. This procedure provides for proximal diversion and for access to the distal bowel through the small mucous fistula. (The mucous fistula stoma is a small lumen because only the corner of the distal limb of bowel is opened and brought to the surface; the remainder of the lumen of the distal bowel remains sutured closed and rests in the subcutaneous tissue layer.) One advantage of this approach is that closure is simplified.

The loop colostomy usually is opened and matured at the time of the operative procedure.[4] The colostomy may be opened longitudinally or transversely; a longitudinal incision is usually recommended because it provides more complete diversion of the fecal stream. This is because a longitudinal incision takes advantage of the haustrations in the bowel wall to provide almost complete separation of the proximal and distal bowel. The longitudinal incision is made 2 to 3 cm above the skin level so that when the stoma is matured there will be some protrusion of the stoma, which facilitates pouching and skin care. An alternative to opening and maturing the stoma at the time of surgery is to wait 2 to 3 days after surgery and then open the colostomy by cautery in the patient's hospital room. This alternative usually is not recommended because the delay causes partial obstruction and crampy abdominal pain and because the patient may be psychologically disturbed by having the stoma opened at the bedside.

**Double-Barrel Colostomy.** A double-barrel colostomy may be performed when the surgeon believes it is necessary for complete diversion of the fecal stream. More commonly a double-barrel colostomy is constructed when segmental resection is required in cases of perforation or necrosis. In these situations anastomosis usually is contraindicated, so both

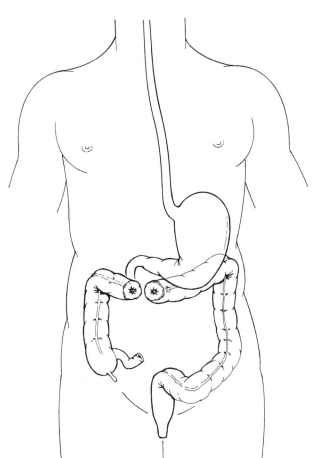

**Fig. 11-16** Abdominal view of double-barrel colostomy.

ends of the bowel are brought to the abdominal wall as stomas. A double-barrel colostomy usually is intended to be a temporary diversion.

In the construction of a double-barrel colostomy a loop of the bowel is completely divided, and the two ends are brought out to the surface and are sutured to the skin (Fig. 11-16). The skin and fascia usually are closed between the proximal and distal ends to provide separation of the stomas and a more suitable pouching surface.

**End Colostomy.** The most frequent site for an end colostomy is the left or sigmoid colon, and usually this procedure is performed after an APR (Fig. 11-13). If for some reason the entire sigmoid and left colon are removed, the transverse colon is used for the end colostomy. An end colostomy also may be constructed in conjunction with a Hartmann's pouch, in which the distal bowel segment is oversewn and left in place.

The stoma site should be marked before the surgical procedure, as described earlier in this chapter and in Chapter 1. The surgical construction of an end colostomy involves the same considerations and principles as those described for construction of an end ileostomy (see pp. 358 and 359).

For years, flush colostomy stomas were advocated; however, slight protrusion of the colostomy stoma is beneficial. Generally, left colon contents are formed, which minimizes the risk of leakage and skin problems. Also, some patients with colostomies are able to regulate bowel function by routine irrigations; these patients may not require a pouch at all times but can simply wear a dressing or a stoma cap over the stoma. However, not all colostomy patients have formed stool, for a variety of reasons. In addition, bowel patterns and management preferences change as one ages. Therefore a slightly protruding stoma is considered ideal; it remains inconspicuous but drains well into a pouching system if needed.

## STOMAL COMPLICATIONS

### Necrosis

Ischemia and necrosis of the stoma occur because of inadequate blood supply. This condition may be due to removal of too much of the mesentery when the stoma is constructed (more than 3 to 4 cm) or to tension on the mesentery. In the obese patient the abdominal wall is thick, and it sometimes is difficult to obtain enough length of bowel without tension and interference with the blood supply. Ischemia usually is noticeable within 12 to 24 hours. If the stoma and the bowel immediately proximal to the stoma (below fascial level) become necrotic, immediate revision is necessary.

### Retraction

Retraction may be caused by insufficient stomal length, tension on the mesentery, or inadequate fixation of the bowel to the parietal peritoneum. Obesity contributes to this problem. Mild retraction usually can be managed with firm convexity. If significant retraction occurs, elective revision is usually indicated (see Chapter 3).

### Prolapse

Prolapse usually results from inadequate fixation of the bowel to the parietal peritoneum or from an overly large opening in the abdominal wall, which allows the bowel to protrude. Colostomy prolapse also can result from a redundant sigmoid and left colon.

Mild prolapse can be treated conservatively. If, however, it becomes severe, the blood supply may be compromised and surgical correction is then required. In most cases another stoma is constructed, and the bowel is anchored to the parietal peritoneum. If the prolapse resulted from a redundant sigmoid and left colon, surgical correction involves resection of the redundant bowel (see Chapter 3).

### Stenosis

Stenosis may result if the stoma is not matured at the time of initial surgery or if mucocutaneous separation of the stoma develops. These situations commonly are associated with serositis, infection around the stoma, and scarring, which result in stenosis. If stenosis becomes severe, the scar tissue around the stoma can be removed with the patient under local anesthesia and the end of the bowel resutured to the dermis. Severe stenosis at the fascial level necessitates open laporotomy and stomal revision.

## Parastomal Hernia

Parastomal hernia usually is due to the placement of the stoma lateral to the rectus fascia where the abdominal wall is weak; the muscle and fascia stretch, allowing the bowel to enter the parastomal space. A parastomal hernia also can occur as a result of an overly large opening in the fascial-muscle layer, or in a debilitated patient whose tissues are weak. If the parastomal hernia is large, it should be repaired. Generally, it is not wise to repair the hernia around the stoma. Instead, the stoma should be taken down, the defect in the abdominal wall closed primarily, and the stoma moved to another site.

## Perforation and Fistulae

Perforation can occur when a patient with a parastomal hernia forces an irrigating catheter through the bowel wall. The perforation usually occurs in the abdominal wall, resulting in an abscess. Occasionally a perforation can be the result of a foreign body that injures the wall of the colon. When the abscess is drained, a colocutaneous fistula results.

Fistulae also can be caused by inflammatory bowel disease or by a suture incorrectly placed through the wall of the bowel during maturation of the stoma. If the fistula does not heal with conservative treatment, the stoma is taken down and another stoma is constructed.

## SUMMARY

In recent years three major developments have led to improved care of the stoma patient. The first is improvements in the techniques for stomal construction; the second is the development of new pouching systems; and the third is the team approach in caring for the patient with a stoma—the physician, the nurse, and the ET nurse.

Construction of the ideal stoma is a critical factor that influences the patient's ability to return to an optimal life-style. Technical construction essentially dictates the patient's stoma care after surgery in terms of the type of pouch used, the accessory products required, and the frequency of pouch change. Stoma construction requires a high standard of knowledge, technical competence, and collaboration among members of the medical team.

# SELF-EVALUATION

## QUESTIONS

1. Which of the following stomas is always constructed as a permanent diversion?
   a. Loop ileostomy
   b. End colostomy with Hartmann's pouch
   c. Double-barrel colostomy
   d. End colostomy with abdominoperineal resection of the rectum

2. Permanent ileostomy is most commonly performed for:
   a. Crohn's disease involving the entire colon and rectum
   b. Diverticular disease
   c. Necrotizing enterocolitis
   d. Cancer of the colon

3. A Brooke ileostomy refers to:
   a. A temporary loop ileostomy
   b. A continent ileostomy
   c. An end ileostomy that is matured at the time of surgery
   d. A double-barrel ileostomy

4. Mucocutaneous separation may lead to development of:
   a. Stomal stenosis
   b. Stomal prolapse
   c. Parastomal hernia
   d. Intestinal obstruction

5. Which of the following complications occurs only in the patient with an ileostomy?
   a. Mucocutaneous separation
   b. Stomal necrosis
   c. Food blockage
   d. Stomal stenosis

6. Identify common indications for a temporary colostomy.

7. Permanent colostomy is most commonly performed for management of:
   a. Penetrating trauma of the rectosigmoid
   b. Carcinoma of the rectum
   c. Crohn's disease
   d. Diverticulitis

8. Cecostomy is the procedure of choice for decompression of the right colon.
   a. True
   b. False

9. External support devices for loop stomas usually can be removed:
   a. When peristalsis resumes, as evidenced by bowel sounds
   b. 6 weeks after surgery
   c. About 1 week after surgery
   d. 3 to 4 weeks after surgery

10. Loop colostomies usually provide almost complete diversion of the fecal stream, especially if the loop is opened longitudinally.
    a. True
    b. False

11. Identify indications for construction of a double-barrel ostomy.

12. Hartmann's pouch refers to which of the following?
    a. Continent ileostomy (internal pouch)
    b. Proximal stoma with distal mucous fistula
    c. End stoma with distal segment oversewn and left in place
    d. Ileoanal reservoir
13. Identify four principles for construction of an end stoma (such as an end sigmoid colostomy).
14. Explain why a descending or sigmoid colostomy stoma can be constructed so that it is almost flush with the skin, whereas an ileostomy must be constructed so that it protrudes above skin level.
15. Which of the following mandates emergent surgical intervention?
    a. Stomal necrosis extending to fascial level
    b. Parastomal hernia
    c. Mucocutaneous separation
    d. Stomal retraction
16. Which of the following helps to prevent stomal prolapse and parastomal hernia formation?
    a. Preoperative stoma site selection
    b. Avoiding an overly large opening in the fascial muscle layer
    c. Limiting the amount of mesentery that is removed
    d. Maturing the stoma at the time of surgery

# SELF-EVALUATION

## ANSWERS

1. **d.** End colostomy with abdominoperineal resection of the rectum
2. **a.** Crohn's disease involving the entire colon and rectum
3. **c.** An end ileostomy that is matured at the time of surgery
4. **a.** Stomal stenosis
5. **c.** Food blockage
6. Indications:
   Congenital disorders such as Hirschsprung's disease or atresia of the rectum
   Trauma, such as stab wound or gunshot wound, to the colon
   Conditions affecting the colon, such as diverticulitis, obstruction, perforation, or volvulus
7. **b.** Carcinoma of the rectum
8. **b.** False
9. **c.** About 1 week after surgery
10. **a.** True
11. Indications:
    When complete diversion of the fecal stream is required
    When segmental resection is required for perforation or necrosis and reanastomosis is contraindicated because of sepsis or ischemia
12. **c.** End stoma with distal segment oversewn and left in place
13. Four principles:
    Placement of stoma in a favorable site
    Location of exit wound within the rectus muscle
    Sufficient mobilization of bowel to provide a tension-free anastomosis
    Immediate maturation of the stoma
14. The stool from a descending or sigmoid colostomy is much easier to contain because it usually is soft and formed, and it is much less damaging to the skin because it contains no proteolytic enzymes. Ileostomy output is fluid to mushy in consistency and is extremely damaging to the skin as a result of its proteolytic enzymes. Therefore it is important for the ileostomy stoma to protrude above skin level and to project into the pouch.
15. **a.** Stomal necrosis extending to fascial level
16. **b.** Avoiding an overly large opening in the fascial muscle layer

## REFERENCES

1. Brooke BN: The management of an ileostomy including its complications, *Lancet* 2:102, 1952.
2. Bryant J, Boarini J: Gastrointestinal surgical procedures, *J Enterostom Ther* 13(1):34, 1986.
3. Ellis H: Abdominoperineal resection. In Schwartz S, Ellis H, editors: *Maingot's abdominal operations*, ed 9, vol 2, Norwalk, Conn, 1989, Appleton-Century-Crofts.
4. Jagelman D: Ileostomy and colostomy. In Schwartz S, Ellis H, editors: *Maingot's abdominal operations*, ed 9, vol 2, Norwalk, Conn, 1989, Appleton-Century-Crofts.
5. McGarity WC, Broadwell DC, Goode PS: Complications following abdominoperineal resection: sexual and bladder dysfunction, *Ostomy Management* 3:4, 1980.
6. Miller JS et al: Ileal pouch-anal anastomosis: the Emory University experience, *Am Surg* 57(2):89, 1991.
7. Nemer FD, Rolstad B: The role of the ileoanal reservoir in patients with ulcerative colitis and familial polyposis, *J Enterostom Ther* 12(3):74, 1985.
8. Pemberton J: Surgery for ulcerative colitis, *Surg Clin North Am* 67:633, 1987.
9. Smith D, Johnson D: *Ostomy care for the cancer patient*, New York, 1986, Grune & Stratton.
10. Tretbar L: The use of flexible catheters for constructing, bridging, and pouching loop ileostomies, *J Enterostom Ther* 13(3):111, 1986.

# Index